D0386500

EXERCISE IN HEALTH AND DISEASE

Evaluation and Prescription for Prevention and Rehabilitation

MICHAEL L. POLLOCK, Ph.D.

Director, Cardiac Rehabilitation Program and Human Performance
Laboratory, Universal Services Rehabilitation and Development, Inc.,
Texas Heart Institute, Houston, Texas

JACK H. WILMORE, Ph.D.

Professor, Department of Physical Education and Director, Exercise and
Sport Sciences Laboratory, University of Arizona, Tucson, Arizona

SAMUEL M. FOX III, M.D.

Professor of Medicine and Director, Preventive Cardiology Program,
Georgetown University School of Medicine, Washington, D.C.

W. B. SAUNDERS COMPANY

Philadelphia, London, Toronto, Mexico City, Rio de Janeiro, Sydney, Tokyo

W. B. Saunders Company: West Washington Square
Philadelphia, PA 19105

1 St. Anne's Road
Eastbourne, East Sussex BN21 3UN, England

1 Goldthorne Avenue
Toronto, Ontario M8Z 5T9, Canada

Apartado 26370 - Cedro 512
Mexico 4, D.F., Mexico

Rua Coronel Cabrita, 8
Sao Cristovao Caixa Postal 21176
Rio de Janeiro, Brazil

9 Waltham Street
Artarmon, N.S.W. 2064, Australia

Ichibancho, Central Bldg., 22-1 Ichibancho
Chiyoda-Ku, Tokyo 102, Japan

Library of Congress Cataloging in Publication Data

Pollock, Michael L.
    Exercise in health and disease.

    1. Exercise therapy.   2. Exercise—Physiological
aspects.   I. Wilmore, Jack H., 1938–   . II. Fox,
Samuel M. (Samuel Mickle), 1923–   . II. Title.
[DNLM: 1. Exertion.   2. Physical fitness.   3. Preven-
tive medicine.   4. Rehabilitation. QT 255 P777e]
RM725.P64   1984   615.8'2   83-15270
ISBN 0-7216-1147-8

Exercise in Health and Disease   ISBN   0-7216-1147-8

© 1984 by W. B. Saunders Company.   Copyright under the Uniform Copyright Convention.
Simultaneously published in Canada.   All rights reserved.   This book is protected by copyright.   No part of it may be reproduced, stored in a retrieval system, or transmitted in any form
or by any means, electronic, mechanical, photocopying, recording, or otherwise, without written permission from the publisher. Made in the United States of America.   Press of W. B.
Saunders Company.   Library of Congress catalog card number 83-15270.

Last digit is the print number: 9   8   7   6

This book is dedicated to our families:

Rhonda and Jonathan
Dottie, Wendy, Kristi, and Melissa
Mary Alice, Elizabeth, John, Samuel, and Emily

CONTENTS

PHYSICAL ACTIVITY IN HEALTH AND DISEASE

Since the time of the Industrial Revolution, technology has advanced at an astounding rate. From that time to today, there has been a remarkable transformation of a basically hard-working, physically active, rural-based society into a population of anxious and troubled city dwellers and suburbanites with little or no opportunity for physical activity. These advances in modern technology have enabled our present-day society to live a life of relative comfort. Hand or push lawn mowers have been replaced by power lawn mowers, the most advanced having seats to support the person's body weight. Even grass itself is being replaced by synthetic turf! Elevators and escalators have replaced stairs—just try to find an open stairway in a modern high rise. The walk to the corner market has been replaced by a short drive to the supermarket in the neighborhood shopping center. Life *is* getting easier—easier, that is, from the viewpoint of conserving effort and human energy. But can "easier" be equated with a better and more productive life? In short, do we profit from this newly acquired sedentary existence, or does the sedentary lifestyle contribute in its own way to a totally new set of problems?

1

To answer this last question, it is necessary only to reflect on the simple but intricate manner in which the body functions and the delicate manner in which the body systems are so consistently in perfect harmony. Disrupt that harmony in even a simple way (e.g., the common cold or the tension headache), and the whole person suffers. There is a growing body of evidence that is beginning to demonstrate without question that physical inactivity and the increased sedentary nature of our daily living habits pose a serious threat to the body, causing major deterioration in normal body function. Such common and serious medical problems as coronary artery disease, hypertension, obesity, anxiety and depression, and lower back problems have been either directly or indirectly linked with a lack of physical activity. In addition to physical inactivity, a number of other factors are associated with these diseases or medical problems, including smoking, overeating, improper diet, excessive alcohol consumption, and emotional stress. These factors are all complications of the modern lifestyle, and they are interactive. Thus, to make the most significant impact on improving general health and reducing the risk of disease and disability, it is imperative to deal with the total person, altering the total lifestyle to achieve good health habits.

The first two chapters of this book will discuss those diseases and associated health problems that are attributable, at least in part, to physical inactivity, with the major focus on cardiovascular disease and obesity. Following a brief introduction, each chapter will focus on the pathophysiology of the disease or condition, discuss the associated risk factors, and then summarize the current knowledge concerning the role of physical activity in the prevention and treatment of that disease or condition. The underlying theme of both chapters is that physical fitness is more than the absence of disease. Rather, physical fitness represents a means to attain optimal health.

Chapter 1

CARDIOVASCULAR DISEASE

INTRODUCTION

Cardiovascular diseases constituted the leading cause of deaths in the United States in 1980, accounting for 1,012,150 deaths, or 51 per cent of the total annual mortality.[1] Stated in a slightly different manner, deaths from cardiovascular diseases *alone* outnumbered the combined total of all other causes of death! Cardiovascular diseases include coronary artery disease, hypertension, stroke, congestive heart failure, peripheral vascular disease, congenital heart defects, valvular heart disease, and rheumatic heart disease. See Figure 1–1.

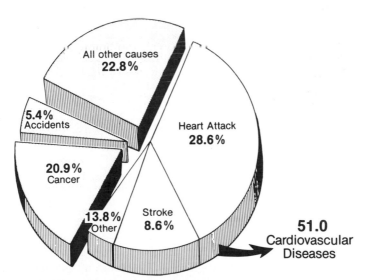

FIGURE 1–1. Leading causes of death in the United States: 1980 estimate. (Data from National Center for Health Statistics, U.S. Public Health Service, Department of Health and Human Services.)

Coronary artery disease (CAD), also referred to as coronary heart disease (CHD), is the major form of cardiovascular disease, accounting for 56 per cent of all cardiovascular disease deaths in 1980.[1] Nearly one of every three deaths is the result of CAD, making CAD the single leading cause of death in the United States. CAD is almost always the result of atherosclerosis, which is a narrowing and hardening of the arteries. The actual process of atherosclerosis will be discussed in detail in the following section. As the coronary arteries, i.e., the arteries that supply the myocardium, become narrowed and hardened, an imbalance between oxygen demand and delivery can develop. This is most likely to occur during periods of emotional stress or during exercise, when the heart is beating at a rate well above resting levels. The oxygen and energy demands of the heart are highly related ($r = 0.88$) to the heart rate; i.e., the higher the heart rate, the higher the oxygen and energy demands of the heart.[2] When the coronary arteries become narrowed to a certain critical point, it is no longer possible to supply sufficient oxygen to the heart at the higher heart rates; thus the demand exceeds the supply (see Fig. 1–2). When this occurs, the individual will typically feel chest pressure, a sharp pain, or a dull ache, sometimes radiating up into the neck and left shoulder and down the left arm. This transient chest discomfort is referred to as angina pectoris and is the result of localized ischemia, i.e., lack of adequate blood flow, in that section of the myocardium distal to the narrowed section of the coronary artery. This narrowed section of the coronary artery may close totally, or a blood clot may lodge in this area, resulting in a myocardial infarction or heart attack. Another form of heart attack that frequently leads to death is a disturbance in the heart's rhythm, or an arrhythmia. A fatal arrhythmia can occur in the presence of normal coronary arteries.

Hypertension is the most prevalent of the cardiovascular diseases. Over

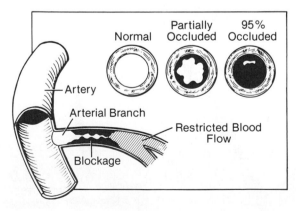

FIGURE 1–2. Gradual narrowing of a coronary artery through the progression of atherosclerosis.

37 million Americans were estimated to have hypertension in 1980.[1] Hypertension is simply a condition in which the blood pressure is chronically elevated above levels considered desirable for the person's age and size. For the adult, a systolic blood pressure between 140 and 160 mm Hg and/or a diastolic blood pressure between 90 and 95 mm Hg is considered to be borderline hypertension. A systolic pressure of 161 or greater and/or a diastolic pressure of 96 or greater is considered to be absolute hypertension.[3] These standards are reduced in the pediatric population, with the absolute standard traditionally defined as the 95th percentile of the normative data for a specific age.[4]

Stroke is the result of obstructions in, or hemorrhages of, blood vessels in and around the brain, which lead to the death of brain tissue.[5] The most common cause of stroke leading to the death of brain tissues is cerebral infarction resulting from atherosclerosis of the cerebral vessels. Cerebral infarction can also result from a cerebral embolism, in which an embolus or blood clot breaks loose from another site in the body and lodges in a cerebral artery, reducing or restricting blood flow distal to the clot. Cerebral hemorrhage is the other principal cause of stroke and is the result of a ruptured artery that bleeds into the substance of the brain or into the fluid-filled spaces over the surface of the brain.

Congestive heart failure describes the situation in which the heart is unable to deliver adequate blood to satisfy the oxygen and nutritional needs of the body at rest and during normal physical activity.[5] With chronically reduced blood delivery (reduced cardiac output), there is an excessive accumulation of fluids in the body. The excess fluid retention combined with failure of the heart is called congestive heart failure. Three kinds of impairment of heart function can lead to congestive heart failure: a diminished force of contraction of the ventricles, a mechanical failure in filling of the ventricles during diastole, and an overloading of the ventricles during systole.[5]

Peripheral vascular diseases involve both the arterial and venous blood vessels. Peripheral arterial diseases are primarily of four kinds: occlusive, in which blood flow is blocked; vasospastic, in which small arteries constrict or go into spasm; functional, in which the small arteries dilate; and aneurysm, in which the arterial wall balloons or bulges because of wall weakness.[5] Arteriosclerosis obliterans, a chronic, progressive arterial disease, is one of the major peripheral artery diseases and includes intermittent claudication, which is an ischemic pain in the lower extremities resulting from narrowed arteries. Of the peripheral venous diseases, varicose veins and phlebitis are the most common. In varicose veins, the wall of the vein weakens and may become dilated, or the valves in the vein that prevent backward flow fail to function normally. This results in venous pooling and a discoloration of the vessels from the stagnating blood. With phlebitis, a clot or thrombus forms in the vein, partially or completely stopping the flow of blood. This can be fatal if the clot dislodges and travels to the lungs, i.e., pulmonary embolus.

Congenital heart defects occur in approximately one out of every 100 births, and the cause can be determined in only about 3 percent of the cases.[5] These defects can include narrowed heart valves (stenosis), constriction of the aorta (coarctation), septal defects, and abnormal shunts of blood. Valvular heart disease involves one or more of the four valves that control the direction of blood flow from each of the four chambers of the heart. Valvular disease has numerous causes, but in all cases the heart is forced to do more work to deliver the same amount of blood, which can lead to serious cardiac complications. Rheumatic heart disease is the result of rheumatic fever, a disease caused by a streptococcal infection of the upper respiratory tract. Rheumatic fever most frequently strikes children of school age. Patients with rheumatic heart disease are prone to develop infection of the heart valves or the lining of the heart (endocarditis).[5]

The remainder of this chapter will focus on the two major cardiovascular diseases, coronary artery disease and hypertension. Although the other cardiovascular diseases are of considerable importance, relatively little is known concerning the role of physical activity in altering their course of development.

PATHOPHYSIOLOGY OF CORONARY ARTERY DISEASE AND HYPERTENSION

How do CAD and hypertension evolve or develop? What factors predispose one to atherosclerosis and myocardial infarction at an early age? What physiological changes occur that lead to a narrowing of the coronary arteries? What causes blood pressure to increase and to remain elevated throughout one's life? These and similar questions will be addressed in this section in an attempt to understand the disease processes that lead to CAD and hypertension.

Coronary artery disease is now recognized as a pediatric disease, even though the clinical manifestations of the disease appear much later in life.[6] It is now recognized that there are three basic periods of disease development.[7] First, the incubation period occurs between infancy and adolescence. During this period, mesenchymal cushions form on the intima, or inner layer of the arterial wall, particularly at points of bifurcation. These consist of a meshwork of embryonic connective tissue, with an increase in ground substance, disordered elastic fibers, and possibly some lipid deposits. In the second phase of this period, fatty flecks or streaks begin to appear. There is a slight focal thickening of the intima, an increased number of fibroblasts, and possible precursors of smooth muscle cells. The end result is a small round or oval plaque that is visible to the naked eye. Fatty streaks are found in the aorta in the first years of life and almost universally by the age of three years.[7] Second, the latent period occurs between adolescence and early adulthood. During this period, the fatty streaks are found in the coronary arteries. Although these are considered to be the precursors of the atherosclerotic lesions, they are certainly reversible at this stage.[7] Likewise, the presence of fatty streaks in children or adolescents is not a good forecaster of adult lesions. The fatty streak, however, does precede the fibrous plaque, which is generally considered irreversible, and leads to a complicated lesion. The final period is referred to as the clinical period, in which the clinical manifestations of the disease become apparent, i.e., angina pectoris, myocardial infarction, cerebral infarction, peripheral vascular disease, and sudden death. The fibrous plaque progresses to produce a substantial narrowing of the coronary artery lumen, thus reducing the coronary flow reserve (Fig. 1–2).

The normal artery is composed of three distinct layers: the intima, or inner layer; the media, or middle layer; and the adventitia, or outer layer. The media is composed of large numbers of smooth muscle cells, each surrounded by small amounts of collagen, small elastic fibers, and other connective tissue matrix components. The adventitia consists mainly of fibroblasts and loosely arranged collagen. The intima is the critical layer relative to the formation of atherosclerotic lesions and will be discussed in much greater depth.

The intima, although the innermost layer of the arterial wall, is protected from the blood and its constituents by a layer of endothelial cells. The endothelium normally provides a barrier to the passage of plasma proteins from the blood to the intima.[8] Local injury to the endothelium increases the concentration of plasma proteins in the intima, which can eventually lead to the migration of smooth muscle cells from the media into the intima. At this point, the smooth muscle cells can either proliferate or undergo cellular destruction depending on the internal milieu, or internal environment. Within a favorable environment, the smooth muscle cells will undergo destruction and the affected area will be repaired. Within an unfavorable environment (e.g., hypertension, increased blood lipid concentration, and hormonal imbalances), the smooth muscle cells will proliferate and the newly formed plaque will increase in size.[8]

In a recent review article on the genesis of atherosclerosis, Ross[8] provides an excellent summary of research supporting his current theory on plaque formation. Findings of both experimental research and autopsy studies show that atherosclerotic plaques are the result of proliferated smooth muscle cells in the intima, not lipid degeneration and accumulation as had previously been thought. It is now recognized that three cellular changes are involved in this process. First, smooth muscle cells proliferate or multiply within the intima. Second, these smooth muscle cells synthesize and release substances associated with connective tissue, including collagen, elastic fibers, and carbohydrate-containing proteins. Last, there is a deposition of lipids within the proliferated smooth muscle cells. Thus, the plaque is not a mass of fat, but a mass of smooth muscle cells that provide a repository for fats (see Fig. 1–3).

With this current theory, it is necessary to explain how the smooth muscle cells migrate from the media to the intima and how, once in the

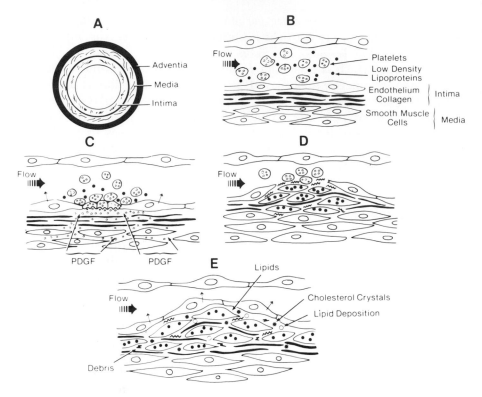

FIGURE 1–3. Changes in the arterial wall with injury, illustrating the disruption of the endothelium and the subsequent alterations.

intima, they are able to continue to proliferate. As was stated earlier, injury to the endothelium appears to be the necessary first step. Endothelial cells at the site of the injury are shed into the blood stream, exposing subendothelial connective tissue. Blood platelets adhere to the arterial wall and to each other at the site of the injury. These platelets degranulate and release a mixture of products that interact to promote the migration and proliferation of smooth muscle cells to the damaged portion of the arterial wall. One of these products is a mitogen, a substance essential for growth, that is referred to as a platelet-derived growth factor and is known to induce smooth muscle cell proliferation.

One final aspect of this process that needs to be better defined is the actual mechanism by which the arterial wall is injured. Texon[9] has proposed a hemodynamic basis for arterial wall injury. Applying the laws of fluid mechanics, he has demonstrated that atherosclerosis may be considered the reactive biological response of blood vessels to the effects of the mechanics of fluid flow, namely diminished lateral pressure that creates a suction or pulling effect in certain areas of vessels, e.g., areas of curvature, branching, bifurcation, and tapering. Ross[8] discusses experiments in which both mechanical injury and diet to increase plasma levels of LDL-cholesterol can

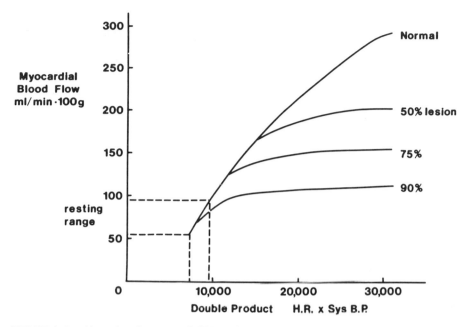

FIGURE 1–4. Alterations in myocardial blood flow with increasing exercise are plotted on this graph; the influence of luminal narrowing of the coronary vessels is evident.

induce arterial wall injury to initiate the atherosclerotic process. There may well be multiple factors that initiate or contribute to the injury process.

The end result of the atherosclerotic process in the coronary arteries is a progressive narrowing of the vessel lumen. This will eventually lead to a reduction in the peak flow to the myocardium. Figure 1–4 illustrates the influence of vessel narrowing on the myocardial flow during rest and exercise. Myocardial blood flow becomes increasingly limited for the same level of work, as indicated by the double product (HR X SBP), as the vessel lumen decreases with atherosclerotic narrowing.

As was discussed earlier in this section on the pathophysiology of atherosclerosis, the disease process begins at an early age. The actual pathological changes begin in infancy and progress during childhood.[6] This is exemplified in the work of Enos et al.,[10] who demonstrated that 70 per cent of autopsied Korean War casualties, with an average age of 22.1 years, already had at least moderately advanced coronary atherosclerosis. In a later study, McNamara et al.[11] found evidence of atherosclerosis in 45 per cent of Vietnam War casualties, with 5 per cent demonstrating severe coronary atherosclerosis. Mason[12] and Rigal et al.[13] reported similar findings in groups of young men. It is important to recognize the early onset of this disease, for prevention is preferable to rehabilitation and must be initiated at an early age.

The pathophysiology of hypertension is not nearly so well defined. In fact, Kaplan[14] has stated that the overwhelming majority of all hypertensive cases are idiopathic, i.e., of unknown origin. In a randomly chosen group of 689 hypertensive men between 47 and 54 years of age in Göteborg, Sweden, the disease was found to be idiopathic in nearly 95 per cent of the cases. Secondary causes of hypertension were chronic renal disease (4%), renovascular disease (1%), coarctation of the aorta (0.1%), and primary aldosteronism (0.1%).[15] Idiopathic hypertension, sometimes referred to as essential hypertension, may be the result of genetic factors, high levels of sodium in the diet, obesity, psychological stress, a combination of these factors, or other factors yet to be substantiated or determined.

CORONARY ARTERY DISEASE AND HYPERTENSION RISK FACTORS

While the pathophysiology of CAD and hypertension has been determined by experimental research and autopsy studies, another branch of medicine has been actively investigating the disease through observation of large population samples. Epidemiology is that branch of medicine which studies the relationships of various factors that determine frequencies and distributions of a disease. With respect to CAD and hypertension, epidemiology has attempted to isolate or identify those factors that are *associated* with the disease. These identified factors, when present, place that particular individual at an increased risk for the premature or early development and subsequent manifestation of the disease.

Epidemiological studies can be either retrospective, i.e., looking back on data previously collected to observe relationships, or prospective, i.e., planned well in advance of the period of data collection. The Framingham Study exemplifies the prospective epidemiological approach to the study of coronary artery disease. In 1947, the United States Public Health Service began to initiate plans for a major prospective epidemiological study of cardiovascular disease, with the focus on atherosclerosis and hypertension. Framingham, Massachusetts, a small community 21 miles west of Boston, was selected for this monumental study. Framingham had also been selected in the first community study of tuberculosis in 1917. Following several years of preparing the community and the staff for such a major undertaking, the study was begun in 1952. From the age group of 30 to 59 years, 6,600 individuals were randomly selected from a potential population of approximately 10,000. It was anticipated that this would yield approximately 2,150 new cases of cardiovascular disease by the end of the twentieth year of the study. Periodically, those who were selected and who elected to participate in the study were given extensive medical examinations and medical histories. This study has become one of the most productive of its kind in the history of medicine. As individuals developed cardiovascular disease, it was possible to group those individuals by disease and determine what factors they shared in common. These became recognized as CAD and hypertensive disease risk factors.

At the present time, CAD risk factors are classified into two categories, primary risk factors and secondary, or contributing, risk factors. The primary risk factors are those that have been shown without question to be implicated as contributory to the genesis of atherosclerosis. The secondary risk factors are not necessarily of any lesser importance but may simply need additional research support to elevate them to the level of being primary factors. To date, hypertension, cigarette smoking, and elevated blood cholesterol levels have been identified as the primary risk factors for CAD. Secondary risk factors include those factors that can be altered, i.e., diabetes, emotional stress, personality type, obesity, and physical inactivity. Unalterable contributing risk factors include age, race, sex, and family history. Since hypertension can be diagnosed rather simply with multiple blood pressure determinations, little attention has been given to the concept of risk factors for hypertensive disease. However, overweight and diet, particularly a diet high in sodium intake, appear to be the major factors; age, race, and family history are also important.

PRIMARY RISK FACTORS

According to the U.S. Health and Nutrition Examination Survey (HANES) of 1971 to 1974, 18 per cent of the adult population in the United States are hypertensive.[16] Although hypertension can be identified by blood pressure screening, it is important to recognize that multiple determinations of blood pressure should be taken and that care should be used in the selection of the proper blood pressure cuff. Frequently, individuals are misdiagnosed as hypertensive on the basis of only a single blood pressure measurement or the selection of a cuff that is too short or too narrow for that particular individual.

Hypertension has become one of the most powerful predictors of CAD, and the risk increases markedly when hypertension is coupled with other risk factors. Studies to date have demonstrated the following:

- **The risk of premature cardiovascular disease and death rises sharply with increased resting levels of systolic or diastolic blood pressure.**

- **Even within the "statistically normal" level of blood pressure, there are a greater number of heart attacks and strokes among the so-called high normal than in persons with lower blood pressure readings.**

- **There are indications that the incidence of strokes and heart failure can be reduced in groups of patients whose high blood pressure is lowered by medication.[5]**

Cigarette smoking is undoubtedly the single most important health hazard in the United States today. The total mortality from all causes of death combined is twice as high in smokers as in nonsmokers. Of this excess mortality, 19 per cent is due to lung cancer and 37 per cent to CAD. The

Surgeon General's report on smoking and health, issued in 1964, addressed the issue of cigarette smoking, disease, and death and contributed to a general reduction in the prevalence of cigarette smokers in certain subsets of the total population. For example, the prevalence of cigarette smokers among adult males declined from 53 per cent in 1964 to 38 per cent in 1978. However, the overall percentage of adult female smokers remained unchanged at about 30 per cent, and the percentage for younger women, particularly older teenage girls, increased.[17]

The research literature concerning smoking and increased risk for CAD is quite clear. The evidence includes the following:

- **The risk and frequency of heart attacks are greater in persons who smoke and increase according to the number of cigarettes smoked.**

- **The rate of heart attacks is lower among those who have given up smoking compared with current smokers.**

- **Mechanisms have been identified linking the components of tobacco smoking with arterial damage and the subsequent development of atherosclerosis.[5]**

Of recent concern has been the effect of tobacco smoke on the nonsmoker. The passive or involuntary smoker is one who is exposed to the smoke of others. An excellent study by White and Froeb[18] concluded that chronic exposure to tobacco smoke in the work place is deleterious to the nonsmoker and significantly reduces small-airways function. Spirometry tests showed the passive smoker to have the same profile as smokers who do not inhale or light smokers.

Increased levels of blood cholesterol have been linked with a substantial increase in risk for CAD. For a number of years, it was recognized that CAD is low in populations that subsist on low-fat, low-cholesterol diets or diets that are low in saturated fats and high in populations consuming high saturated fat and/or high cholesterol diets.[5] However, it is now acknowledged that the relationship of cholesterol to CAD is not simple, but very complex. Lipids, being insoluble in the blood plasma, must be packaged or combined with protein molecules. This combination of lipid with protein is termed a lipoprotein. Lipoprotein molecules are of different sizes and densities but are generally classified into one of four major categories: chylomicrons, very low density lipoproteins, low density lipoproteins (LDL), and high density lipoproteins (HDL). HDL-cholesterol (HDL-C) contains the highest proportion of protein and carries approximately 20 per cent of the plasma cholesterol. HDL-C is thought to be responsible for carrying cholesterol away from the arterial wall back to the liver, where it is metabolized and excreted. High levels of HDL-C have been associated with a low risk for CAD, which would be expected on the basis of its proposed function. LDL-cholesterol (LDL-C), on the other hand, is associated with a high risk for CAD when present in high concentrations. LDL is responsible for transporting approximately 65 per cent of the plasma cholesterol. Monkeys subjected to a diet high in cholesterol leading to increased LDL-C levels have been shown to develop atherosclerosis within a period of two years.[8]

The Framingham Study and other epidemiological studies have presented rather convincing evidence that both elevated total cholesterol and LDL-C levels place the individual at increased risk for CAD.[5] Conversely, these studies and others have shown that elevated levels of HDL-C provide some degree of protection from CAD.[5] Recently, clinicians have expressed HDL-C relative to total cholesterol, i.e., HDL-C/total cholesterol, with a ratio of 5.0 or greater indicating high risk and a ratio of 3.5 and lower indicating low risk. In addition, the only way to produce atherosclerosis in animals is to feed them diets high in cholesterol. Also, cholesterol is predominant in the atherosclerotic plaques. Reducing cholesterol in the diet has led to a reduction in the degree of atherosclerosis in animals and similar anecdotal reductions in humans.

SECONDARY, OR CONTRIBUTING, RISK FACTORS

With respect to the unalterable risk factors, it is obvious that the older the individual the greater the risk of death from CAD. Race also appears to be a distinct factor. With respect to hypertension, the black population is at approximately twice the risk of the white population. Family history, or the genetic component, is much more difficult to quantify. It is nearly impossible to divorce the influence of environment from family history. A family typically eats together, is exposed to similar stresses in the home, and shares many common experiences that may either increase or decrease the risk for CAD. Still, it is fairly clear that, if CAD manifests itself at an early age in one or two close relatives, the individual is placed in an elevated risk category. Finally, males appear to be at a substantially increased risk compared with females, at least up to the time of menopause in the female.[5] It was at one time thought that hormonal differences were the major cause of the reduced risk for women. Studies investigating this possibility showed just the opposite of what was expected. Men given female hormones were actually found to have an increased risk for CAD.[5] Thus, this differential in rates of CAD between men and premenopausal women has yet to be adequately explained.

With respect to the alterable secondary risk factors, obesity is one that has become quite controversial. Keys et al.[19] investigated the relationship of relative weight and of skinfold thickness to the 5-year incidence of CAD in men 40 through 59 years of age. When the other risk factors were disregarded, an excessive incidence of CAD was associated with overweight and obesity. However, when the other risk factors were taken into consideration, overweight and obesity were found to be unrelated to future CAD. Gordon and Kannel,[20] however, reporting data from the Framingham Study, demonstrated that a higher relative weight was associated with an increased risk for CAD. At 35 per cent above ideal weight, the odds of CAD were 1.6 and 1.4 times the risk for men and women, respectively, who were at their ideal weight. Recent data from Framingham over a longer period of follow-up indicate that without question overweight or obesity is a distinct risk factor, independent of the other risk factors for both men and women. Also, weight gain after age 25 resulted in increased risk of CAD in both sexes, independent of initial weight or other risk factors.[21]

With respect to diabetes, the Framingham Study reported that diabetic men were at twice the risk of nondiabetic men, and diabetic women were at three times greater risk.[22] Unfortunately, the pathogenesis of CAD in the diabetic is not well understood, but there does appear to be something unique about the diabetic that accelerates the atherosclerotic process.

Emotional stress has been suggested as a possible risk factor for CAD. This would appear obvious, but the relationship is not so simple. As an example, corporate executives have a relatively low incidence of CAD, whereas those who are on their way up the ladder have a relatively high incidence. Also, the prevalence of CAD decreased considerably in those individuals who were held prisoner in German World War II concentration camps, yet the stress levels had to be very high. Another area that has received considerable attention over the past ten years is the coronary-prone behavior pattern. Pioneered by Friedman and Rosenman,[23] the coronary-prone behavior pattern is characterized by excesses of aggressiveness, hurrying, and competitiveness; such individuals are often deeply committed to their vocation or profession to the exclusion of other aspects of their lives and have a sense of restlessness and guilt during leisure hours or periods of relaxation. Although there is a growing body of research to support the concept of the coronary-prone behavior pattern, the concept is not without its critics. Some feel that to try to classify all individuals into either a coronary-prone (Type A) or non–coronary-prone (Type B) behavior pattern is a great oversimplification. Additional research will be necessary before any conclusions can be drawn.

Physical inactivity as a risk factor for CAD will be discussed in considerable detail in the following section. Other factors have been proposed as risk factors, with little or no supporting evidence. At one time, coffee drinking was considered to be a risk factor, but subsequent studies were unable to confirm this.[5] Soft water has also been proposed as a risk factor, but the evidence is not conclusive.[5]

PHYSICAL ACTIVITY, CORONARY ARTERY DISEASE, AND HYPERTENSION

It is extremely difficult to ascertain directly the role of physical activity in the prevention of CAD and hypertension. The ideal study would necessitate a large population of infants randomly assigned to either a sedentary or an active lifestyle. Following 60 years or more of close and detailed observation, accurate conclusions could, ideally, be drawn. Obviously, such a study will never be conducted. Thus, to gain some insight into the basic relationship between physical activity, CAD, and hypertension, it has become necessary to accept indirect lines of inquiry into this problem.

Several indirect approaches have been used. First, epidemiologists have investigated the prevalence of CAD in active versus inactive populations, predominantly using occupation and/or leisure time as the index of activity level. Second, epidemiologists have compared the prevalence of CAD in former athletes versus nonathletes. Third, researchers have observed the influence of physical training, usually of a cardiorespiratory endurance nature, on the reduction of certain CAD risk factors. Fourth, researchers have attempted to use animal models to investigate physical activity, CAD, and hypertension. Last, several studies have attempted to determine the influence of physical activity on the long-term outlook of those patients who have documented CAD, i.e., angina pectoris, myocardial infarction, and coronary artery bypass surgery. Each of these five areas will be discussed separately to determine if a consistent pattern emerges across all lines of evidence.

EPIDEMIOLOGICAL STUDIES: ACTIVE VS. SEDENTARY POPULATIONS

A number of studies have been published in which the prevalence of CAD has been compared between active and sedentary populations. The first of these, conducted by Morris et al.[24] and published in 1953, compared "sedentary" bus drivers with "active" conductors who worked on double-decked buses for the London Transport Executive. They found the more physically active conductors to have a 30 per cent lesser occurrence of all manifestations of CAD and 50 per cent fewer myocardial infarctions. Mortality from CAD was less than half as frequent in the conductors. A similar finding was reported by the same investigators in a companion study of postal workers, comparing active mail carriers with less active postal service clerks.[24] Interesting, and somewhat difficult to explain, is the fact that in both studies the more active populations, i.e., the bus conductors and the postal mail carriers, had approximately twice the frequency of angina pectoris.

Morris and his associates followed their initial publication with a 1956 report entitled "Physique of London Busmen: The Epidemiology of Uniforms."[25] For any given height, the drivers, upon entry into the Transport Executive, were fitted with trousers that had at least a one-inch greater waist circumference than those of the conductors, and the drivers had higher serum cholesterol and blood pressure levels.[26] Because the groups were already different upon entry into the Transport Executive, it is difficult to determine if the greater physical activity of the conductors helped lower their CHD risk or if the conductors were simply different, even before entry into the Transport Executive.

These initial studies by Morris and his colleagues led to a number of similar studies, most confirming the early work of Morris et al. These studies were summarized in 1977 in a comprehensive review by Froelicher.[27] With only several exceptions, most of these observational studies showed a lower age-specific rate of CAD in the more active groups. The disease, when present, was found to be less severe in the more active groups, and the mortality was also lower.

These early studies suggested several interesting points. First, it does not appear to require considerable amounts or high intensities of exercise in order to achieve some degree of protection from coronary artery disease. Second, the protection gained from an active lifestyle appears to be transient, unless the activity is a lifelong pursuit. The results from several studies dealing with these specific issues will be briefly reviewed.

Zukel et al.[28] demonstrated a significant relationship between the incidence of CAD and hours of heavy labor. Their data revealed that people who engaged in from one to two hours of heavy physical labor per day had less than one fifth the incidence of coronary events as those whose life pattern included no heavy work. Unfortunately, this data did not permit an analysis for heavy work of less than one hour per day. Frank et al.,[29] in their report of the large (55,000 men) study of the Health Insurance Program of urban New York, found that the main difference in the incidence of heart attack deaths occurred between the least active and the moderately active groups. The few extra blocks of walking, extra stair climbing, and other activities of the moderately active group appeared to help protect them from heart attack deaths, which suggests potential benefits for "useful" increased activity without a great change in lifestyle.

It has been proposed by Bassler that the marathon runner's lifestyle is necessary to provide immunity from CAD.[30] However, a relatively small percentage of the population of the United States could rise to the level of commitment necessary to complete a 26.2-mile race. Further, this theory has not been substantiated. In fact, Skinner et al.[31] calculated that daily caloric expenditure increases of only 400 to 500 Kcal above the normal sedentary level were associated with a significantly lower prevalence of CAD in the multiracial communities of Evans County, Georgia. Rose[32] reported that walking 20 minutes or more to work was associated with a one-third lower incidence of ischemic-type electrocardiographic abnormalities.

Brown et al.[33] found the manifestations of coronary disease in men over 65 years of age to be fewer among those whose lifetime activity patterns placed them in a relatively more active group as compared with their more sedentary colleagues. With respect to the transient nature of the protection afforded by an active lifestyle, Kahn's review of postal workers in Washington, D.C., suggests that the difference in the incidence of CAD became indistinguishable within five years after an individual left the physically more active occupational status.[34] Thus, it appears that the potential benefits from physical activity cannot be stored, to be drawn from throughout the remainder of one's life. Rather, exercise habits should be continued regularly if benefits are to be retained.

Almost all of these early studies concentrated on defining a physically active or sedentary group solely on the basis of occupation. However, it is important to recognize that many very active individuals are employed in sedentary jobs. For example, from mid-1970 to the present, thousands of individuals have been attracted to participate in marathon races. However, by occupation, most of these individuals would have to be classified as sedentary. Recognizing this inherent weakness of previous study designs and realizing that work in advanced societies is increasingly light and sedentary, Morris et al.[35] attempted to study leisure-time activity and the incidence of CAD in a group of executive-grade civil servants, thus holding occupation constant. They studied the leisure activity patterns of 16,882 men over a Friday and Saturday, between the years 1968 and 1970. In their first follow-up report of 1973,[35] they found that men who had recorded vigorous exercise during this two-day period had a relative risk of developing CAD that was approximately 33 per cent of that in comparable men who did not record vigorous exercise. In a more recent follow-up, Morris et al.[36] reported that they had observed 1,138 first clinical episodes of CAD in their original sample. They concluded that men who engaged in vigorous sports and kept fit in the initial survey in 1968 to 1970 had an incidence of CAD in the next 8½ years that was somewhat less than half that of their colleagues who recorded no vigorous exercise. They concluded that "the generality of the advantage suggests that vigorous exercise is a natural defense of the body, with a protective effect on the aging heart against ischemia and its consequences."

Holme et al.[37] studied the association between physical activity at work and at leisure, coronary risk factors, social class, and mortality in approximately 15,000 Oslo men of age 40 to 49 years. The four-year total mortality and CAD mortality showed a decrease in risk with an increasing degree of *leisure* activity but an increase in risk with an increasing *work* activity. There was no immediate explanation for this apparent paradox.

Finally, the work of Paffenbarger and his associates on San Francisco Bay area longshoremen and Harvard alumni are certainly deserving of mention. In 1977, Paffenbarger et al.[38] reported on a 22-year follow-up of 3,686 San Francisco longshoremen. They found that higher energy output on the job reduced the risk of fatal heart attack, especially sudden death, in the two younger age groups, with the less active workers at a threefold increased risk. They estimated that combined low-energy output, heavy smoking, and high blood pressure increased risk by as much as 20 times. Most important, they indicated that by the elimination of these three adverse influences, the population under study might have had an 88 per cent reduction in its rate of fatal heart attack during the 22 years (Fig. 1–5). In their study of 16,936 Harvard male alumni, 35 to 74 years of age, Paffenbarger et al.[39] reported that men with an index below 2,000 kilocalories per week of physical activity were at 64 per cent higher risk for first heart attack than classmates with a higher index. Exercise remained a significant risk factor even when other risk factors were controlled for statistically. There were, however, no differences with respect to sudden death.

FORMER ATHLETES VS. NONATHLETES

Numerous studies have observed differences in life expectancy between former athletes and nonathletes. These studies have been adequately sum-

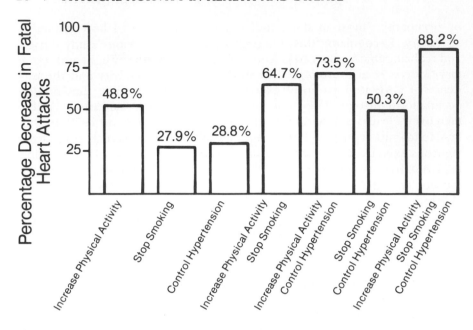

FIGURE 1–5. Percentage reduction in fatal heart attack by increasing physical activity, stopping smoking, and controlling hypertension. (Data from Paffenbarger, R. S., et al.: Am. J. Epidemiol. *105:*200–213, 1977.)

marized by Yamaji and Shephard,[10] and by Olson et al.[41] Generally, little difference has been found between former athletic vs. nonathletic populations relative to total mortality as well as to mortality from CAD. Olson et al. have concluded that there is no clear evidence for a long-term protective effect of athletics on health (Fig. 1–6).[41] As Yamaji and Shephard[40] have noted, athletic competition occupies too short a portion of the total life span to have a significant effect on longevity. They believe that the important question may well be *not* the kind of sport pursued or the intensity of activity during the required training, but whether the activity was continued to an advanced age. The data on Harvard graduates support this finding.[39] As was stated earlier, the benefits of physical activity are transient and are lost rapidly once the individual assumes a sedentary life. Whether one was active as a youngster, teenager, or young man or woman probably plays far less a role in disease protection than the present lifestyle of that individual.

PHYSICAL ACTIVITY AND CAD RISK FACTORS

The specific changes that result from physical training are covered in considerable detail in Section B. However, because of the importance of many of these changes to the CAD risk profile of the individual, several of the more important studies will be discussed. These studies fall into one of

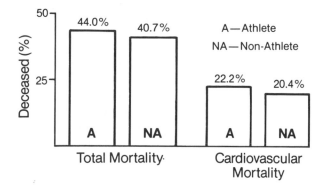

FIGURE 1–6. Comparison of percentages of deceased athletes and nonathletes. (Data from Olson, H. W., et al.: Physician Sportsmed. 6:62–65, 1978.)

two major categories: cross-sectional or longitudinal. In cross-sectional studies, a large number of individuals are usually observed only once, and comparisons are made between those considered to be physically fit and those considered to be unfit. Fitness is typically determined on the basis of the individual's actual or predicted maximal oxygen uptake ($\dot{V}O_2$ max). In longitudinal studies, individuals are assessed initially, placed on a physical training program for a certain interval of time, and then re-evaluated at the conclusion of the training period. For a number of reasons, longitudinal studies are to be preferred. However, they are expensive to conduct and usually involve small numbers of subjects. With cross-sectional studies, large numbers of individuals can be observed in a relatively short period of time.

Cooper et al.[42] observed the relationship between physical fitness, as determined by the length of time the subject could remain on the treadmill using the Balke protocol, and various CAD risk factors. They reported a consistent inverse relationship between physical fitness and resting heart rate, body weight, per cent body fat, serum levels of cholesterol and triglycerides, glucose, and systolic blood pressure. They interpreted their results to imply that physical fitness is related to a lower coronary risk profile. This study was cross-sectional in nature, with approximately 3,000 males constituting the data base, numbers that would have been clearly impossible to obtain with a longitudinal format. More recently, similar findings have been shown with females.[43]

With respect to the major risk factors, numerous studies have been conducted. Cardiorespiratory endurance training is known to have a rather profound influence on plasma lipids and lipoproteins. Athletes who participate in cardiorespiratory endurance sports such as cross country skiing and long distance running have a very characteristic plasma lipid and lipoprotein pattern. Further, endurance training of nonathletes leads to the same characteristic profile. In 1979, Wood and Haskell published a comprehensive review addressing the issue of lipid and lipoprotein alterations with endurance activity.[44] Both cross-sectional studies of endurance-trained individuals and longitudinal studies of individuals before and following an extended period of endurance training suggest that endurance training results in low plasma VLDL concentrations, relatively low LDL concentrations, and high HDL concentrations. In addition, plasma triglyceride concentrations are typically low, and total cholesterol is often but not always low. The ratio of total cholesterol/HDL-C is reduced considerably, an alteration that is associated with a reduction in risk for CAD.[44, 45] Although these represent impressive alterations in lipid and lipoprotein profiles and present a solid link between endurance activity and reduced risk for CAD, the data must be interpreted cautiously. First, not all studies have been able to demonstrate these changes. Second, it is not clear whether these changes are directly the result of the exercise or the physiological concomitants of an active lifestyle. Leanness, or reduction in body fat, has been suggested as a potential mechanism leading to these alterations in plasma lipids and lipoproteins. Williams et al.[46] have recently shown that running approximately 10 miles a week may be a minimum threshold at which to expect changes in HDL-C.

Hypertension, the second of the three major risk factors, also appears to respond positively to chronic physical activity of an endurance nature. Much of the early work in this area was confounded by the use of subjects with normal blood pressures. Endurance training of individuals with normal blood pressure failed to reduce that pressure to lower, or subnormal, levels. In retrospect, a reduction in pressure below normal would not have been expected. Endurance training of hypertensive individuals does appear to result in moderate to substantial reductions in blood pressure, with systolic pressure being reduced by the greatest magnitude.[47] Again, as with the area of blood lipids and lipoproteins, there have been studies that have failed to demonstrate blood pressure reductions in hypertensive patients with endurance exercise. The bulk of the evidence, however, appears to favor endurance exercise as an effective intervention for reducing blood pressure, particularly when combined with reductions in total body weight and salt intake. The mechanisms by which chronic endurance training lowers blood pressure are not clear at the present time, but they could include any one or more of the following: reductions in resting sympathetic tone; decreases in baroreceptor sensitivity; changes in myogenic structures, tone, or relationships; and decreases in resting cardiac output.[47]

With respect to cigarette smoking, the third of the three primary risk factors, exercise may play a significant role. First, those who adopt an active lifestyle soon find that cigarette smoking is not compatible with their new goals and priorities, and many are able to withdraw from their dependency on tobacco. Second, and somewhat related, several of the more popular smoking control or cessation programs are using endurance activity, e.g., long brisk walks or jogging, as a substitute behavior for smoking.

Chronic endurance activity also appears to reduce the risk of CAD through alterations in the secondary, or contributing, risk factors. Endurance activity is an important component of any weight loss program, for exercise combined with modest reductions in the total number of calories consumed will result in substantial decreases in total body fat and will prevent the losses in lean body mass that usually accompany weight loss through low-calorie diets.[48] Brownell and Stunkard have recently completed a comprehensive review of the area of physical activity and obesity; they conclude that physical inactivity is associated with an increased risk for obesity and CAD and that physical activity is an important component of a weight reduction program.[49] Body composition alterations with physical conditioning are extensively reviewed in Chapter 4. With diabetes, physical activity is now recognized as a critical part of the total treatment program. A recent conference on exercise and diabetes provided considerable insight into the role of exercise in the management of the diabetic patient.[50] With respect to emotional factors, endurance activity appears to be a potent tranquilizer, reducing stress and anxiety and facilitating recovery from episodes of depression.[51] There are also many changes in cardiorespiratory function resulting from endurance training that would lead to a more favorable CAD risk profile. These will be the focus of Chapter 3.

Thus, with respect to CAD risk factors, physical activity of a cardiorespiratory endurance nature does facilitate positive changes in the CAD risk profile, apparently reducing the overall risk for heart attack, stroke, and hypertension. Although there are isolated reports to the contrary,[52] the evidence overwhelmingly supports the prophylactic benefits of chronic endurance activity.

ANIMAL STUDIES: PHYSICAL ACTIVITY AND CAD

Animal models have become quite popular in the study of many diseases. However, considerable care must be taken when translating results from the animal model to humans. Some results and concepts obtained from animal work are directly transferable to humans, but others need considerable interpretation and possible modification before they are applied to man.

Several excellent review articles by Froelicher et al.[27,53,54] have summarized the knowledge in this area through 1980. The animal research has demonstrated a number of physiological and morphological alterations with exercise training that would imply a general reduction in risk for CAD. First, numerous animal studies have demonstrated cardiac hypertrophy induced by vigorous endurance exercise. This enlarged heart is typically the result of increases in chamber size, predominantly in the left ventricle. This adaptation is considered important to improved myocardial contractility and increased cardiac work capacity. Within the myocardium, there appears to be a hyperplasia and lengthening of muscle fibers, without fiber thickening. Also, there is consistent evidence that endurance training leads to an increased capillary/fiber ratio. When infarction is induced experimentally, there is a decrease in myocardial infarct size in the exercised animal.

Changes in the coronary circulation with chronic endurance exercise have also been demonstrated in animals. Using corrosion-cast techniques to determine the size of the coronary arterial tree, several studies have demonstrated increased coronary tree size and increased luminal cross-sectional area of the main coronary arteries. These alterations would lead to an increased capacity for myocardial blood flow, even in the presence of atherosclerosis of the coronary arteries. The collateral circulation has also been studied, the theory being that as the major coronary arteries become narrowed as a result of atherosclerosis, chronic endurance exercise would facilitate the development of the coronary collateral circulation. In one of the earliest studies, Eckstein[55] studied the effects of exercise and artifical coronary artery narrowing on coronary collateral flow. He surgically induced a constriction in the circumflex artery of approximately 100 dogs. Various degrees of narrowing were induced, and only dogs that developed changes in their electrocardiogram were included in the study. The dogs were divided into two groups, one receiving regular exercise on the treadmill and the other remaining sedentary. The study demonstrated that moderate and severe arterial narrowing resulted in collateral flow proportional to the degree of narrowing and that exercise led to even greater collateral flow. Further studies failed to confirm these initial results of Eckstein.[27,54]

Several animal studies have observed mechanical and metabolic performance changes of the heart with chronic endurance activity. Trained animals demonstrate higher levels of cardiac work and cardiac output. In addition, they have a greater myocardial oxygen uptake at or near maximal capacity and produce less lactate and pyruvate. In short, the heart of the trained animal is a more efficient pump.[27,53,54]

Finally, several studies have attempted to induce atherosclerosis in experimental animals through atherogenic diets, observing the effects of chronic endurance exercise on the subsequent arterial narrowing and plaque formation. Although many of the initial studies were equivocal,[27] a recent study by Kramsch et al.[56] demonstrated rather remarkable differences between an exercise group and a sedentary control group. They studied the effect of moderate conditioning with treadmill exercise on the development of CAD in monkeys on an atherogenic diet. Although the total serum cholesterol was the same in the exercising and nonexercising monkeys, the exercise group had significantly higher HDL-cholesterol levels and much lower levels of triglycerides and LDL plus VLDL-triglyceride. Ischemic changes in the electrocardiogram and sudden death attributable to CAD were observed only in the nonexercising group. Exercise was associated with substantially reduced overall atherosclerotic involvement, lesion size, and collagen accumulation. It also produced larger hearts and wider coronary arteries (Fig. 1–7), further reducing the degree of luminal narrowing. Kramsch and associates concluded that moderate exercise may prevent or retard CAD in primates.

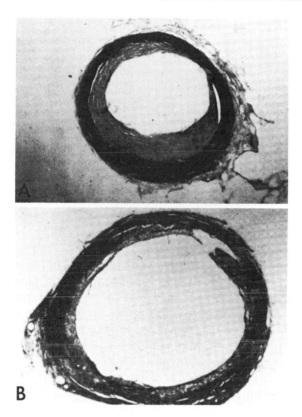

FIGURE 1-7. Comparison of the left main coronary artery in sedentary (**A**) vs. exercising (**B**) monkeys. (From Kramsch, D. M., et al.: N. Engl. J. Med. 305:1483, 1981. Reprinted by permission of the New England Journal of Medicine.)

SECONDARY/TERTIARY PREVENTION OF CAD: ROLE OF PHYSICAL ACTIVITY

Finally, the role of chronic endurance activity has been observed in those individuals who are symptomatic for CAD or who have sustained a myocardial infarction in order to determine if an active lifestyle will improve their general prognosis. Although this has classically been referred to as secondary prevention, Froelicher and Brown[57], in a recent review article, have redefined this terminology. By their new definition, tertiary prevention is now that area which deals with the minimization of disability, morbidity, and mortality once the disease is clinically manifest.

With respect to cardiac morphology, little or no change has been demonstrated in left ventricular mass and volume following six months of exercise training. Similarly, coronary angiography has not been able to demonstrate significant changes in atherosclerotic lesions or collateral vessels. However, recent studies have indicated that certain patients may show considerable improvement in left ventricular function and in indices of myocardial blood flow with training, but that, when these patients are averaged in with those who demonstrate no improvement or who actually have decreased capacity, the positive results are masked.[58,59]

The electrical and hemodynamic function of the heart appears to be improved in some patients undergoing exercise training. In some cases, those with S-T segment depression have a normalization of their electrocardiogram following training. Anginal threshold is also increased in certain patients following training when expressed relative to the exercise heart rate. In addition, even if the absolute threshold is not altered, i.e., angina occurs at the same submaximal heart rate, there is an increase in the actual work level achieved before the onset of angina. There have been isolated reports of increased ejection fraction following training, but the evidence is not convincing at this time.

Several studies have attempted to observe morbidity and mortality in CAD patients, comparing those who exercise with those who remain sedentary. Although some of the early studies showed marked differences in both CAD morbidity and mortality favoring the exercising groups, the results must be viewed with caution, because those patients too sick to exercise were often the patients who were assigned to the sedentary control group. In more highly controlled studies, in which all patients included in the study were considered to be fit enough to exercise, the patient population has been randomly assigned to either the exercise or sedentary control groups. Although the results of these studies have not demonstrated dramatic differences between the exercise and control groups, the trend indicates that a substantial differential in both morbidity and mortality may be evident over a longer period of follow-up and with a larger patient population.[60]

SUMMARY

For more than 30 years, coronary artery disease has been the single greatest cause of death in the United States. Nearly one of every three deaths is the result of CAD. However, death rates for CAD reached their peak during the mid-1960s and have steadily declined since then, for a total reduction that has exceeded 25 per cent (Fig 1–8).[61] The reasons for this decrease are not totally clear, but it does seem evident that an increasing concern for disease prevention and the subsequent modification of unhealthy lifestyles have made a major contribution to this decline. Although a significant portion of this decrease has resulted from better treatment, e.g., pharmacological intervention and coronary artery bypass surgery, treatment is very expensive and represents a substantial portion of total health care costs. Thus, the major thrust for combating CAD must be focused on the area of primary prevention, an area in which exercise must play a significant part.

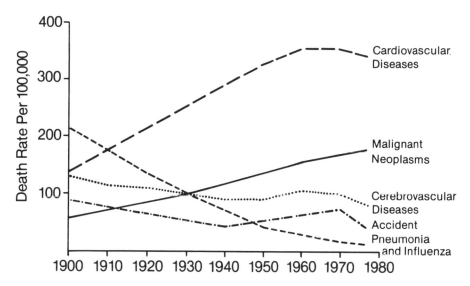

FIGURE 1–8. Alterations in the major causes of death from the years 1900 to 1976. (Data from Stallones, R. A.: Sci. Am. *243:*53–59, 1980.)

Does exercise prevent or reduce the risk for CAD? The review presented in this chapter, although not conclusive, provides strong evidence for the importance of exercise. The recent "Statement on Exercise," prepared by the American Heart Association's Subcommittee on Exercise/Cardiac Rehabilitation, states our present knowledge in this area most succinctly:

> **Exercise training can increase cardiovascular function capacity and decrease myocardial oxygen demand for any given level of physical activity in normal persons as well as most cardiac patients. Regular physical activity is required to maintain the training effects. The potential risk of vigorous physical activity can be reduced by appropriate medical clearance, education and guidance. Exercise may aid efforts to control cigarette smoking, hypertension, lipid abnormalities, diabetes, obesity, and emotional stress. Evidence suggests that regular, moderate, or vigorous occupational or leisure-time physical activity may protect against coronary heart disease and may improve the likelihood of survival from a heart attack.[62]**

REFERENCES

1. American Heart Association: Heart Facts 1983. Dallas, American Heart Association, 1982.
2. Kitamura, K., Jorgensen, C. R., Gobel, F. L., Taylor, H. L., and Wang, Y.: Hemodynamic correlates of myocardial oxygen consumption during upright exercise. J. Appl. Physiol. *32:*516–522, 1972.
3. Kannel, W. B., Sorlie, P., Castelli, W. P., and McGee, D.: Blood pressure and survival after myocardial infarction: the Framingham Study. Am. J. Cardiol. *45:*326–330, 1980.
4. Lauer, R. M., and Shekelle, R. B., editors: Childhood Prevention of Atherosclerosis and Hypertension. New York, Raven Press, 1980.

5. American Heart Association: Heart Book: A Guide to and Treatment of Cardiovascular Disease. New York, E. P. Dutton, 1980.
6. Kannel, W. B., and Dawber, T. R.: Atherosclerosis as a pediatric problem. J. Pediatr. *80:* 544–554, 1972.
7. McMillan, G. C.: Development of arteriosclerosis. Am. J. Cardiol. *31:* 542–546, 1973.
8. Ross, R.: The genesis of atherosclerosis. In National Research Council: 1980 Issues and Current Studies. Washington, D.C., National Academy of Sciences, 1981.
9. Texon, M.: The hemodynamic basis of atherosclerosis. Bull. N.Y. Acad. Med. *52:* 187–200, 1976.
10. Enos, W. F., Holmes, R. H., and Beyer, J.: Coronary disease among United States soldiers killed in action in Korea. J.A.M.A. *152:* 1090–1093, 1953.
11. McNamara, J. J., Molot, M. A., Stremple, J. F., and Cutting, R. T.: Coronary artery disease in combat casualties in Vietnam. J.A.M.A. *216:* 1185–1187, 1971.
12. Mason, J. K.: Asymptomatic disease of coronary arteries in young men. Br. Med. J. *2:* 1234–1237, 1963.
13. Rigal, R. D., Lovell, F. W., and Townsend, F. M.: Pathologic finds in the cardiovascular systems of military flying personnel. Am. J. Cardiol. *6:* 19–25, 1963.
14. Kaplan, N. M.: The control of hypertension: a therapeutic breakthrough. Am. Sci. *68:* 537–545, 1980.
15. Berglund, G., Anderson, O., and Wilhelmsen, L.: Prevalence of primary and secondary hypertension: studies in a random population sample. Br. Med. J. *2:* 554–556, 1976.
16. U.S. Department of Health and Human Services, Public Health Service, National Center for Health Statistics: Hypertension in Adults 25–74 Years of Age: United States, 1971–75. Vital and Health Statistics. Series 11–No. 221. DHHS Pub. No. (PHS)81–1671. Washington, D.C., U.S. Government Printing Office, April 1981.
17. U.S. Department of Health and Human Services: Promoting Health/Preventing Disease: Objectives for the Nation. Washington, D.C., U.S. Government Printing Office, (331–699) 1980.
18. White, J. R., and Froeb, H. F.: Small-airways dysfunction in nonsmokers chronically exposed to tobacco smoke. N. Engl. J. Med. *302:* 720–723, 1980.
19. Keys, A., Aravanis, C., Blackburn, H., VanBuchem, F.S.P., Buzine, R., Djordjevic, B. S., Fidanza, F., Karvonen, M. J., Menotti, A., Puddu, V., and Taylor, H. L.: Coronary heart disease: overweight and obesity as risk factors. Ann. Intern. Med. *77:* 15–27, 1972.
20. Gordon, T., and Kannel, W. B.: The effects of overweight on cardiovascular disease. Geriatrics *28:* 80–88, 1973.
21. Hubert, H. A., Feinleib, M., McNamara, P. M., and Castelli, W. P.: Obesity as an independent risk factor for cardiovascular disease. A 26-year follow-up of participants in the Framingham heart study. Circulation *67:* 968–977, 1983.
22. Kannel, W. B., and McGee, D. L.: Diabetes and cardiovascular risk factors: the Framingham Study. Circulation *59:* 8–13, 1979.
23. Friedman, M., and Rosenman, R. H.: Type A Behavior and Your Heart. Greenwich, Conn., Fawcett Publications, Inc., 1974.
24. Morris, J. N., Heady, J. A., Raffle, P. A. B., Roberts, C. G., and Parks, J. W.: Coronary heart-disease and physical activity of work. Lancet II: 1053–1057, 1111–1120, 1953.
25. Morris, J. N., Heady, J., and Raffle, P. A. B.: Physique of London busmen: the epidemiology of uniforms. Lancet II: 569–570, 1956.
26. Morris, J. N., Kagan, A., Pattison, D. C., Gardner, M., and Raffle, P.: Incidence and prediction of ischemic heart disease in London busmen. Lancet II: 553–559, 1966.
27. Froelicher, V. F. Does exercise conditioning delay progression of myocardial ischemia in coronary atherosclerotic heart disease? *In* Corday, E., and Brest, A., editors: Controversy in Cardiology (Cardiovascular Clinics series, vol. 8, no. 1). Philadelphia, F. A. Davis, 1977.
28. Zukel, W. J., Lewis, R., Enterline, P., Painter, R. C., Ralston, L. S., Fawcett, R. M., Meredith, A. P., and Peterson, B.: A short-term community study of the epidemiology of coronary heart disease. Am. J. Public Health *49:* 1630–1639, 1959.
29. Frank, C. W., Weinblatt, E., Shapiro, S., and Sager, R. V.: Physical inactivity as a lethal factor in myocardial infarction among men. Circulation *34:* 1022–1033, 1960.
30. Bassler, T. J.: Marathon running and immunity to heart disease. Physician Sportsmed. *3:* 77–80, 1975.
31. Skinner, J. S., Benson, H., McDonough, J. R., and Hames, C. G.: Social status, physical activity and coronary proneness. J. Chronic Dis. *19:* 773–783, 1966.
32. Rose, G. Physical activity and coronary heart disease. Proc. R. Soc. Med. *62:* 1183–1187, 1969.

33. Brown, R. G., Davidson, A. G., McKeown, T., and Whitfield, A. G. W.: Coronary artery disease: influences affecting its incidence in males in the seventh decade. Lancet II: 1073–1077, 1957.
34. Kahn, H. A.: The relationship of reported coronary heart disease mortality to physical activity of work. Am. J. Public Health 53:1058–1067, 1963.
35. Morris, J. N., Adam, C., Chave, S. P. W., Sirey, C., Epstein, L., and Sheehan, D. J.: Vigorous exercise in leisure-time and the incidence of coronary heart-disease. Lancet I: 333–339, 1973.
36. Morris, J. N. N., Pollard, P., Everitt, M. G., Chave, S. P. W., and Semmence, A. M.: Vigorous exercise in leisure-time: protection against coronary disease. Lancet II: 1207–1210, 1980.
37. Holme, I., Helgeland, A., Hjermann, I., Leren, P., and Lund-Larson, P. G.: Physical activity at work and at leisure in relation to coronary risk factors and social class. Acta Med. Scand. 209:277–283, 1981.
38. Paffenbarger, R. S., Hale, W. E., Brand, R. J., and Hyde, R. T.: Work-energy level, personal characteristics, and fatal heart attack: a birth cohort effect. Am. J. Epidemiol. 105:200–213, 1977.
39. Paffenbarger, R. S., Wing, A. L., and Hyde, R. T.: Physical activity as an index of heart attack risk in college alumni. Am. J. Epidemiol. 108:161–175, 1978.
40. Yamaji, K., and Shephard, R. J.: Longevity and cause of death of athletes. J. Human Ergol. 6:15–27, 1977.
41. Olson, H. W., Montoye, H. J., Sprague, H., Stephens, K., and Van Huss, W. D.: The longevity and morbidity of college athletes. Physician Sportsmed. 6(8):62–65, 1978.
42. Cooper, K. H., Pollock, M. L., Martin, R. P., White, S. R., Linnerud, A. C., and Jackson, A.: Physical fitness levels vs. selected coronary risk factors: a cross-sectional study. J.A.M.A. 236:166–169, 1976.
43. Gibbons, L. W., Blair, S. N., Cooper, K. H., and Smith, M.: Association between coronary heart disease risk factors and physical fitness in healthy adult women. Circulation 67: 977–983, 1983.
44. Wood, P. D., and Haskell, W. L.: The effect of exercise on plasma high density lipoproteins. Lipids 14:417–427, 1979.
45. Kannel, W. B.: High-density lipoproteins: epidemiologic profile and risks of coronary artery disease. Am. J. Cardiol. 52:98–128, 1983.
46. Williams, P. T., Wood, P. D., Haskell, W. L., and Vranizan, K.: The effects of running mileage and duration on plasma lipoprotein levels. J.A.M.A. 247:2674–2679, 1982.
47. Tipton, C. M., Matthes, R. D., Bedford, T. B., Leininger, J. R., Oppliger, R. A., and Miller, L. J.: Exercise, hypertension, and animal models. In Lowenthal, D. T., Bharadwaja, K., and Oaks, W. W., editors: Therapeutics through Exercise. New York, Grune & Stratton, 1979.
48. Zuti, W. B., and Golding, L. A.: Comparing diet and exercise as weight reduction tools. Physician Sportsmed. 4:49–53, 1976.
49. Brownell, K. D., and Stunkard, A. J.: Physical activity in the development and control of obesity. In A. J., Stunkard, editor: Obesity. Philadelphia, W. B. Saunders Co., 1980.
50. Vranic, M., Horvath, S. M., and Wahren, J., editors: Proceedings of a Conference on Diabetes and Exercise. Diabetes 28:Suppl. 1, 1979.
51. Greist, J. H., Klein, M. H., Eischens, R. R., and Faris, J. T.: Running out of depression. Physician Sportsmed. 6:49–56, 1978.
52. Sedgwick, A. W., Brotherhood, J. R., Harris-Davidson, A., Taplin, R. E., and Thomas, D. W.: Long-term effects of physical training programme on risk factors for coronary heart disease in otherwise sedentary men. Br. Med.J. 2:7–10, 1980.
53. Froelicher, V. F.: Animal studies of effect of chronic exercise on the heart and atherosclerosis: a review. Am. Heart J. 84:496–506, 1972.
54. Froelicher, V., Battler, A., and McKirnan, M. D.: Physical activity and coronary heart disease. Cardiology 65:153–190, 1980.
55. Eckstein, R. W.: Effect of exercise and coronary artery narrowing on coronary collateral circulation. Cir. Res. 5:230–235, 1957.
56. Kramsch, D. M., Aspen, A. J., Abramowitz, B. M., Kreimendahl, T., and Hood, W. B.: Reduction of coronary atherosclerosis by moderate conditioning exercise in monkeys on an atherogenic diet. N. Engl. J. Med. 305:1483–1489, 1981.
57. Froelicher, V. F., and Brown, P.: Exercise and coronary heart disease. J. Cardiac Rehab. 1:277–288, 1981.
58. Jensen, D., Atwood, J. E., Froelicher, V., McKirnan, M. D., Battler, A., Ashburn, W., and

Ross, J.: Improvement in ventricular function during exercise studied with radionuclide ventriculography after cardiac rehabilitation. Am. J. Cardiol. *46:*770–777, 1980.
59. Froelicher, V., Jensen, D., Atwood, J. E., McKirnan, D., Gerber, K., Slutsky, R., Battler, A., Ashburn, W., and Ross, J.: Cardiac rehabilitation: evidence for improvement in myocardial perfusion and function. Arch. Phys. Med. Rehab. *61:*517–522, 1980.
60. Naughton, J.: Physical activity for myocardial infarction patients. Cardiovasc. Rev. Rep. *3:*237–242, 1982.
61. Stallones, R. A. The rise and fall of ischemic heart disease. Sci. Am. *243:*53–59, 1980.
62. American Heart Association, Subcommittee on Exercise/Cardiac Rehabilitation: Statement on Exercise. Circulation *64:*1302–1304, 1981.

Chapter 2

OBESITY AND WEIGHT CONTROL

INTRODUCTION

Overweight and obesity constitute two of the most significant health problems in the United States today.[1] They are either directly or indirectly associated with a wide variety of diseases that collectively account for 15 to 20 per cent of the annual U.S. mortality. Further, in developed countries, 35 per cent of the adult population is obese, with evidence that the prevalence is increasing.[1] Before beginning a detailed discussion of prevalence data, it is first important to define the terms *overweight* and *obesity,* since they are frequently used incorrectly.

Overweight is simply defined as that condition in which an individual's weight exceeds the population norm or average, which is determined on the basis of gender, height, and frame size. The standardized height/weight tables had their genesis in the 1912 publication of the "Medico-Actuarial Mortality Investigation," by the Association of Life Insurance Medical Directors and the Actuarial Society of America.[2] The original tables gave the average values for men and women of specific ages who obtained life insurance policies between the years of 1888 and 1905. The data was obtained mostly from urban centers on the Eastern seaboard. Heights and weights were recorded with shoes and clothing, with a one- and two-inch allowance for heels for men and women, respectively, and a four- to nine-pound allowance for clothing.[3] Over the years, this same data has been reanalyzed and subsequently placed into a format that provides weight ranges for each of three frame sizes according to each one-inch increment in height.[4] As an example, a 6 ft 2 in male with a "large" frame size would be allowed to weigh between 173 and 194 pounds. Any weight below 173 pounds would be classified as underweight, and any weight over 194 pounds would be considered overweight. The tables look very scientific and accurate, but they contain basically the same data that was published in 1912, with the categorization into frame size done in a rather arbitrary manner. In fact, no indication is given as to how to estimate frame size. Many people determine their frame size on the basis of the column in which they find their weight!

The problems of using standard normative data for determining one's desired or ideal weight* were illustrated by Welham and Behnke in 1942.[5] In a study of professional football players, they found that these men were grossly overweight, yet they had very high specific gravities, indicating low levels of body fat and high levels of lean tissue, i.e., muscle and bone. Thus, it is possible to be overweight but of normal or below normal levels of body fat. Likewise, it is also possible to be excessively fat, yet to fall within the normal weight range for height and frame size. Since the original work of Welham and Behnke, many other studies have confirmed the fact that the standard tables do not provide accurate estimates of ideal or desirable weight for a large segment of the population.

The major problem associated with the use of the standard tables is that these tables do not take into consideration the composition of the body. Although the body is composed of numerous elements, scientists have categorized the total body into four component parts: the fat mass, the bone mass, the muscle mass, and the remainder. The last category is a catch-all category that includes the skin and various organs of the body. To simplify this categorization even further, two component parts have been identified: the fat mass and the lean body mass. Procedures have been developed that allow for a relatively accurate fractionization of the total body weight into its two component parts, the fat and lean weights. The most accurate of these procedures involves weighing the individual while he or she is submerged underwater. The difference between scale weight and the underwater weight, when corrected for trapped air volumes, is equal to the volume of the body.[6] Dividing the body mass or weight by the body volume provides an accurate estimate of the density of the body, i.e., $M/V = $ density. The density of fat has been determined to be approximately 0.900, and it varies little between and within individuals. The density of the lean tissue is much more variable, but the constant of 1.100 is typically used in most equations that provide an estimate of relative body fat from body density. Further methodological considerations will be discussed in Chapter 6.

Although the underwater weighing technique is the most accurate laboratory test available to determine the total density of the body and its subsequent composition, i.e., lean and fat weights, it does have its limitations. For those individuals undergoing changes in bone mineral, i.e., increasing bone mineral in the youngster as he or she matures or decreasing bone mineral in the aging individual, the equations used to estimate relative fat from body density will be inaccurate, providing an overestimation of the actual fat concentration. For those individuals with a larger preponderance of bone or bone that is denser than the population average, the estimate of relative fat will also be inaccurate, with an underestimation of the actual fat

---

*Desired or ideal weight refers to that weight which represents an optimal balance between lean and fat weight. Fat weight should not exceed 20% and 27% of total body weight for men and women, respectively.

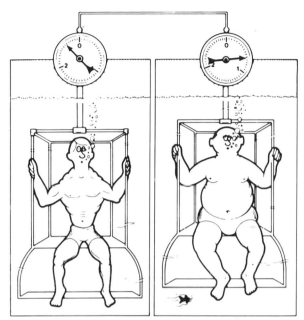

FIGURE 2–1. Illustration of the underwater weighing technique to determine body density, from which total body fat can be determined. The two individuals have the same total body weight, but the individual on the left weighs more underwater because of a higher percentage of lean tissue and a lower percentage of fat tissue.

concentration. The authors of this book have observed this phenomenon in children, adolescents, and senior or master athletes, who are all overestimated, and in young male athletes with large bone structure, who are estimated to be 3 per cent body fat or less, values that are physiologically impossible. Fortunately, these inaccuracies occur infrequently, but the fact that they do occur should be recognized.

Although the underwater weighing technique, despite its limitations, is considered the "gold standard" for evaluating body composition, the procedure is time consuming, requires considerable space and equipment, and must be conducted by someone who is highly trained in body composition assessment. As a result, most body composition evaluations, particularly in nonresearch clinical settings, are derived through anthropometric techniques. Using skinfold thickness measurements, girths, and diameters, either singly or in combination, it is possible to derive accurate estimates of body composition.[6] For many years it was assumed that the equations to predict the various components of body composition—e.g., lean weight, fat weight, and relative fat—were population specific, i.e., that they were accurate only for a population similar to the population from which the equations were derived. Recently, Jackson and Pollock[7] and Jackson, Pollock, and Ward[8] have derived a series of equations for men and women, respectively, that are generalized equations applicable for men and women of varying age and body composition. The actual application of these equations will be discussed in Chapter 6.

Understanding that there is a definite distinction between overweight and obesity, it is possible to better understand the data now available regarding the prevalence of overweight and obesity in the United States. According to the U.S. Public Health Service, obesity has become a health problem of epidemic proportions, with approximately 20 per cent of the adult population overweight to a degree that may interfere with optimal health and longevity. After age 40, this figure increases to 35 per cent.[9] These figures are impressive, but they are derived on the basis of variations in weight from the standard height and weight tables. Thus, they reflect only the extent of the problem relative to overweight and not obesity. More recent surveys have attempted to differentiate between overweight and obesity by using skinfold measurements in addition to total body weight. The Ten-State Nutrition Survey, conducted between 1968 and 1970, identified between 9 and 25 per cent of the black and white male and female teenage population evaluated as exceeding an established criterion for obesity based on triceps skinfold thickness.[10] The U.S. Health and Nutrition Examination Survey (HANES), conducted between 1971 and 1974, evaluated 12,900 individuals in the 20- to 74-year-old age range, and found the following. With respect to the appropriate weight for height, 18 per cent of men and 13 per cent of women were from 10 to 19 per cent in excess of their desired values, and an additional 14 per cent of men and 24 per cent of women were 20 per cent or more above their desired value. It was also found that overweight increases sharply beyond 30 years of age, with the highest values reaching 39 per cent for men and 50 per cent for women who are 10 per cent or more overweight. Using skinfold analyses, and projecting to the total population, it was estimated that 10 to 50 million Americans are overweight or obese, and 2.8 million men and 4.5 million women are severely obese.[11]

The problems associated with obesity are considerable. In 1973, it was estimated that $10 billion per year were invested in the diet industry. Of this total, it was estimated that $14.9 million went to Weight Watchers International, $220 million to health spas and reducing salons, $100 million to exercise equipment, $54 million to the "legal" diet pill market, and $1 billion to the diet food market.[12] In addition, it is not unusual to find at least one diet book on the list of the top ten selling books in the United States at any one time. Hannon and Lohman[13] speculate on the economic costs of obesity in a totally different manner. Using the data from the National Health Survey for 18- to 79-year-olds,[14] in which skinfold fat data were available, they calculated the body composition and the excess body fat for the adult U.S. population, assuming a population data base of 146.8 million people in 1975. They calculated 377 million kg of excess fat in men and 667 million kg of excess fat in women, for a total adult excess fat in the United States of 1.044 billion kg, or 2.3 billion pounds! The energy saved by dieting to achieve desirable weight in these individuals would be equal to 1.3 billion gallons of gasoline. The savings accrued from the fact that persons would eat less to maintain this new weight would equal 750 million gallons of gasoline per year, or enough to fuel 900,000 average U.S. autos at 12,000 miles per year at 14 miles per gallon! Similarly, such savings would provide the total electrical demands of the cities of Boston, Chicago, San Francisco, and Washington, D.C., for a full year. The economic consequences of obesity are truly staggering.

There are also a series of medical problems that are associated with obesity. These have been recently reviewed by Angel and Roncari.[15] As was discussed in the previous chapter, obesity is a risk factor for cardiovascular disease, particularly coronary artery disease (CAD) and hypertension. With respect to CAD, the data is generally considered equivocal. The seven-country study reported by Keys et al.[16] indicated that overweight and obesity were unrelated to CAD risk when all other risk factors were statistically controlled. However, the Framingham data, reported by Hubert et al.,[17] indicate that obesity is a discrete risk factor independent of the other CAD risk factors. Thus, obesity may be a primary risk factor for CAD, or it may exert its influence through the other known risk factors, such as hypertension, diabetes, reduced plasma HDL concentrations, and hypercholesterolemia.[15] Hypertension, on the other hand, is clearly related to obesity in a causal manner, with both imparting considerable risk for stroke and congestive heart failure. Weight reduction has been demonstrated to be one of the most effective measures for reducing and controlling high blood pressure.[1]

Obesity is a major factor in diabetes, particularly late-onset diabetes. With obesity, there appears to be an increase in insulin secretion of well over 100 to 200 per cent, and yet there is still a relative insulin deficiency, as indicated by elevated blood glucose levels.[18] It appears that as one becomes obese, there is a reduction in insulin receptor sites. This leads to an overproduction of insulin in an attempt to control blood glucose levels. As the obese individual undergoes weight loss, there is a subsequent return of receptor sites and blood glucose levels are brought under control. Whether receptor sites are actually increased or decreased, or whether they simply become active or inactive, is not well understood at this time.

Abnormal plasma lipid and lipoprotein concentrations are commonly associated with obesity.[15] Most common are elevated levels of plasma triglycerides, usually due to increased rates of production of very low density lipoproteins by the liver. Total cholesterol and low density lipoprotein cholesterol are typically elevated, and high density lipoprotein cholesterol is reduced in the obese patient. This lipid and lipoprotein profile is characteristic of the individual at high risk for CAD; however, weight reduction does tend to normalize these abnormal values.

Gallstones, gout, and carcinoma have also been associated with obesity.[19] Other diseases and disorders associated with obesity include respiratory insufficiency, thromboembolic disease, congestive heart failure, and increased risk from surgery.[20] Obesity also has serious social and psychological consequences. The obese population is a prime target group of the mass media, which promote the image of thinness and the undesirability of being fat. The cosmetic and clothing industries also perpetuate this image.[12] Society frequently looks on the obese individual as lacking self-control and practicing overindulgence. They see obesity as a self-inflicted disability. Obesity may actually be the cause of downward mobility in society, and it may adversely influence acceptance into college, job hiring, and promotion.[12, 21] There are also practical considerations, such as impaired heterosexual relations, the fact that a higher percentage of one's income must go for food and clothing, and even the fact that most seats are too small to comfortably accommodate the obese individual.

The above discussion implies serious consequences for those who become obese. The most serious would appear to come in the area of increased morbidity and mortality from various diseases.[15] However, there have been recent challenges to this assumption. Andres, following an extensive review of epidemiological studies, concludes that the major population studies of obesity and mortality fail to show that, overall, obesity leads to a greater risk. He even suggests that new research be initiated to look into the possible benefits of moderate obesity![22] Fitzgerald, in a 1981 review article, presents three theses for consideration.[23] First, obesity may be more an aesthetic and moral problem than one of physical health. Second, the therapy for obesity may be, in some circumstances, more detrimental than fatness. Finally, there may be some advantages, in medical and other senses, to being fat. She contends that when such a high percentage of the population is overweight, or exceeds the normal values, then the standards should be raised so that "normal" truly reflects normal. She states:

> **A well-adapted animal has the ability to store fat during periods of abundant food supply in preparation for the inevitable intervals of famine. It may be, then, that the prevalence of obesity in the United States is due to the conjunction of millions of years of evolutionary thrust with a remarkable sufficiency of food available at minimal exertion. The fat may be the most highly evolved among us. And should food become scarce through natural disaster, war, or shortages of energy, the fat may be the most likely survivors.[23]**

These views, however, appear to represent only a minority opinion.

PATHOPHYSIOLOGY OF OBESITY

To understand the pathophysiology of obesity, it will be necessary to review first the morphology of adipose tissue and then the various factors that lead to the obese state, i.e., the etiology of obesity. With a basic appreciation for both the morphology of adipose tissue and the etiology of obesity, the role of physical inactivity as a contributing factor, and of physical activity as a means of dealing with the problem, can be more clearly delineated.

First, what is adipose tissue? It is a form of connective tissue composed

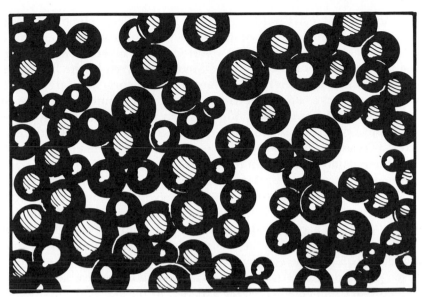

FIGURE 2–2. Illustration of fat cells taken from a fat biopsy in the gluteal region.

of cells (adipocytes) that are separated from each other by a matrix of collagenous fibers and yellow elastic fibers. Fat accumulates by the filling of existing adipocytes (hypertrophy) and by the formation of new fat cells (hyperplasia). The normal, nonobese individual will increase fat stores from birth to maturity by a combination of hypertrophy and hyperplasia. At maturity, the obese individual has 90 to 150 billion fat cells, compared with 20 to 30 billion for the nonobese, or 3 to 5 times more. Obese individuals also typically have more fat per cell.

How does the obese individual become obese? This may vary depending on whether the obesity was of early or late onset. Knittle,[24] in an article reviewing much of the initial work in this area, proposed several possibilities in the genesis of obesity. Early work suggested that fat increases steadily for the first nine months of life and then levels off or increases slightly until the age of seven years, when it once again increases. A final spurt of fat deposition occurs during adolescence. Using the needle biopsy technique, Knittle and his associates were able to determine the actual changes in fat-cell size and number during these critical periods of fat deposition. In their studies, they were able to obtain samples of subcutaneous fat from obese and nonobese subjects between 2 and 26 years of age. At all age levels studied, the obese children had larger cells, attaining adult size by the age of 11 years, and a greater number of fat cells, often attaining the adult cell number at an early age. He concluded that it is reasonable to assume that subjects who have exceeded normal adult values for cellularity will most likely retain their obesity, whereas those who are within the normal range or below may outgrow their "baby fat."

Much of the early work indicated that fat cell number increased markedly during the first year of life, increased gradually until puberty, and then increased markedly again for a period of several years, with the maximum number of fat cells becoming stabilized or fixed by the late teens or early twenties.[25] Apparently, according to this theory, adult-onset obesity could only be the result of hypertrophy, since fat cell number became fixed before adulthood was reached. These findings seemed to be at odds with both clinical observation and subsequent scientific studies. Clinicians reported increases in total body fat in patients who were lean in early adulthood; these could not be accounted for only on the basis of an increase in the size of the existing cells, for adipocytes are known to have a maximum size that cannot be exceeded. In an extremely interesting study of piglets, Widdowson and Shaw[26] took litters of pigs with a normal complement of fat cells at 10 days of age and fed half of the pigs a normal diet while starving the other half. At the end of the first year, those pigs that had been starved weighed only 5 to 6 kg, compared with 200 kg for the control group. The starved pigs had no detectable fat cells at the end of the year, although they had a normal complement at 10 days of age. At the end of the first year, the starved pigs were allowed to eat freely, and were soon of normal or above normal body fat. This study and others raised serious questions regarding the stability of fat cell number at a specific age and cast doubts on the methodology that had been used to assess fat cell number.[25,27]

The potential problem of methodological error in fat cell counting is an important issue. If fat cell number is increased only to a certain age, i.e., maturity, at which point it becomes fixed, then the first twenty years of one's life are extremely critical with respect to preventing or controlling obesity. Entering adulthood with a lower number of fat cells should ensure one a life free of extreme obesity, since the existing fat cells cannot enlarge beyond a certain size. On the other hand, those who enter adulthood with an elevated number of cells will be doomed to a life of obesity. Recently, it has been suggested that the initial methods used to determine fat cell number may have, in fact, underestimated the true number of fat cells.[25] Using an automated cell counter for counting osmium-fixed fat cells, the early studies probably were not able to measure cells with a diameter of less than 25 microns. Also, early studies were unable to detect preadipocytes and undifferentiated cells that were destined to become adipocytes. Sjöström[25] provides an excellent discussion of these methodological considerations in a recent review. Current evidence suggests that fat cells can be increased throughout life, and that the achievement of some mean adipocyte size triggers the events that culminate in an increase in the number of adipocytes.[28] Whether this cell increase is the result of newly formed cells or simply the use of existing preadipocytes or undifferentiated cells has yet to be resolved.

With respect to the developmental aspects of adipose tissue, Sjöström and his colleagues conducted a longitudinal study on 16 healthy, nonobese infants from the first through the eighteenth month of life.[25] Six biopsies from gluteal adipose depots were taken throughout this 18-month period. Fat weight increased from 0.7 to 2.8 kg during the first 12 months, an increase that was the result of increases in fat cell size, with little increase in fat cell number. Fat weight increased another 0.5 kg during the next six months, with cell size remaining constant and cell number increasing. At 12 months of age, the existing fat cells had reached adult size. This would tend to confirm the hypothesis that increases in cell number are triggered by the attainment of a certain maximum cell size.

A number of studies have been conducted in an attempt to manipulate fat cell size and number. Faust et al.[29] placed newborn rat pups into either small litters (4 pups/litter) or large litters (20 pups/litter). Following weaning, half of the rats from the small litters and half from the large litters were placed on ordinary stock diet for nearly a year, while the remaining halves of the large and small litters were placed on the stock diet for the first six months and then switched to a highly palatable high-fat diet for the remaining six months. The average body weights of the four groups at the end of the experiment were 704 vs. 956 g for the large and small litter rats fed the high-fat diet, and 584 vs. 749 g for the large and small litter rats fed the stock diet throughout the study. Fat cell size was not influenced by the size of the litters, but fat cell number was greater in rats raised in small litters. The high-fat diet resulted in increases in both cell size and cell number. The authors pointed to the importance of early nutrition in establishing a basis for obesity later in life.

Studies have also been conducted on experimental obesity in humans. Sims[30] has conducted several studies on experimental weight gains in both college students and inmates from a state prison. First, he found that it was difficult to add even 10 per cent to the normal body weight when the activity of the subject was not restricted. He reported data on 22 volunteers who achieved a weight gain of 20 per cent or more of their initial weight.[30] Interestingly, he found that once a desired experimental overweight was achieved, it took a considerable number of calories consumed to maintain that weight, i.e., 3,100 Kcal maintained their initial weight, but 5,100 Kcal were necessary to maintain their experimental overweight. He found that the initial weight gain and the subsequent weight loss back to the original weight were accomplished without a change in the number of fat cells; i.e., fat cells did not increase with weight gain or decrease with weight loss. Salens et al.[31] reported similar results with a 3-to-4–month period of weight gain. Their six subjects had a mean gain of 16.2 kg, 10.4 kg of which being fat. This gain in fat and the subsequent reduction back to normal values were not accompanied by changes in fat cell number, just changes in fat cell size.

From the preceding discussion, it appears that fat cell size can vary throughout life. Fat cell number also appears to vary throughout life, although it is relatively stable once maturity is reached. Increases in cell number are probably the result of the existing fat cells' attaining a certain maximum cell size, which then acts to trigger an increase in cell number.

Hypercellularity leads to a permanently elevated cellular mass, making weight loss in the obese an extremely difficult task and possibly explaining the high rate of failure of obese subjects on weight reduction programs.

ETIOLOGY OF OBESITY: RISK FACTORS

How does obesity develop? What factors contribute to its development? Society has been both kind and cruel in its perception of the obese individual, swinging like a pendulum from the one extreme of "glandular problems" to the other extreme of gluttony. In the first, all blame is removed from the individual; in the second, the individual must accept full responsibility. Fox, in his classic article entitled "The Enigma of Mass Regulation," states that to dispose of obesity as being due to overeating is about as helpful as attributing alcoholism to the consumption of too much alcohol.[32] It is now clear that obesity is the result of a number of causes, an observation that has led to the formation of several classification systems for obesity.

One of the first classifications systems was proposed by von Noorden in the early 1900s.[18] He classified obesity into two major types: endogenous, including metabolic abnormalities, endocrine abnormalities, and brain lesions; and exogenous, which comprised basically everything from outside the body, including overeating and physical inactivity. Bray proposes an anatomical classification (i.e., hypertrophic vs. hyperplastic, or obesity due to increases in cell size vs. increases in cell number)[33] as well as an etiological classification.[34] In his etiological classification, Bray lists the following factors: genetic, nutritional, inactivity, endocrine, hypothalamic, and drugs.[34] Five of these six factors will be discussed briefly here. Drugs will not be reviewed.

Genetic Factors

The genetic aspects of obesity are difficult to discern. There are certain genetic disorders that predispose one to obesity, such as the Laurence-Moon-Bardet-Biedl syndrome, Alstrom's syndrome, and Morgagni's syndrome.[34] Of greater concern, however, is the familial aspect of obesity. Is there a genetic link between the obese parent and the obese child, or is the obesity the result of their eating at the same table and living under the same environmental conditions? These are not easy questions to answer. Foch and McClearn[35] have completed a recent review of the literature in this area. Studies on various species of animals indicate that there is a definite genetic component to obesity. With humans, investigations are much more difficult to control and the results are not as definitive. Typical models used include observing identical twins raised in the same or in different environments and observing adopted children compared with their biological parents (genetic) and their adoptive parents (environmental). Foch and McClearn concluded that twin studies and family studies implicate a heritable component in the development of obesity, but the evidence is far from unequivocal.[35] The magnitude of the genetic contribution varied considerably with the criterion of obesity, e.g., weight vs. skinfolds, and depended on age and sex.

Nutritional Factors

With respect to nutritional factors, in the previous section on the morphology of adipose tissue several studies were cited that supported the importance of nutritional factors in the development of obesity. Overfeeding, as demonstrated by the rats raised in small litters and by the overfeeding studies in humans, led to major increases in total body fat.[29,30] Rats placed on high-fat diets also gained substantially more body fat than similar rats fed standard stock diets.[29] The size and number of meals per day also influence the development of obesity, with frequent small meals resulting in smaller gains in adipose tissue.[32] Thus, total calories, the composition of the diet with respect to palatability, and meal size and frequency are all factors that appear to be linked to obesity.

Inactivity

There is strong evidence that between 80 and 86 per cent of adult obesity has its origins in childhood.[36] In addition, many of the early studies that will be reviewed in this section suggest that childhood obesity is associated more with inactivity than with overeating. Mayer has stated: "I am convinced that inactivity is the most important factor in explaining the frequency of 'creeping' overweight in modern Western societies."[37] Bruch studied a group of 160 obese children and found that 76 per cent of the boys and 68 per cent of the girls were abnormally inactive, whereas only 18 per cent of the boys and 22 per cent of the girls fell within the normal range of activity.[38] Rony,[39] Bronstein et al.,[40] Graham,[41] Tolstrup,[42] and Juel-Nielsen[43] observed similar results. Fry[44] found obese children to have average caloric intakes comparable to nonobese children of the same age, but a much higher proportion of the obese were labeled as only moderately active or as inactive. Johnson et al.[45] observed two groups of high school girls—28 obese and 28 nonobese of similar height, age, and grade—with respect to maturation, food intake, and physical activity. The obese girls showed advanced development, with an earlier deceleration of growth in height and an earlier menarche. The caloric intake of the obese group was significantly lower than that of the nonobese group, and although both groups were found to be relatively inactive, the obese girls were significantly more so.

Stefanik et al.[46] studied food intake and energy expenditure patterns of 14 obese adolescent boys in relation to a paired control group of nonobese boys during summer camp. The energy intake of the obese boys was significantly less than that of the nonobese boys. In addition, although little difference was noted in the amount of time scheduled for light, moderate, and very active exercise, the degree of participation in active exercise was generally less for the obese. Bullen et al.[47] employed a motion picture technique for comparing activity levels of obese and nonobese adolescent girls while they engaged in three sports at a summer camp. Three-second shots were taken at regular intervals, and were analyzed for the time spent motionless and for energy expenditure calculated on the basis of type and speed of locomotion and intensity of movement. On the basis of nearly 30,000 observations, it was concluded that the obese girls were far less active than the nonobese girls. Corbin and Pletcher[48] observed the caloric intake and physical activity patterns of obese and nonobese elementary school children; they found the groups to have similar energy intakes, but the obese had significantly lower activity levels.

However, to the contrary, Durnin[49] observed energy intake and expenditure in approximately 100 boys and girls, 13 to 15 years of age. Although energy intake was not specified by classification of obesity, he found that there was no difference in the number of minutes per day spent in moderate or heavy physical activity between lean, normal, and obese subjects. Watson and O'Donovan[50] studied 85 17-to-18–year-old school boys and found no relationship between relative leanness and fatness and the level of habitual physical activity. Wilkinson et al.[51] reported on the energy intake and physical activity levels of obese and matched nonobese 10-year-old boys and girls and found no significant differences between the groups for energy intake or expenditure. Bradfield et al.[52] reported no significant differences in energy expenditure between nonobese and obese girls during physical education classes, school classroom activities, and afterschool work or play. Three-day activity assessments showed that both groups were very inactive, 70 per cent of their time being spent either in sleep or in very light activities. Waxman and Stunkard[53] converted measures of activity into caloric expenditure by measuring oxygen consumption and found that obese boys actually expended more calories through activity than did nonobese boys.

In the adult population, Brownell and Stunkard[54] conclude that obese adults are less active than are those of normal weight on the basis of studies that have used self-report, pedometers, spontaneous use of stairs in place of escalators in public places, and a device that discriminates standing from sitting. They suggest that caution be used in interpreting this data, since lower levels of activity may not represent lower levels of energy expenditure because of the greater cost of activities for the obese person. Also, it is not clear whether the inactivity is a cause of obesity or the result of it. Thus, for the population of both children and adults, the role of physical inactivity in predisposing one to obesity is still not resolved. Additional research is needed. Such research must approach this problem from a fresh perspective, using tight controls and taking advantage of recent developments in monitoring equipment.

Endocrine Factors

Three different endocrine manipulations can produce obesity: administration of insulin, administration of glucocorticoids, and castration.[33] Also, approximately 12 substances, which either are hormones or have hormone-like activity, have been identified as being involved in stimulating lipogenesis, and an additional nine stimulate lipolysis.[32] Thus, it is not surprising that the endocrine system is implicated in weight control and obesity. With respect to the three endocrine manipulations, the experimental elevation of insulin produces hyperphagia, or overeating. This hyperphagia is in response either to lowered blood glucose levels or to the direct effect of insulin on the brain.[33] Glucocorticoids administered experimentally to animals often will result in increases in body fat with little or no increase in body weight. Evidently, steroid administration modifies the metabolism of adipose tissue toward increased fat storage.[33] Castration of animals results in substantial redistributions of body fat, undoubtedly mediated through altered estrogen and testosterone levels in the blood plasma

Hypothalamic Factors

The hypothalamus is implicated in obesity primarily through lesions in specific areas of the lower anterior portion of the ventromedial nucleus.[19] Most lesions are experimentally induced in animals to determine changes in feeding behavior. From a considerable body of research in this area, two centers have been identified that regulate food intake. The lateral hypothalamus has been determined to induce eating when stimulated, and the ventromedial region is responsible for turning off the appetite. Thus, these areas have been termed the "feeding" and "satiety" centers, respectively. This information is important in trying to better understand what controls eating behavior, but actual lesions of the hypothalamus in the human population are extremely rare.

PREVENTION AND TREATMENT OF OBESITY

Ideally, obesity should be prevented. However, realistically, millions of Americans are obese and many are desperately seeking help. Although prevention is basically a matter of balancing caloric expenditure with caloric intake, treatment of the obese person involves a much more complex plan of action. For those who are moderately obese, i.e., no more than 20 to 30 pounds above ideal weight as determined by body composition assessment, a modest reduction in caloric intake of approximately 250 Kcal per day and an equally modest increase in activity levels of 250 Kcal per day, e.g., 2.5 miles of walking, should result in a 1 pound weight loss per week. This 500 Kcal deficit per day would total 3,500 Kcal per week, which is approximately the energy equivalent of one pound of fat. Over a 20-to-30–week period of time, weight would return to desirable levels. For those who are grossly obese, more drastic measures are often taken. The forms of treatment generally used include diet; drugs; surgery; behavioral modification, self-help groups, psychoanalysis, and psychotherapy; and physical activity. Two textbooks have reviewed each of these areas in considerable detail.[55,56] A very brief review will be conducted in this chapter on the areas of diet, drugs, surgery, and the behavioral aspects. Physical activity will be discussed in considerable detail in Chapter 5.

Once obesity has been identified, it is important to start treatment as soon as possible. Generally, the greater the degree of obesity, the more difficult it is to treat successfully. Three key factors in any treatment program are motivation, expectation, and self-responsibility. Providing information to the obese individual is not sufficient by itself. Motivation can take many forms, but it can be illustrated by the general program used in behavior modification, in which a system of goals and rewards is established. There must also be a well-defined reason for the weight loss, one that will truly be motivational for the individual. For many, the reason may be cosmetic, i.e., they want to look better. For others, e.g., the hypertensive or diabetic patient, health may be the reason. Regarding expectation, the obese person must have a realistic weight goal established. When this goal is a considerable distance from the present weight, intermediate goals must be established, along with designated times for accomplishing them. If weight loss does not follow the patient's expectations, he or she will typically become discouraged and discontinue the treatment program. The patient should also be warned about plateaus or periods of decreased rate of weight loss. If these are expected, they will not produce serious anxiety, guilt, and discouragement.

In the dietary treatment of obesity, several levels of treatment are possible: starvation and fasting; semistarvation or low-calorie diets; and diets that are moderately deficient in calories, i.e., 500 Kcal or less below maintenance levels. Starvation and fasting are usually considered to be synonymous terms, but with starvation vitamins and minerals are not typically supplemented. In total fasting, the amount of glucose stored in the muscles and liver can suffice for only relatively short periods of time, after which amino acids from muscle protein are used for gluconeogenesis. Thus, protein loss does occur, and there are accompanying losses of nitrogen. During fasting, the major fuel for most tissues is derived from free fatty acids, with the release of ketone bodies into the blood. These are referred to as ketoacids, and include acetone, which imparts a characteristic odor to the breath. In a 24-hour fast, a normal man lying down will use 1800 Kcal of energy, including 360 Kcals from 75 g of protein. The remaining energy comes from triglycerides. The contribution of protein decreases to 18 to 24 g per day with prolonged fasting. The initial loss of 75 g of protein per day can be reduced to 15 g per day by having the subject consume 1 liter of dextrose water (10 per cent solution).[19,56]

With a total fasting regime, the typical 300-pound patient will average a weight loss of approximately 1 pound per day for the first two months.[19] Up to 20 pounds of this weight loss can come from the lean tissues, and an additional 26 pounds can come from body water stores, leaving a loss of body fat of approximately 14 to 16 pounds, or only 23 to 25 per cent of the total weight loss. Most of the water loss (67 per cent) comes from the extracellular fluid compartment, with a plasma volume loss of from 400 to 700 ml. There are a number of potential complications to total fasting, including nausea, diarrhea, persistent vomiting, postural hypotension, nutritional deficiencies, menstrual irregularities, and sudden death. There is, however, a general loss of appetite within the first two days which remains throughout the period of fasting; this is considered to be a positive aspect of this approach to weight loss.

The long-term benefits of fasting, evaluated on the basis of follow-up studies, are disappointing.[19] The large amounts of weight lost during the fast are quickly regained. It is important to evaluate any treatment regimen on the basis of long-term follow-up studies. Although the immediate results are of interest, the real test is in the follow-up data of five years or more.

Semistarvation, or low-calorie, diets result in changes similar to those seen in total fasting, although to a lesser degree. Water losses are considerable during the first several weeks of dieting, but the protein losses are of a much lower magnitude. In both fasting and semistarvation diets, ketone bodies are formed from the increased metabolism of free fatty acids. High blood and urine levels of ketone bodies (ketosis) may be responsible for loss of appetite, but they may also have undesirable side effects. Thus, many diets suggest monitoring urine on a daily basis for the presence of ketosis, so that modifications can be made if ketone levels are too high.

More recently, traditional low-calorie diets have been modified to reduce the loss of protein, i.e., protein-sparing diets. In addition, supplements have been added to some of these diets to ensure adequate intake levels of the essential vitamins and minerals. Finally, small amounts of glucose have been suggested to increase even more the protein-sparing aspects of the diet. A fairly standard low-calorie diet includes 15 to 25 g of high biological value protein, such as egg albumin, and 45 g of carbohydrate.

Moderate decreases in caloric intake can be achieved without major alterations in the individual's diet. Simply cutting down on portion sizes, reducing the intake of high-density caloric foods, and eliminating between-meal snacking can lead to reductions in total caloric intake of from 200 to 500 Kcal. Although this is a much slower approach, the individual is learning a new pattern of eating that, ideally, will result in a more permanent loss of weight. Also, the losses in lean tissue and body water are much less, resulting in larger percentage decreases in body fat; i.e., the percentage of the weight lost from fat is increased.

Although common sense is probably the best guide to dieting for optimal weight loss, many individuals feel that they must follow one or more of the popular diets currently in vogue. Most of these diets have far more similarities than differences, but some can be potentially dangerous. The reader is referred to an excellent review of 16 popular diets written by Dwyer.[57]

Drugs have become a very popular means for treating obesity. Drugs presently used include anorexigenic agents, thyroid preparations, digitalis, diuretics, bulking agents, and human chorionic gonadotropin. Anoretic drugs, by definition, are those agents that act to decrease appetite, and they are usually classified as amphetamines and nonamphetamines.[58] The mechanisms through which these drugs act are quite complex and well beyond the scope of this chapter.[59] The anoretic drugs do appear to result in weight loss, but the loss is usually only temporary, with weight being quickly regained following the cessation of drug therapy. There are moderate to serious side effects associated with anoretic drugs, including the potential for drug abuse or addiction. Thyroid preparations have been used in the treatment of obesity, but this practice is not a very effective form of drug therapy, and it is no longer popular. Similarly, digitalis was at one time a popular drug for the treatment of obesity, but it is seldom used by physicians today. Diuretics have also been popular in weight loss programs in which large weight losses are desired. These lead to major losses in total body water, however, with little loss in body fat. With certain individuals, diuretics may aggravate the loss of electrolytes, which is certainly an undesirable side effect. Bulking agents are usually calorically inert bulk materials that lead to feelings of fullness in the stomach. They have been used with little or no success. Finally, about 25 years ago, a new treatment was proposed in which the subject was injected with human chorionic gonadotropin, a compound obtained from the urine of pregnant women. Daily injections coupled with a 500-Kcal diet were supposed to lead to major losses of body fat. Controlled studies have failed to demonstrate that these injections are any more effective than the 500-Kcal diet alone.[58,59]

Surgery has become an increasingly popular means of dealing with the grossly obese patient, when all other forms of treatment have failed. The first form of surgery was jejunoileal bypass surgery, in which the jejunum is connected with the terminal ileum, bypassing a substantial portion of the gastrointestinal tract. Although this procedure resulted in substantial weight loss for most patients, the side effects were typically major. In addition to a high operative mortality (up to 6 per cent), complications have included pulmonary embolization, serious wound infection, and renal failure. Liver failure is an occasional complication, and persistent diarrhea is almost always present. Gastric bypass surgery has become the more accepted surgical approach in recent years. Referred to as gastric stapling, the stomach is stapled together, dividing it into a proximal and distal portion. The proximal portion is small and becomes the functional portion of the stomach. The distal portion is much larger and becomes nonfunctional. This procedure has resulted in rather marked weight losses, and the complications appear to be far less serious when compared with those of the intestinal bypass procedure.[55] Finally, jaw wiring has drawn considerable attention because of the uniqueness of the procedure. Through the use of mandibular fixation, the jaws are wired together, preventing the ingestion of solid food. Unlike gastric stapling and intestinal bypass surgery, jaw wiring weight losses are transitory, with weight being quickly regained following the removal of the wires.

A great deal of attention has been focused on the behavioral treatment of obesity and eating disorders. Pioneered by Stuart in 1967[60] and made popular by Stuart's and Davis's book, *Slim Chance in a Fat World: Behavioral Control of Obesity,* [61] this rather practical approach to the treatment of obesity became very popular in the 1970s and 1980s. Based on an approach to weight loss that focused on the patient's feeding behavior, a major goal was to achieve a permanent change in lifestyle patterns. Attention was given to the patient's ingestive behavior, by looking at pace or speed of eating, bite size, bite frequency, pause time between bites, and length of chewing time. Organismic variables such as the state of hunger, mood state, and the physical state were also evaluated. Behavioral factors such as the physical position while eating and the activities associated with eating, and the stimuli preceding or concurrent with eating, were also important input variables associated with the individual's total eating behavior profile. Once these variables were determined, the individual's behavior was "shaped," making gradual changes in eating behavior. Thus, the individual learned those problem areas in his or her eating behavior that were responsible for the weight problem. Then, eating patterns were altered, or shaped, to produce a more favorable eating behavior that would lead to weight loss and control of weight at desirable levels. Although the early research on behavior modification was highly favorable, and the technique was considered superior to other treatment modalities, long-term studies have indicated that it too is not immune from a return to prior eating behaviors and, thus, a return to pretreatment body weight.[62]

From the above, it appears that all present forms of treatment of obesity are confronted with either potential major complications associated with the treatment, e.g., surgery, or with problems of poor compliance, e.g., diet and behavior modification. It is evident that far more research effort must go into two major areas: prevention and compliance. First, it is far easier to prevent obesity than to be challenged with its treatment, and it is far easier to treat obesity if it is identified in its early stages. Second, very little is known about how to deal with problems of noncompliance. This is true not only of treatment programs for obesity, but also of treatment programs for hypertension, diabetes, or any other diseases that are treated pharmacologically. Research directed toward gaining a better understanding of those factors that influence compliance is essential. This is a problem that is universal in almost all areas of medicine.

SUMMARY

Overweight and obesity constitute serious health problems in the United States. Overweight refers to any weight that exceeds the range of weights for a specific height, frame size, and gender—a range that was determined on the basis of population averages. Obesity refers to being overfat. Although overweight and obesity are related, there is a sizable percentage of individuals who are "overweight" but of normal or below normal body fat, or who are of "normal" weight but excessively fat. A body composition assessment is essential to determine obesity and to estimate a reasonable, desirable, or "ideal" body weight.

The average individual will gain approximately one pound of weight per year during each year beyond the age of 25 years. At the same time, there is a loss of approximately one-quarter to one-half pound per year of lean body tissue, predominantly from muscle and bone. The loss in lean tissue is closely associated with reductions in physical activity; i.e., if you do not use it you will lose it! The net result is a gain of 1.5 pounds per year of fat weight, or a total of 45 pounds of extra body fat by the age of 55 years. To reiterate, these values represent mean values for the U.S. population. This increase in body fat has economic, medical, social, and psychological consequences. In a single year, billions of dollars are spent, thousands of people are dying, and millions are suffering, all the result of our present epidemic of obesity. What is the basic cause of obesity? Unfortunately, the answer to this question is complex and undoubtedly involves genetic, nutritional, endocrine, hypothalamic, and pharmacological factors, in addition to physical inactivity. The end result is an increased fat cell size and probably an increased number of fat cells, or adipocytes. Knittle[24] believes that individuals are probably endowed with a certain range of adipose tissue cellularity that can be modified by a variety of environmental influences. The final depot size will in all likelihood depend upon the interaction of a genetic template with all the environmental and hormonal factors that influence number and size. Several new theories that tie in both genetic and environmental factors have been proposed to explain obesity. Newsholme[63] has proposed disruption of substrate cycling as a potential basis for obesity. Substrate cycling involves an obligatory loss of chemical energy as heat, and it may be important in burning off excess energy. In obesity, hormonal and nervous control of substrate cycles may be impaired. DeLuise et al.[64] have found the number of sodium-potassium pump units in erythrocytes to be reduced by 22 per cent in obese persons as compared with nonobese controls. The cation-transport activity of the pump was also reduced, and an increased concentration of sodium was found in the red cells. This would be considered a thermogenetic defect resulting in a decrease in cellular thermogenesis. These and other theories are being explored, and it is hoped that within the near future we will have a better understanding of the etiology of obesity.

The treatment of obesity is equally complex. Present forms of treatment include diet, drugs, surgery, behavior modification, and increased physical activity. With all forms of treatment, the major problem involves a lack of total commitment on the part of the obese patient. Although rather spectacular decreases in weight can occur with just about any form of treatment, the true success of any treatment is in the long-term follow-up. In all cases, with the exception of surgery, the follow-up results are not encouraging. Thus, attention must be given first to the prevention of the problem. Second, for those who become obese, the condition should be diagnosed as soon as possible. Third, once obesity has been diagnosed, an acceptable plan of treatment should be outlined, and considerable effort should be placed on seeing the patient follow through with that plan, including long-term follow-up well beyond the period of treatment.

REFERENCES

1. Craddock, D.: Obesity and its Management, 3rd ed. New York, Churchill Livingston, 1978.
2. Keys, A., and Grande, F.: Body weight, body composition and nutritional status. In Wohl, M. G., and Goodhart, R. S., editors: Modern Nutrition in Health and Disease. Philadelphia, Lea & Febiger, 1968.
3. U.S. Department of Health, Education and Welfare, Public Health Service: Obesity and Health. PHS Pub. No. 1485. Washington, D.C., U.S. Public Health Service, 1966.
4. Metropolitan Life Insurance Company: New weight standards for men and women. Stat. Bull. Metropol. Life Insur. Co. 40:3, 1959.
5. Welham, W. C., and Behnke, A. R.: The specific gravity of healthy men; body weight divided by volume and other physical characteristics of exceptional athletes and of naval personnel. J.A.M.A. 118:498–501, 1942.
6. Behnke, A. R., and Wilmore, J. H.: Evaluation and Regulation of Body Build and Composition. Englewood Cliffs, N.J., Prentice-Hall, 1974.
7. Jackson, A. S., and Pollock, M. L.: Generalized equations for predicting body density of men. Br. J. Nutr. 40:497–504, 1978.
8. Jackson, A. S., Pollock, M. L., and Ward, A.: Generalized equations for predicting body density of women. Med. Sci. Sports Exer. 12:175–182, 1980.
9. U.S. Department of Health, Education and Welfare, Public Health Service: Facts About Obesity. DHEW Pub. No. (NIH) 76–974. Washington, D.C., U.S. Public Health Service, 1976.
10. Centers for Disease Control: Ten-State Nutrition Survey 1968–70. DHEW Pub. No. (HSM) 72–8134. Atlanta, Centers for Disease Control, 1972.
11. Abraham, S., and Johnson, C. L.: Prevalence of severe obesity in adults in the United States. Am. J. Clin. Nutr. 33:364–369, 1980.
12. Allon, N.: The stigma of overweight in everyday life. In Bray, G. A., editor: Obesity in Perspective. DHEW Pub. No. (NIH) 75–708. Washington, D.C., U.S. Department of Health, Education, and Welfare, 1975.
13. Hannon, B. M., and Lohman, T. G.: The energy cost of overweight in the United States. Am. J. Pub. Health 68:765–767, 1978.
14. Stoudt, H. W., Damon, A., McFarland, R., and Roberts, J.: Weight, height and selected body dimensions of adults. Washington, D.C., U. S. Government Printing Office, 1965.
15. Angel, A., and Roncari, D. A. K.: Medical complications of obesity. Can. Med. Assoc. J. 119:1408–1411, 1978.

16. Keys, A., Aravanis, C., Blackburn, H., Van Buchem, F. S. P., Buzine, R., Djordjevic, B. S., Fidanza, F., Karvonen, M. J., Menotti, A., Puddu, V., and Taylor, H. L.: Coronary heart disease: overweight and obesity as risk factors. Ann. Intern. Med. 77:15–27, 1972.
17. Hubert, H. B., Feinleib, M., McNamara, R. M., and Castelli, W. P.: Obesity as an independent risk factor for cardiovascular disease: A 26-year follow-up of participants in the Framingham heart study. Circulation 67:968–977, 1983.
18. Sims, E. A. H.: Syndromes of obesity. In DeGroot, L. J., editor: Endocrinology, vol. 3. Baltimore, Williams & Wilkins, 1979.
19. Powers, P. S.: Obesity: The Regulation of Weight. Baltimore, Williams & Wilkins, 1980.
20. Petit, D. W.: The ills of the obese. In Bray, G. A., and Bethune, J. E., editors: Treatment and Management of Obesity. New York, Harper and Row, 1974.
21. Hirsch, J.: The psychological consequences of obesity. In Bray, G. A., editor: Obesity in Perspective. DHEW Pub. No. (NIH) 75–708. Washington, D.C., U.S. Department of Health, Education, and Welfare, 1975.
22. Andres, R.: Effect of obesity on total mortality. Int. J. Obesity. 4:381–386, 1980.
23. Fitzgerald, F. T.: The problem of obesity. Ann. Rev. Med. 32:221–231, 1981.
24. Knittle, J. L.: Obesity in childhood: a problem in adipose tissue cellular development. J. Pediatr. 81:1048–1059, 1972.
25. Sjöström, L.: Fat cells and body weight. In Stunkard, A. J., editor: Obesity. Philadelphia, W. B. Saunders Co., 1980.
26. Widdowson, E. M., and Shaw, W. T.: Full and empty fat cells. Lancet II:905, 1973.
27. Gurr, M. I., Kirtland, J., Phillip, M., and Robinson, M. P.: The consequences of early overnutrition for fat cell size and number: the pig as an experimental model for human obesity. Int. J. Obesity. 1:151–170, 1977.
28. Faust, I. M., Johnson, P. R., Stern, J. S., and Hirsch, J.: Diet-induced adipocyte number increase in adult rats. Am. J. Physiol. 235:E279–E286, 1978.
29. Faust, I. M., Johnson, P.R., and Hirsch, J.: Long-term effects of early nutritional experiences on the development of obesity in the rat. J. Nutr. 110:2027–2034, 1980.
30. Sims, E. A.: Studies in human hyperphagia. In Bray, G. A., and Bethune, J. E., editors: Treatment and Management of Obesity. New York, Harper and Row, 1974.
31. Salens, L. B., Horton, E. S., and Sims, E. A. H.: Experimental obesity in man: cellular character of the adipose tissue. J. Clin. Invest. 50:1005–1011, 1971.
32. Fox, F. W.: The enigma of mass regulation. S. Afr. Med. J. 48:287–301, 1974.
33. Bray, G. A.: The varieties of obesity. In Bray, G. A., and Bethune, J. E., editors: Treatment and Management of Obesity. New York, Harper and Row, 1974.
34. Bray, G. A.: Experimental models for the study of obesity: introductory remarks. Fed. Proc. 36:137–138, 1977.
35. Foch, T. T., and McClearn, G.E.: Genetics, body weight, and obesity. In Stunkard, A. J., editor: Obesity. Philadelphia, W. B. Saunders Co., 1980.
36. Wilson, N. L., editor: Obesity. Philadelphia, F. A. Davis Co., 1969.
37. Meyer, J.: Exercise and weight control. Postgrad. Med. 25:325–332, 1959.
38. Bruch, H.: Obesity in childhood. IV. Energy expenditure of obese children. Am. J. Dis. Child. 60:1082–1109, 1940.
39. Rony, H. R.: Obesity and Leanness. Philadelphia, Lea & Febiger, 1940.
40. Bronstein, I. P., Wexler, S., Brown, A. W., and Halpern, L. J.: Obesity in childhood. Psychologic studies. Am. J. Dis. Child. 63:238–251, 1942.
41. Graham, H. B.: Corpulence in childhood and adolescence: a clinical study. Med. J. Aust. 2:649–658, 1947.
42. Tolstrup, K.: On psychogenic obesity in children IV. Acta Pediatr. 42:289–303, 1953.
43. Juel-Nielsen, N.: On psychogenic obesity in children II. Acta Pediatr. 42:130–145, 1953.
44. Fry, P. C.: A comparative study of "obese" children selected on the basis of fat pads. Am. J. Clin. Nutr. 1:453–468, 1953.
45. Johnson, M. L., Burke, B., and Mayer, J.: Relative importance of inactivity and overeating in the energy balance of obese high school girls. Am. J. Clin. Nutr. 4:37–44, 1956.
46. Stefanik, P. A., Heald, F. P., and Mayer, J.: Caloric intake in relation to energy output of obese and non-obese adolescent boys. Am. J. Clin. Nutr. 7:55–62, 1959.
47. Bullen, B. A., Reed, R. B., and Mayer, J.: Physical activity of obese and nonobese adolescent girls appraised by motion picture sampling. Am. J. Clin. Nutr. 14:211–223, 1964.
48. Corbin, C. B., and Pletcher, P.: Diet and physical activity patterns of obese and nonobese elementary school children. Res. Q. 39:922–928, 1968.

49. Durnin, J. V. G. A.: Physical activity by adolescents. Acta Paediatr. Scand. [Suppl.] *217:* 133–135, 1971.
50. Watson, A. W. S., and O'Donovan, D. J.: The relationship of level of habitual activity to measures of leanness-fatness, physical working capacity, strength and motor ability in 17 and 18 year-old males. Eur. J. Appl. Physiol. *37:*93–100, 1977.
51. Wilkinson, P. W., Parklin, J. M., Pearlson, G., Strong, H., and Sykes, P.: Energy intake and physical activity in obese children. Br. Med. J. *1:*756, 1977.
52. Bradfield, R. B., Paulos, J., and Grossman, L.: Energy expenditure and heart rate of obese high school girls. Am. J. Clin. Nutr. *24:*1482–1488, 1971.
53. Waxman, M., and Stunkard, A. J.: Caloric intake and expenditure of obese children. J. Pediatr. *96:*187–193, 1980.
54. Brownell, K. D., and Stunkard, A. J.: Physical activity in the development and control of obesity. *In* Stunkard, A. J., editor: Obesity. Philadelphia, W. B. Saunders Co., 1980.
55. Stunkard, A. J., editor: Obesity. Philadelphia, W. B. Saunders Co., 1980.
56. Munro, J. F., editor: The Treatment of Obesity. Baltimore, University Park Press, 1979.
57. Dwyer, J.: Sixteen popular diets: brief nutritional analyses. *In* Stunkard, A. J., editor: Obesity. Philadelphia, W. B. Saunders Co., 1980.
58. Lasagna, L.: Drugs in the treatment of obesity. *In* Stunkard, A. J., editor: Obesity. Philadelphia, W. B. Saunders Co., 1980.
59. Blundell, J. E., and Burridge, S. L.: Control of feeding and the psychopharmacology of anorexic drugs. *In* Munro, J. F., editor: The Treatment of Obesity. Baltimore, University Park Press, 1979.
60. Stuart, R. B.: Behavioral control of overeating. Behav. Res. Ther. *5:*357–365, 1967.
61. Stuart, R. B., and Davis, B.: Slim Chance in a Fat World: Behavioral Control of Obesity. Champaign, Ill., Research Press, 1972.
62. Wilson, G. T.: Behavior modification and the treatment of obesity. *In* Stunkard, A. J., editor: Obesity. Philadelphia, W. B. Saunders Co., 1980.
63. Newsholme, E. A.: A possible metabolic basis for the control of body weight. N. Engl. J. Med. *302:*400–405, 1980.
64. DeLuise, M., Blackburn, G.L., and Flier, J. S.: Reduced activity of the red-cell sodium-potassium pump in human obesity. N. Engl. J. Med. *303:*1017–1022, 1980.

PHYSIOLOGY OF EXERCISE RELATED TO FITNESS DEVELOPMENT AND MAINTENANCE

The next three chapters will summarize the research findings concerning the effects of physical activity on the major components of health-related fitness. Since relaxation and emotional stability, as well as risk factor reduction, have already been covered, this section will deal primarily with cardiorespiratory function, body composition, muscular strength and endurance, and flexibility.

Even though the various components of physiological function will be discussed as separate entities, it is important to emphasize that the body functions as a whole, and often something that affects one bodily system has an effect on the whole. For example, a person who is participating in a jogging program generally would be trying to develop or maintain cardiorespiratory fitness. Jogging would also have an effect on the musculoskeletal system of the legs and trunk, i.e., some muscular strength and endurance would be developed in these areas with a possible reduction in flexibility. Body composition would also be affected, resulting in weight and fat loss and maintenance or increase in lean body weight. This particular jogging program may increase bone den-

51

sity in the lower extremity; on the other hand, if too strenuous, it may cause injury. The mind would also be at work during the jog and could perceive the effort in a positive or negative manner. Hence, one can see the complexity involved in trying to quantify the effects of physical activity on the various bodily systems.

Chapter 3

CARDIORESPIRATORY
FUNCTION

INTRODUCTION

Cardiorespiratory function is dependent upon efficient respiratory and cardiovascular systems, adequate blood components (red blood cell count, hemoglobin, hematocrit, and blood volume), and specific cellular components that help the body utilize oxygen during exercise.[1-3]

The oxygen transport system comprises the lungs, which bring in fresh air from the external environment and permit oxygen to move across a membrane system (by diffusion) into the circulation. When oxygen reaches the blood, it is picked up within the red blood cells and transported through the arterial portion of the circulatory system to the working cells (diffusion and utilization). End products of cellular metabolism (carbon dioxide and lactic acid) are then transported back through the veins of the circulatory system to the heart and lungs. Various buffering and biochemical reactions are also taking place in the liver, kidney, and cells in an attempt to maintain bodily homeostasis and replenish energy supplies for continued work. The heart is the key to the oxygen transport system, since it must continually pump blood to all bodily systems as well as larger quantities to the more active tissues.

Pulmonary factors, such as total lung volume, maximum breathing capacity, pulmonary diffusion capacity, vital capacity, pulmonary ventilation, and breathing rate, do not limit endurance performance unless one has significant pulmonary disease or is training at altitude.[1,4] That is, under most conditions and at sea level, arterial blood leaving the heart is approximately 97 per cent saturated with oxygen, and therefore most of the limitation to endurance performance depends on the capacity of the heart and circulation and on cellular function.

As shown in Table 3–1, important components of the oxygen transport system improve with endurance training. Cardiac output is the amount of blood pumped out of the heart per minute and is determined by multiplying

TABLE 3-1. THE EFFECTS OF CHRONIC PHYSICAL ACTIVITY
ON CARDIORESPIRATORY FUNCTIONS

VARIABLES	UNIT	CHANGES WITH ENDURANCE TRAINING
Maximal values		
Oxygen uptake	$ml \cdot kg^{-1} \cdot min^{-1}$	Increase
Cardiac output	L/min	Increase
Heart rate	beats/min	Unchanged—decrease
Stroke volume	ml	Increase
Arteriovenous oxygen difference	ml/100 ml blood	Increase
Systolic blood pressure	mm Hg	Unchanged
Rate pressure product	beats/min $\times$ mm Hg $\times$ 10^3	Unchanged
Endurance performance	sec	Decrease*
Submaximal values†		
Oxygen uptake	$ml \cdot kg^{-1} \cdot min^{-1}$	Unchanged—decreased
Cardiac output	L/min	Unchanged
Heart rate	beats/min	Decrease
Stroke volume	ml	Increase
Systolic blood pressure	mm Hg	Decrease
Diastolic blood pressure	mm Hg	Unchanged—decreased
Rate pressure product	beats/min $\times$ mm Hg $\times$ 10^3	Decrease
Resting values		
Oxygen uptake	$ml \cdot kg^{-1} \cdot min^{-1}$	Unchanged
Cardiac output	L/min	Unchanged
Heart rate	beats/min	Decrease
Stroke volume	ml	Increase
Systolic blood pressure	mm Hg	Unchanged—decrease
Diastolic blood pressure	mm Hg	Unchanged—decrease
Rate pressure product	beats/min $\times$ mm Hg $\times$ 10^3	Decrease

*The performance will improve, i.e., performance at a given distance will decrease, and performance time on a treadmill or cycle ergometer will increase.

† Same absolute load.

heart rate (HR) by stroke volume (amount of blood pumped out of the heart per beat). The arteriovenous oxygen difference (A-V O_2 difference) represents the amount of oxygen being utilized by the cells from the arterial blood. Maximum oxygen uptake ($\dot{V}O_2$ max), or aerobic capacity, is the largest amount of oxygen that one can utilize under the most strenuous exercise.[5-7] See Figure 3-1. It correlates highly with cardiac output.[1] Because maximum oxygen uptake generally summarizes what is going on in the oxygen transport system (including cellular utilization) during maximum or exhaustive exercise and can be measured rather easily, it has been used as the measure most representative of cardiorespiratory fitness.[1,2,8]

Because a larger person generally has more muscle mass, and thus the capability of burning more oxygen per unit of time, aerobic capacity is often expressed relative to body weight, i.e., milliliters of oxygen per kilogram of body weight per minute ($ml \cdot kg^{-1} \cdot min^{-1}$). More specifically, if one's efficiency to move the body from one place to another is important, $\dot{V}O_2$ max should be expressed as $ml \cdot kg^{-1} \cdot min^{-1}$, as mentioned previously. If efficiency of the heart and oxygen transport system is more important, $\dot{V}O_2$ max should be expressed in milliliters per kilogram of lean body weight

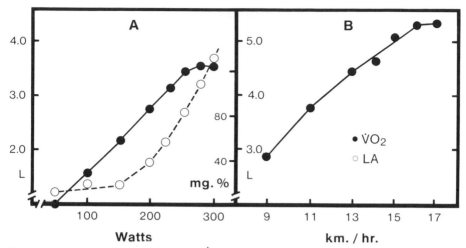

Figure 3–1. Increase in oxygen uptake ($\dot{V}O_2$, continuous line) and blood lactate concentration (HLA, interrupted line) in relation to work load. The subjects were working *(A)* on a bicycle ergometer and *(B)* on a treadmill. In both cases, a definite plateau for the oxygen uptake was obtained. (Originally published in Åstrand, P. O.: Measurement of maximal aerobic capacity. Canadian Medical Association Journal, Vol. 96, March 25, 1967, pp. 732–735.)

(LBW) per minute ($ml \cdot kg^{-1} \, LBW \cdot min^{-1}$).[9] Because most often it is important to evaluate aerobic capacity in respect to moving one's body weight, $\dot{V}O_2$ max expressed as $ml \cdot kg^{-1} \cdot min^{-1}$ is preferred. When an individual gains or loses a large amount of body weight by diet, exercise, or some combination thereof, the per cent change in $\dot{V}O_2$ max expressed as $ml \cdot kg^{-1} \cdot min^{-1}$ will be biased as a result of change in body weight. In this case, looking at the change in $\dot{V}O_2$ max expressed as L/min would provide better information about the improved aerobic capacity.

The effects of physical training on the cardiorespiratory functions listed in Table 3–1 are based on results from healthy adults who were free from overt signs of heart disease. How these functions may differ in patients with cardiovascular disease will be discussed later in this chapter and in Chapter 8. Maximum oxygen uptake and cardiac output almost always improve with endurance training. This improvement is most related to increases in stroke volume and A-V O_2 difference.[1-3] Maximum heart rate (HR_{max}) generally remains constant after training or is reduced by approximately 5 to 7 beats/min.[1,10]

An indirect measure of coronary blood flow is the rate pressure product: HR (beats/min) × systolic blood pressure (mm Hg).[11,12] Thus, since HR_{max} and maximum systolic blood pressure are not altered as a result of training, maximum coronary blood flow does not change when ventricular function and the coronary anatomy are normal.

When standard submaximal tests are administered before and after an endurance training regimen, for activities that require little skill, such as walking, running, and bicycling, $\dot{V}O_2$ and cardiac output remain relatively constant, whereas HR and systolic blood pressure are significantly re-duced.[1,13] Stroke volume is increased and is the important factor in main-taining cardiac output or $\dot{V}_{O_2}$ at submaximal levels. The lower HR and systolic blood pressure at a standard submaximal workload indicate lower myocardial blood flow (reduced rate pressure product) and, thus, improved efficiency of the cardiorespiratory system. For activities that require a lot of skill, such as swimming and cross-country skiing, $\dot{V}_{O_2}$ and cardiac output will also be reduced at a standard work task as the skill improves.[1]

Increased efficiency of cardiorespiratory fitness is also reflected in a reduced HR and rate pressure product at rest. In normotensive individuals, blood pressure at rest is usually not affected by aerobic training.[10] However, studies show significant reductions in resting blood pressure with hyperten-sive patients after aerobic training.[14,15] Usually systolic and diastolic blood pressures are affected equally. Some of this reduction in blood pressure is associated with a concomitant decrease in body weight. Although weight loss by exercise or diet, or both, and other dietary manipulations, such as salt restriction, significantly affect blood pressure, aerobic exercise has been shown to be effective as an independent factor.[15,16] Although the effect of exercise on blood pressure can be significant with hypertensive patients, most often blood pressure cannot be normalized without the added dietary controls. If diet and exercise do not normalize blood pressure, more aggres-sive medical management would be recommended. Caution is necessary for persons who are on blood pressure medication and plan to begin an exercise regimen. Once a participant begins a program, the medication may have to be reduced in order to offset the effect of the training program.

AEROBIC CAPACITY

Because it is easily measured and highly correlated with cardiac output and endurance performance, $\dot{V}_{O_2}$ max or its equivalent in multiples of metabolic units above resting (METs) is being used as the "gold standard" for classification of aerobic capacity.[1-3,8] Oxygen uptake at rest equals ap-proximately 3.5 ml $\cdot$ kg^{-1} $\cdot$ min^{-1}; thus, 1 MET = 3.5, 2 METs = 7, and so forth.

Figure 3–2 shows a champion distance runner taking a treadmill test for determination of $\dot{V}_{O_2}$ max. More details on treadmill test procedures and protocols will be discussed in Chapter 6. Figure 3–3 shows a comparison of $\dot{V}_{O_2}$ max values of young and middle-aged men of various fitness levels. The illustration clearly shows the difference in aerobic capacity as related to status of fitness and age. Values for women are approximately 10 to 20 per cent lower.[17-19]

Is there a level of aerobic capacity necessary to attain and maintain an optimal level of cardiorespiratory fitness? It is difficult to set a standard for optimal fitness because a specific level of aerobic capacity for optimal health has not been determined. As shown in Figure 3–3, $\dot{V}_{O_2}$ max for sedentary

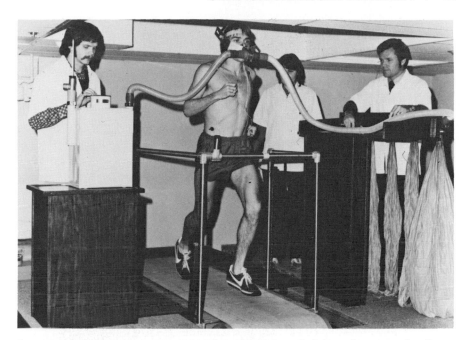

Figure 3–2. The maximum oxygen uptake test is being administered to a premier distance runner, the late Steve Prefontaine. At the time of this test, Prefontaine held 10 American distance running records. His maximum oxygen uptake was 84.4 ml · kg^{-1} · min^{-1}, one of the highest values ever recorded for a runner.[19–21] Breathing valve channels all expired air into a series of bags, which were later analyzed for oxygen and carbon dioxide content. The nose was blocked with a noseclip. Prefontaine was also attached to an electrocardiogram machine by a special 20 foot cable lead system. In this way, the electrical action of the heart (electrocardiogram, or ECG) and HR could be continually monitored throughout the run. It should be noted that more automated systems for determining maximum oxygen uptake are now available.[2] See Chapter 6 for more details concerning graded exercise testing for functional capacity and for diagnostic purposes. (From Pollock, M. L., Wilmore, J. H., and Fox, S. M.: Health and Fitness Through Physical Activity. New York, copyright © John Wiley and Sons, 1978, with permission.)

middle-aged men characteristically falls below 40 ml · kg^{-1} · min^{-1}. This value drops to 30 ml · kg^{-1} · min^{-1} by age 50 to 60. The values of 35 to 50 ml · kg · min^{-1} would seem a reasonable estimate for an adequate aerobic capacity for ages 20 to 60, i.e., values of 45 to 50 ml · kg^{-1} · min^{-1} for the 20 year old and 35 to 40 ml · kg^{-1} · min^{-1} for the 60 year old.[8,22]

Figure 3–4 shows differences in resting HR between sedentary and trained groups of men. This information shows that the endurance runner has a slower, stronger, and thus more efficient heart.[21] The slower HR is accompanied by a greater stroke volume.[1,2]

A critical exception to the fact that a lower resting HR is characteristic of the trained and healthy heart occurs in the case of certain pathologically diseased hearts. In such cases, the heart may beat more slowly, permitting a decrease in the metabolic needs of the heart muscle.[23] Another problem in using resting HR as a criterion for fitness is its wide variability within the population.[8,24] For example, Jim Ryun, once world record holder for the

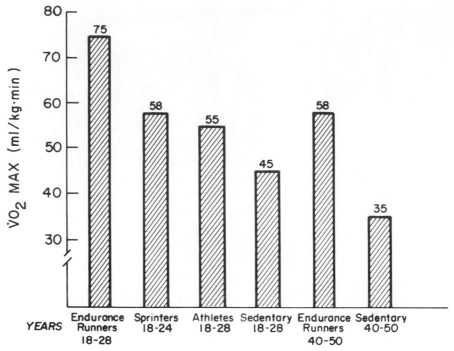

Figure 3–3. Comparison of maximum oxygen uptake of young and middle-aged men of various fitness levels. Values for women average 5 to 10 ml · kg^{-1} · min^{-1} lower. (From Pollock, M. L., Wilmore, J. H., and Fox, S. M.: Health and Fitness Through Physical Activity. New York, copyright © John Wiley and Sons, 1978, with permission.)

one-mile run, had a high resting HR compared with other distance runners (unpublished data: Jack Daniels, University of Texas, Austin, Texas, 1966). Therefore, caution should be taken when using resting HR as a measure of physical fitness. Although women adapt to training in the same manner as men, their resting HRs average 5 to 10 beats/min higher than those in men.[8,25] Elite women endurance athletes who train as much as men may have similar resting HRs.

QUANTIFYING THE RESULTS OF ENDURANCE TRAINING PROGRAMS

Improvement in cardiorespiratory fitness is a result of many factors. Generally, the magnitude of improvement is dependent on the total work or energy cost of the exercise regimen.[8,10,26,27] Energy cost can be measured by the number of kilocalories (Kcal) expended, and improvement in cardiorespiratory fitness is dependent upon the frequency, intensity, and duration of the exercise program. Improvement is also related to initial status of health and fitness; mode of exercise, such as walking, running, swimming,

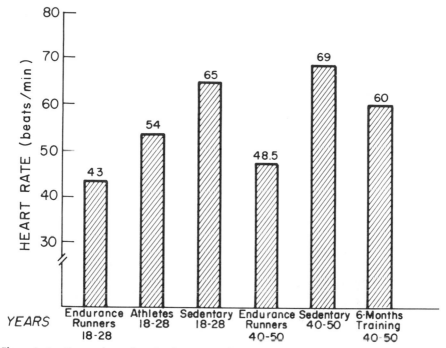

Figure 3–4. Comparison of resting heart rate of young and middle-aged men of various fitness levels. Values for women average 5 to 10 beats/min higher. (From Pollock, M. L., Wilmore, J. H., and Fox, S. M.: Health and Fitness Through Physical Activity. New York, copyright © John Wiley and Sons, 1978, with permission.)

and cycling; regularity of exercise; and age.[8,10,27] These factors, as well as individual interests, should be considered in designing an exercise program to meet the needs and abilities of the person or group involved in the training regimen.

Although much of the data from various training studies and subsequent recommendations for training programs to be presented in this chapter as well as Chapters 4 (body composition) and 5 (muscular strength and endurance, and flexibility) concern a variety of participants, the main target population will be for average adults 15 to 70 years of age. More specific information on the training of high-performance athletes can be found elsewhere.[1,2,28] Recommendations for cardiac patients will be presented in Chapter 8.

Needs and goals differ for elementary school children, athletes, and middle-aged men and women. School children need a broad spectrum of sports and activities to kindle their interests and to provide them with a broad educational experience.[29,30] The activities of most elementary school programs should provide for physical development, but many existing physical education classes do not. Athletes' programs are geared to competitive situations in which maximum skill and physiological and psychological effort are necessary. Preparing for such events often requires 2 to 3 hours of rigorous training daily. Adults generally are concerned with developing and maintaining strength and stamina, avoiding increases in body weight and fat, reducing stress and anxiety, and preventing potential health problems that occur with a sedentary lifestyle. Women often exercise for cosmetic reasons, such as weight and figure control.

A recent Harris Poll Survey[31] stated that 59 per cent of Americans of adult age say they are participating in physical activity programs. Of these, probably no more than 15 to 25 per cent are getting adequate amounts of exercise for developing and maintaining proper cardiorespiratory fitness and weight control and body composition. How much exercise is enough? The American College of Sports Medicine, in a position statement, has made the following recommendations.

1. **Frequency of training: 3 to 5 days per week.**

2. **Intensity of training: 60% to 90% of maximum HR reserve or, 50% to 85% of maximum oxygen uptake ($\dot{V}O_2$ max).**

3. **Duration of training: 15 to 60 minutes of continuous aerobic activity. Duration is dependent on the intensity of the activity, thus lower intensity activity should be conducted over a longer period of time. Because of the importance of the "total fitness" effect and the fact that it is more readily attained in longer duration programs, and because of the potential hazards and compliance problems associated with high intensity activity, lower to moderate intensity activity of longer duration is recommended for the nonathletic adult.**

4. **Mode of activity: Any activity that uses large muscle groups, that can be maintained continuously, and is rhythmical and aerobic in nature, e.g., running-jogging, walking-hiking, swimming, skating, bicycling, rowing, cross-country skiing, rope skipping, and various endurance game activities.[27]**

We are in agreement with these guidelines for healthy adults. Earlier, the importance of total energy expenditure of a training program was mentioned. It has been estimated that to improve aerobic fitness to the proper level, approximately 300 Kcal (based on 70 kg, or 154 lb, of body weight) should be expended during an exercise session.[8,22,26] The proper amount of exercise will usually improve a participant's aerobic capacity 15 to 25 per cent over a period of 4 to 6 months.[8,10] Thus, the proper combination of frequency, intensity, and duration of exercise is important in developing and maintaining the training effect. The rationale and research results supporting these notions will be discussed next.

FREQUENCY OF TRAINING

Several studies have placed less importance on frequency of training as a training stimulus than on intensity or duration.[32-36] A couple of these

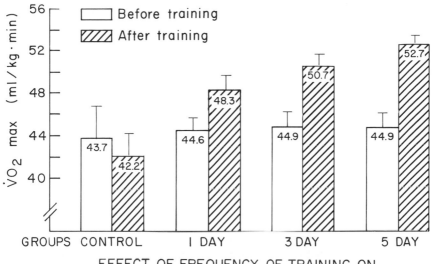

Figure 3–5. Effects of different training frequencies on maximum oxygen uptake ($\dot{V}O_2$ max). Data from Gettman, L. R., et al.: Physiological responses of men to 1, 3, and 5 day per week training programs. Res. Q. *47*, 638–646, 1976. (From Pollock, M. L., Wilmore, J. H., and Fox, S. M.: Health and Fitness Through Physical Activity. New York, copyright © John Wiley and Sons, 1978, with permission.)

investigations have attempted to evaluate frequency by controlling the total number of training sessions or total work output.[34-36] These studies generally show no difference in changes in aerobic capacity with frequency of training. For example, a group of men were trained for either 3 or 5 days per week, and at the end of 8 weeks, both groups were re-evaluated. At that time in the experiment, the 5-day-per-week group showed more improvement than the 3-day group. In an attempt to equalize training sessions (total kilocalorie expenditure), the 3-day-per-week group continued to train another 5 weeks. Upon re-evaluation, the 3-day-per-week group then equaled the improvement of the 5-day group.[34] The results of investigations such as this are not surprising, since total energy expenditures were equalized between groups. However, in prescribing exercise, one should not regard frequency of training in this manner because, in reality, training regimens should not terminate after just a few weeks but should continue throughout life.

When weeks of training are held constant instead of total number of training sessions, results generally show frequency to be a significant factor as a training stimulus.[37-39] Figure 3–5 shows the results of a training study conducted with men 20 to 35 years of age for a period of 20 weeks.[40] The intensity of training was standardized at 85 to 90 per cent of maximum HR range with the men participating for 30 minutes in each exercise session.

Improvement in $\dot{V}O_2$ max was 8, 13, and 17 per cent for the 1-, 3-, and 5-day-per-week training groups, respectively.

There are some inconsistencies in the literature related to frequency of training and improvement in aerobic capacity. These experiments have used frequencies of 2, 3, 4, and 5 days per week for from 5 to 13 weeks of training. Although most of the subjects used were of college age, initially all were generally considered sedentary. In some cases, the investigators found no significant differences in improvement in 2 to 3 days of training per week compared with 5 days per week[35] and in 2 days per week versus 4 days per week.[41] The facts that the subjects used in the investigations were beginners and that the experiments were conducted over such a short time period make interpretation of the results difficult. In training experiments with sedentary subjects, it can take several weeks before adaptation to training transpires. In fact, it often takes several weeks for the subject to recover from the initial fatigue and soreness found in the early stages of training. Further, it is certainly possible that the 4- or 5-day-week regimens were too frequent for the subjects' initial state of fitness and thus left them partially fatigued during the final test period.

Of the points mentioned previously that can affect the interpretation of training studies, the length of a training experiment appears to be a very critical factor. Pollock et al.[37,38] conducted two training experiments with middle-aged men (30 to 45 years of age) who trained either 2 or 4 days per week and found both groups improved in $\dot{V}O_2$ max, HR response to a standard work task, and other variables related to cardiovascular function. Midtest results of the 16-and 20-week programs showed no differences between groups, but subsequent final testing found the 4-day-per-week group to have improved significantly more. Thus, if these experiments would have terminated at their midpoints (8 and 10 weeks), the results would have been similar to the short-term studies mentioned earlier.

In two 2-day-per-week experiments conducted with middle-aged men who trained 3 to 4 miles per workout, approximately a 15 per cent improvement in $\dot{V}O_2$ max was attained.[37,38] If this is the case, why is a 3-day-per-week minimum recommended? Because in these same 2-day-per-week training studies, the subjects never lost body weight or fat. This fact has been replicated in additional studies in which subjects kept diet relatively constant and did aerobic training 2 days per week.[42,43] The exact mechanism for this is not fully understood, but it appears that training 2 days per week at 4.5 miles per workout will give approximately the same improvement in aerobic capacity as training 3 days per week at 3 miles, but the latter program will also affect changes in body composition. Thus, when we look at minimal guidelines for exercise prescription, total fitness should be considered. For further discussion concerning changes in body composition with exercise, see Chapter 4.

Two other factors are important to consider when interpreting the improvement in aerobic capacity through training of 1 or 2 days per week.

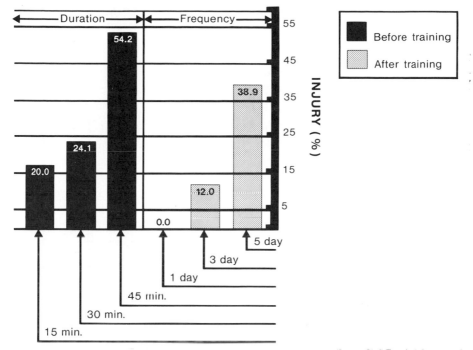

Figure 3–6. Effects of frequency and duration of training on incidence of injury. Data from Pollock, M. L., et al.: Effects of frequency and duration of training on attrition and incidence of injury. Med. Sci. Sports 9: 31–36, 1977. (From Pollock, M. L.: How much exercise is enough? Phys. Sportsmed. 6: 50–64, 1978. Reproduced by permission of the *Physician and Sportsmedicine*, McGraw-Hill Publication.)

First, the studies were jog-run programs of moderate to high intensity (80 to 90 per cent of maximum HR reserve) and may not be suitable or enjoyable for many adults. Second, research has shown that musculoskeletal injuries to the foot, leg, and knee double when beginners jog-run (even with some walking interspersed) 45 minutes per day compared with 30 minutes.[44] See Figure 3–6.

How about training more than 5 days per week? Training more than 5 days per week is possible, but certain factors should be considered first. (1) It has been estimated that more than 95 per cent of the improvement in aerobic capacity can be attained in a jog-run program (or other activities of equivalent intensity) of 4 to 5 days per week.[10] Thus, unless athletic competition is an important factor, added days of training are probably not warranted. (2) Orthopedic injuries appear to increase exponentially with jog-run types of activities in association with increased frequency of training. Figure 3–6 shows data from beginning jogger-runners regarding increased injuries with added frequency of training.[44] The data on beginners who trained 30 minutes daily for 1, 3, or 5 days per week strongly suggest that a day's rest between workouts is advisable to prevent injuries. As a participant gets in better shape, frequency can be increased. The injury

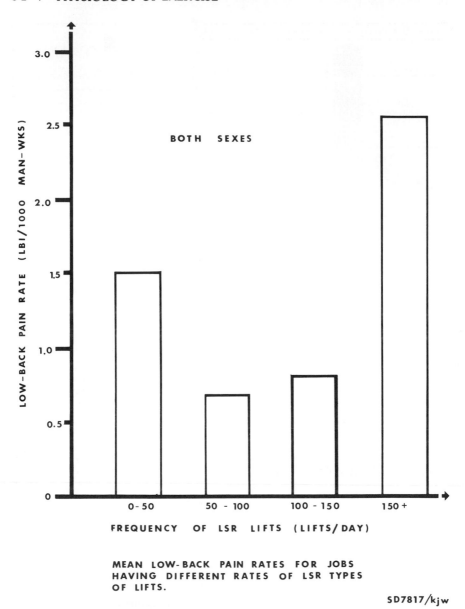

MEAN LOW-BACK PAIN RATES FOR JOBS
HAVING DIFFERENT RATES OF LSR TYPES
OF LIFTS.

SD7817/kjw

Figure 3–7. Mean low-back incidence rates with different frequencies of lifting. LSR refers to a lifting strength ratio. (From Chaffin, D. B., and Park, K. S.: A longitudinal study of low-back pain as associated with occupational weight lifting factors. A.I.H.A.J. *34:*513–525, 1973, with permission.)

problem is generally related to the total volume of work in the program. Other aspects of training, e.g., intensity, duration, and mode of activity, as well as age and initial level of fitness, must be considered. Basic anatomical structure is also important, as are proper shoes, texture of training surface, warm-up, and so on, when discussing the potential of injury. Injury prevention will be discussed further in Chapters 7 and 9. (3) The final point regards being realistic. Most adults cannot fit more than 3 to 4 days of training per week into their busy schedules. Although this observation has not been documented, most of us who have been involved in adult fitness programs know it to be true.

There is no question that more research is necessary to better establish and understand the upper-limit guideline. Individual differences will certainly dictate how much a participant can accomplish before becoming injured. Figure 3–7 illustrates a U-shaped curve relating frequency of lifting and incidence of low-back injury.[46] There appears to be an optimal amount of lifting at which point participants have the fewest injuries, with the two extremes (those rarely lifting and those frequently lifting) showing significantly higher injury rates. Although similar data are not available in the sports medicine literature, these probably best reflect the current trend in our society. Certainly, beginners and marathon training types have the greatest number of injuries, with somewhere between the two being optimal.

Does it make any difference whether a participant divides the training program into two small workout sessions per day rather than one larger one? Other than the extra time it takes to change clothes and so forth, either method is satisfactory. For example, Fisher and Ebisu[47] trained 53 male college students three times per week for 10 weeks at 80 per cent of their maximum HR. Group I ran once a day, group II twice a day, and group III three times a day. The total mileage for all three groups was the same. The authors concluded that it made little difference in aerobic adaptation whether a participant trained one, two, or three times per day.

If an individual trains 3 days in a row compared with spreading the training sessions over the full week, will the same improvement occur? Other than the potential injury factor related to running on consecutive days, a person should expect the same results. This was found in a study in which one group ran every Monday, Tuesday, and Wednesday and was compared with a group who trained Monday, Wednesday, and Friday.[48] Both groups had similar improvements in aerobic capacity.

Closely related to frequency of training is the regularity at which one continues to participate and its subsequent effect on cardiorespiratory fitness. A significant reduction in aerobic capacity has been shown after 1 to 2 weeks of detraining.[49] If training is not continued, the improvements gained in a program diminish rather rapidly. Cureton and Phillips,[50] using equal 8-week periods of training, nontraining, and retraining, found significant improvement, decrement, and improvement, respectively, in cardiorespiratory fitness.

Investigations in which subjects are put to bed for extended periods of time have shown decrements in aerobic capacity and related cardiovascular parameters.[51-53] Saltin et al.[52] confined five subjects to bed for 20 days, followed by a 60-day training period. Cardiovascular efficiency measures

TABLE 3–2. EFFECTS OF BED REST AND SUBSEQUENT TRAINING
ON CARDIOVASCULAR FUNCTION OF YOUNG MEN*

VARIABLE	UNITS	CONTROL	BED REST (20 DAYS)	TRAINING (60 DAYS)
Maximum oxygen uptake	$ml \cdot kg^{-1} \cdot min^{-1}$	43.0	31.8	51.1
Maximum heart rate	beats/min	192.8	196.6	190.8
Maximum cardiac output	liters/min	20.0	14.8	22.8
Maximum stroke volume	ml	104.0	74.2	119.8
Heart volume	ml	860	770	895

*From Saltin, B., Blomqvist, G., Mitchell, J., Johnson, R. L., Wildenthal, D., and Chapman, C. B.: Response to exercise after bed rest and after training. Circulation 37; and 38 (Suppl. 7): 1–78, 1968, by permission of the American Heart Association, Inc.

regressed during bed rest and improved steadily during training. Table 3–2 shows the results of bed rest on selected cardiovascular variables. Two of these subjects were initially trained, and the other three were untrained. It took the trained subjects significantly longer to reach their pre–bed rest fitness level once they began training again (40 days versus 14 days, respectively).

Participants in aerobic training programs who stop training have been shown to regress to pretraining levels after 10 weeks[54] to 8 months.[55] A 50 per cent reduction in improvement of aerobic capacity has been shown in just 4 to 12 weeks of detraining.[49,54,56] These data show that the loss of aerobic capacity is rapid but quite variable in rate among individuals after cessation of training. Factors such as level of fitness, age, and length of time in training add to this variability.

Once areobic fitness has been attained, does a participant have to continue at the same training level to maintain this capacity? The answer to this question is not totally clear. As long as training intensity remains constant, it appears that some reduction in frequency of training over a period of 5 to 15 weeks will not greatly affect aerobic capacity.[49,57,58] Roskamm[49] trained two groups of soldiers 5 days a week for 4 weeks. The results showed that both groups improved significantly during this period. See Figure 3–8. A subsequent decrease in working capacity was found within 2 weeks after cessation of training for one of the two groups that refrained from training (group II). The group members who continued to train at least once every third day maintained their fitness for another 4 weeks (group I). After the eighth week, they stopped training, and cardiorespiratory fitness decreased significantly, but not to the same level as group II, whose members had stopped training for a full 8 weeks.

Siegel et al.[59] trained nine sedentary middle-aged men for 12 minutes 3 days per week for 15 weeks and found an increase in $\dot{V}o_2$ max of 19 per cent. After completion of the program, five subjects continued to train once a week for another 14-week period. At this time, $\dot{V}o_2$ max had decreased to 6 per cent above the initial control level. The remaining four subjects who abstained from training fell below their original control values.

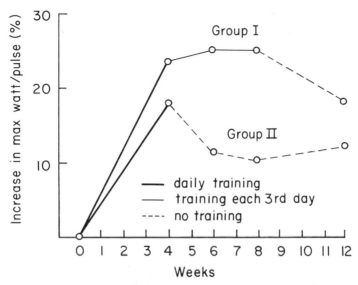

Figure 3–8. The effects of training, reduced training, and detraining on cardiorespiratory fitness (Originally published in Roskamm, H.: Optimum patterns of exercise for healthy adults. Canadian Medical Association Journal Vol. 96, March 25, 1967, pp. 895–899.)

Two studies give important information about reduced training and reduction in aerobic capacity.[57,58] Brynteson and Sinning[57] trained 21 men (age 20 to 38 years) for 30 minutes 5 days per week for 5 weeks at 80 per cent of maximum. They were then divided into four groups that trained one, two, three, or four times per week at the same intensity and duration for an additional 5 weeks. Only the groups that continued to train at least 3 days per week maintained their fitness. In another study, Hickson and Rosenkoetter[58] trained 12 young college-age men and women for 40 minutes 6 days per week for 10 weeks at nearly maximum intensities, i.e., training HR approached maximum by the end of each workout. They were then divided into two groups that trained 2 or 4 days per week for an additional 15 weeks. Intensity and duration remained the same as on the tenth week of training. During the first 10 weeks, $\dot{V}O_2$ max was increased by 20 per cent (treadmill) and 25 per cent (cycle ergometer) and essentially remained the same throughout the additional 15 weeks of reduced training frequencies. The latter results of Hickson and Rosenkoetter were particularly surprising for the 2-day-per-week reduced training group. It is felt that the extreme nature of the experiment (high intensity) was a major contributor to these results. In addition, because of the high-intensity, rigorous nature of the latter investigation, it may not be able to be completely generalized to the average population, who normally train at a significantly lower intensity. Nevertheless, these two studies provide additional important evidence that more exercise is required to increase $\dot{V}O_2$ max than to maintain it. Whether aerobic capacity can be maintained for longer periods of time is only speculative at this time.

INTENSITY OF TRAINING

What is the optimal level of intensity to develop and maintain cardiorespiratory fitness? The levels most frequently mentioned are between 60 and 90 per cent of the maximum HR reserve.[8,27,60,61] The per cent of maximum HR reserve is the per cent difference between resting and maximum HR at which exercise is being performed. The methods for determining and calculating training HR are discussed in Chapter 7.

Two classic studies have been used to describe the minimal intensity threshold for improving cardiorespiratory fitness.[60,61] Karvonen et al.[60] trained young men for 30 minutes 5 times per week on a motor-driven treadmill. They found no significant improvement in maximum working capacity for the group whose sustained HR did not reach 135 beats/min. Subjects whose sustained HRs were above 153 beats/min improved significantly. Hollman and Venrath,[61] in a similar experiment conducted on a cycle ergometer, found that HR values of 130 beats/min or more were needed to stimulate a training response. The group exercising at a rate lower than 130 beats/min increased only slightly in $\dot{V}O_2$ max from 2.90 to 3.07 L/min, whereas the group that trained above this rate increased from 3.07 to 3.57 L/min. The data suggest that young men must exercise at a HR level equal to approximately 60 per cent of their maximum HR reserve. Åstrand et al.[62] state that persons should train at approximately 50 per cent of their $\dot{V}O_2$ max, which is in agreement with Karvonen and with Hollman and Venrath. Figure 3–9 illustrates the relationship between $\dot{V}O_2$ expressed as a percentage of $\dot{V}O_2$ max and simultaneously measured HR as a percentage of maximal HR in men of various ages in the United States and Sweden.[63] As a result of this relationship and ease of measurement, HR has been used as the standard means for quantifying and monitoring the intensity of physical training programs. Although these data are from men, the relationship is the same for women.

It must be remembered that the guideline of 60 per cent of maximum HR reserve to improve aerobic capacity was originally based on healthy young men. Shephard[33] and others[64,65] have since pointed out that this threshold value can fluctuate significantly, depending on level of fitness, i.e., persons with lower initial fitness will have a lower threshold and persons with higher fitness a higher one. This point was well illustrated in a study by Gledhill and Eynon,[66] who trained college students for 20 minutes 5 days per week for 5 weeks. The subjects pedaled cycle ergometers at 120, 135, or 150 beats/min. Although the total group significantly improved their $\dot{V}O_2$ max, when they were divided into low and high fitness levels, the group that initially had high fitness only improved at the higher training HRs,

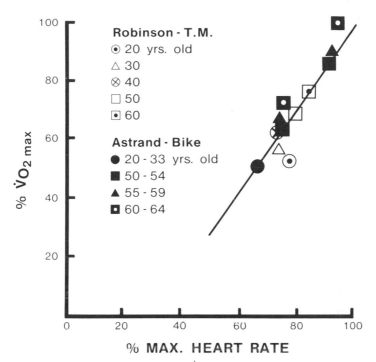

Figure 3–9. The relationship of submaximal $\dot{V}O_2$ expressed as percentage of maximum and simultaneously measured HR as a percentage of maximum HR in men of various ages resident in the United States and Sweden. (From Taylor, H. L., et al.: Exercise tests: a summary of procedures and concepts of stress testing for cardiovascular diagnosis and function evaluation. *In* Blackburn, H., editor: Measurement in Exercise Electrocardiography. Courtesy of Charles C Thomas, Publisher, Springfield, Illinois, pp. 259–305, 1969, with permission.)

whereas the low fitness group improved at all three training intensities. Initial level of fitness and its effect on aerobic capacity will be discussed again later in this chapter.

Kilbom[67] showed a positive relationship between intensity of training and improvement in $\dot{V}O_2$ max. Sharkey and Holleman[68] found similar results when they walked young men on a treadmill 3 days per week at HRs of 120, 150, and 180 beats/min. Faria[69] found no improvement in physical working capacity (PWC_{180}) with young men who bench-stepped at HRs up to 120 to 130 beats/min.

Shephard[33] and Davies and Knibbs[32] designed experiments to look systematically at the training stimulus for improving aerobic capacity. Shephard trained men at 96, 75, or 39 per cent of $\dot{V}O_2$ max, and Davies and Knibbs trained their subjects at 80, 50, or 30 per cent of $\dot{V}O_2$ max. Both studies showed that improvements were in direct relation to intensity of training. In the Shephard study, improvements in $\dot{V}O_2$ max ranged from 5 to 10 per cent (depending on duration and frequency) for the 39 per cent intensity group to approximately 20 per cent for the 96 per cent intensity

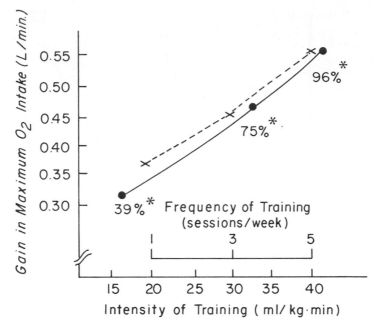

The Influence of Intensity and Frequency
of Training on Improvement in Maximum
Oxygen Intake Capacity·

*Intensity of training expressed as percent
of maximum O_2 intake capacity.

Shephard, R.J. Int. Z. angew. Physiol.
26:272-278, 1968

Figure 3–10. The influence of intensity (●————●) and frequency (x- - - -x) of training on improvement of $\dot{V}O_2$ max.
*Intensity of training expressed as per cent of $\dot{V}O_2$ max (Data from Shephard, R.J.: Intensity, duration, and frequency of exercise as determinants of the response to a training regime. Int. Z. Angew. Physiol. *26:*272–278, 1969, with permission.)

group (see Fig. 3–10). Davies and Knibbs found no improvement in $\dot{V}O_2$ max for their 30 per cent intensity group.

If the total kilocalorie expenditure of the exercise regimen is approximately equal, does it matter whether one trains at a high or a moderate intensity? In general, as long as a person trains above the minimal training intensity threshold, programs that vary in intensity appear to give similar improvements in aerobic capacity.[26,42,70–73] To test this hypothesis, Pollock et al.[73] trained four groups of men who were randomly assigned to a control (no training), continuous, interval, or combination of continuous and interval training group. Training was for approximately 30 minutes, 3 days per week for 20 weeks. The interval training included repetitive nearly all-out bouts of 110- to 330-yd dashes with fast walking of equal distance inter-

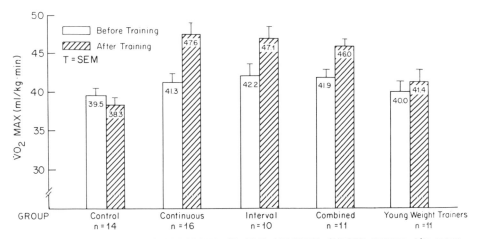

EFFECT OF RUNNING PROGRAMS ON THE MAXIMUM OXYGEN INTAKE ($\dot{V}O_2$MAX)
OF YOUNG POLICE OFFICERS, AGES 21-35

Figure 3–11. Effect of different intensities of running training on $\dot{V}O_2$ max. Total kilocalories of energy expenditure was similar among running groups. (Data from Pollock, M. L., et al.: Physiological comparisons of the effects of aerobic and anaerobic training. Presented to the American College of Sports Medicine. Washington, D.C., May 26, 1978.)

spersed. Total kilocalories among groups were equated on a regular basis. Figure 3–11 shows that improvement in aerobic capacity was similar for each of the three training groups.

In another study, Pollock et al.[42] trained middle-aged men at 80 or 90 per cent of maximum HR reserve for 20 weeks. Distance trained and total kilocalories expended per exercise session were similar between groups, but training HR averaged 15 beats/min lower for the 80 per cent group (175 versus 160 beats/min). Figure 3–12 shows that the improvements in aerobic capacity were similar for both groups.

Many adults—particularly those more than 40 years of age, participants who are injury-prone when jogging, and participants with heart disease—cannot or should not jog or run but can enjoy walking as an exercise program. How does walking compare as a training program? Again, it would depend on the total kilocalories expended and on maintenance of the intensity level above the minimal threshold. Pollock et al.[74] conducted a 20-week fast-walking study with men 40 to 57 years of age. The men walked for 40 minutes 4 days per week. The improvement found in this program (Fig. 3–13) was equal to that found in 30-minute, 3-day-per-week jogging programs for men of similar age.[10,75,76] The lower intensity of the walking program (65 to 75 per cent of maximum HR range) was offset by the increased duration and frequency of training.

The experiments described in the preceding paragraph have important implications for prescribing exercise. First, as long as kilocalorie expenditure is similar, a variety of intensities can elicit approximately the same

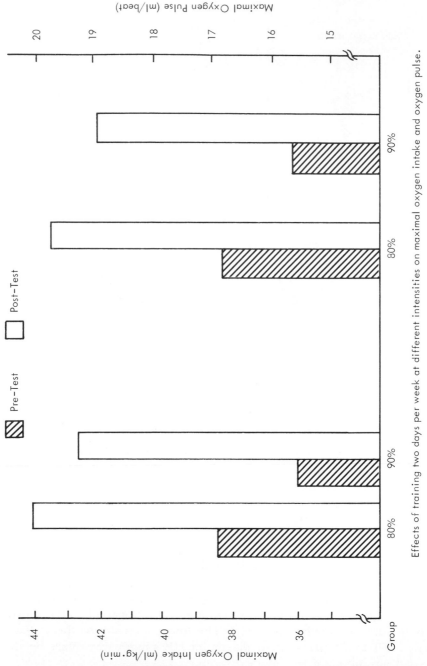

Figure 3–12. Effects of training 2 days per week at different intensities on maximum oxygen intake and oxygen pulse. (From Pollock, M. L., et al.: Effects of training two days per week at different intensities on middle-aged men. Med. Sci. Sports 4:192–197, 1972, with permission.)

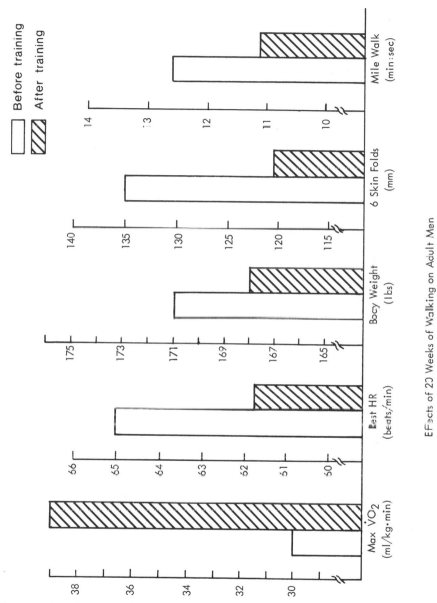

Figure 3–13. Effects of walking on the physical fitness of middle-aged men. Data from Pollock, M. L., et al.: Effects of walking on body composition and cardiovascular function of middle-aged men. J. Appl. Physiol. *30:*126–130, 1971. (From Pollock, M. L., Wilmore, J. H., and Fox, S. M.: Health and Fitness Through Physical Activity. New York, copyright © John Wiley and Sons, 1978, with permission.)

training result. This gives participants latitude in developing their training program. Second, persons can train at a moderately lower intensity without significantly affecting their results, an important factor in long-term adherence to training regimens.

High-intensity effort is often important for high-level competition, but because it is also related to increased musculoskeletal injuries[77,78] and to cardiovascular symptoms and events[79,80] and has been found to be somewhat unattractive psychologically to noncompetitive middle-aged and older adults,[81] it is not generally recommended for the average person. In the study comparing continuous, interval, and combination training, the interval training group had twice the number of dropouts as the continuous training group.[81] This was a result of both more injuries and a dislike for high-intensity effort. At the conclusion of the study, members of the combination group, who had experience in both programs, were queried about which regimen they preferred. Ninety per cent of the group preferred continuous training rather than interval training, with 10 per cent being neutral.

DURATION OF TRAINING

Improvement in aerobic capacity is directly related to duration of training. Improvements in cardiovascular function have been found after 6 to 10 training sessions lasting only 5 to 10 minutes a day.[33] As a rule, the programs of shorter duration (10 to 15 minutes) of moderate intensity show a significantly lower training effect than do programs of 30 to 60 minutes' duration.[8,27,82–85] Figure 3–14 shows the results from a study conducted on men 20 to 35 years of age for a period of 20 weeks.[82] The intensity was standardized at 85 to 90 per cent of maximum HR range, and the men participated 3 days per week. Improvement in $\dot{V}O_2$ max was 8.5, 16.1 and 16.8 per cent for the 15-, 30-, and 45-minute groups, respectively.

In other experiments, Olree et al.[70] trained young men for 20, 40, or 60 minutes and found the longer duration to produce more significant improvements. Their training regimen included a 5-minute warm-up period, followed by a training period in which the resistance on the cycle ergometer was increased to produce a training HR of approximately 180 beats/min. Wilmore et al.[86] conducted a jogging program for middle-aged men three times per week for 10 weeks. Subjects trained either 12 or 24 minutes per exercise session. Both groups improved significantly in most cardiovascular variables, with the latter group showing an advantage in most values. Yeager and Brynteson[87] trained young women on a cycle ergometer for 10, 20, and 30 minutes 3 days per week for 6 weeks. The training HR averaged 144 beats/min. These authors' results were in agreement with the above-mentioned studies. In these experiments, attempts were made to keep the intensity and frequency of training equal among groups.

At this stage in the discussion, it is important to emphasize that duration and intensity are closely interrelated and that the total amount of work

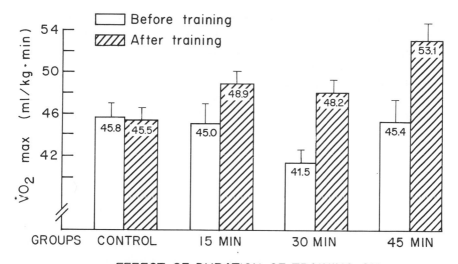

Figure 3–14. Effect of different training durations on $\dot{V}o_2$ max. Data from Milesis, C.A., et al.: Effects of different durations of training on cardiorespiratory function, body composition and serum lipids. Res. Q. *47*, 716–725, 1976, (From Pollock, M. L., Wilmore, J. H., and Fox, S. M.: Health and Fitness Through Physical Activity. New York, copyright © John Wiley and Sons, 1978, with permission.)

(energy cost) accomplished in a training program is an important criterion for fitness development. Sharkey[71] mentioned that previous studies were not designed to separate the effects of intensity from those of duration and and that a cell sample size of only 1 or 2 is often limiting; thus, the interaction effects could not be determined. Therefore, he randomly assigned 36 college men to the cells of a 3 X 2 factorial design that included three intensities (training HRs of 130, 150, and 170 beats/min) and two levels of work (7,500 or 15,000 kpm of total work). The 6-week training program was conducted on cycle ergometers 3 days per week. He concluded that intensity did not significantly influence the extent of training changes when the total amount of work was held constant. In addition, intensity and duration of training did not interact to produce significantly different training changes. These results are supported by the two previously described investigations by Pollock et al.[42,72] (Figs. 3–11 and 3–12) and Blair et al.[88] Although more definitive investigations conducted at other levels of intensity and length of duration are necessary, the current studies appear to point to the importance of the total amount of work (energy cost) accomplished as the important criterion for cardiovascular improvement. That is, as long as training is performed above the minimum threshold of intensity, improvement in aerobic capacity will be similar for activities performed both at a lower intensity and longer duration and at a higher intensity and shorter duration if the total energy expenditure of the activities are equal. For many years, Cureton[26] has hypothesized this concept.

The American College of Sports Medicine guidelines suggest a minimum of 15 minutes per training session.[27] How does this relate to the above-mentioned research findings? In general, most training programs that meet the guideline standards show a 15 per cent to 25 per cent improvement in aerobic capacity. In addition, a 300-Kcal expenditure per training session was recommended. The above-mentioned experiments support these guidelines. Thus, 15 to 20 minutes of high-intensity activity (more than 95 per cent of maximum), 20 to 30 minutes of moderately high-intensity training (80 to 90 per cent of maximum), or 40 to 50 minutes of moderate-intensity training (60 to 80 per cent of maximum) will generally meet these standards. Because of the problems associated with high-intensity programs mentioned earlier, a 20- to 30-minute program is a more realistic minimum standard. In addition, because of the injury factor shown in Figure 3–6, beginning jogger-runners initially should keep their duration to within 30 minutes.

MODE OF TRAINING

There are a multitude of training modes available. They range from individual to group activities requiring different levels of skill and varying degrees of competitiveness. The relative value of these activities in producing changes in cardiorespiratory fitness is in question. Previous parts of this review have shown that certain quantities and combinations of intensity, duration, and frequency are necessary to produce and maintain a training effect. Theoretically, in view of the results from the aforementioned training studies, it would appear that training effects would be independent of mode of activity if the various combinations of intensity, duration, and frequency are the same. Little information comparing the effects of various modes of training is available.

Olree et al.[70] compared the effects of running, walking (treadmill), and cycling (ergometer) training regimens on college men. Each group trained for 20 minutes 5 days per week for 10 weeks, at a HR of 150 to 160 beats/min. In general, they found running and cycling to be superior training modes when compared with walking. Pollock et al.[72] in a similar experiment conducted with middle-aged men, found all three modes of training to be equally effective in producing a significant aerobic effect. In this study, the subjects trained for 30 minutes 3 days per week for 20 weeks, at 85 to 90 per cent of maximum HR reserve (approximately 175 beats/min). See Figure 3–15. These studies agree except for the college-age walkers. This discrepancy is not clearly understood, but may exist because the training intensity level was much less for the younger men and because the HR training data were not expressed as a percentage of maximum. Therefore,

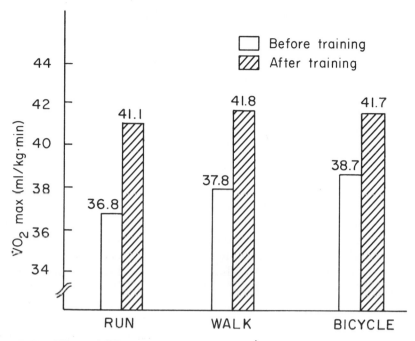

Figure 3–15. Effects of different modes of training on V̇o₂ max. Data from Pollock, M. L., et al.: Effects of mode of training on cardiovascular function and body composition of middle-aged men. Med. Sci. Sports 7:139–145, 1975. (From Pollock, M. L., Wilmore, J. H., and Fox, S. M.: Health and Fitness Through Physical Activity. New York, copyright © John Wiley and Sons, 1978, with permission.)

it is concluded that a variety of aerobic activities can be interchanged for improving and maintaining fitness, i.e., it is not necessarily what you do but how you do it that is important.

A variety of activities have been shown to elicit a significant improvement in aerobic capacity. These are generally known as moderate- to high-energy expenditure activities, e.g., running/jogging,[37,58,75,77,82,86–102] fast walking,[68,70,72,85,103,104] cycling (bicycling),[41,59,70,72,88,99,105,106] swimming,[107–111] cross-country skiing,[1,112] aerobic dance,[113–115] tennis,[116] rope skipping,[117,118] soccer,[119] wheeling (wheelchair) or arm cranking,[120–123] and so on. In contrast, low energy cost or highly intermittent activities (lots of rest breaks) show little or no effect. These activities include moderate calisthenics,[124,125] golf,[126] and weight lifting.[127,128] Tables listing the energy expenditure (Kcal/min and METs) of various activities are shown in Chapter 7.

Are weight lifting and circuit weight training suitable activities to improve cardiorespiratory fitness? In a recent review, Gettman and Pollock[129] showed that traditional weight-lifting and training activities in which a participant lifted heavy weights with few repetitions and long rest periods resulted in no improvement in aerobic capacity. Circuit weight training that used moderately heavy weights and included many repetitions for each exercise (12 to 20 repetitions) with little rest between bouts of exercise showed only modest improvements in aerobic capacity. The average increase in $\dot{V}O_2$ max of the seven studies reported was 5 per cent.[130-136] Kimura et al.,[137] using fit and unfit young men, found no significant improvement in $\dot{V}O_2$ max with the fit subjects and a 6.7 per cent improvement with the unfit subjects. The subjects performed three circuits of eight exercises (45-second training and 15-second rest for each exercise) 3 days per week for 8 weeks, for approximately 24 minutes per session, at approximately 40 to 50 per cent of one-repetition maximum. All of these programs resulted in highly significant improvements in strength and favorable changes in body composition. Strength changes will be discussed in Chapter 5 and body composition in Chapter 4.

The results from weight lifting and circuit weight training studies show the effects of specificity of exercise training. It has been well documented that the muscles are trained and improved in the specific manner and rate that they are exercised.[1,3,138-140] Thus, arm work will favor changes in arm strength and endurance compared with the legs and vice versa.[141] In addition, strength activities are primarily designed to improve strength and aerobic activities to improve cardiorespiratory fitness. Therefore, a well-rounded fitness program will include activities to enhance aerobic fitness, flexibility, and strength. Strength and flexibility programs should consist of a variety of exercises that train all the major muscle groups of the body.[8]

Although the above-mentioned results on circuit weight training are consistent within the literature, certain aspects of the results may seem confusing at first glance. Circuit weight trainers tend to increase their HRs within the acceptable training zone, and the activity uses large muscle groups and is rather continuous in nature. Why then the modest aerobic effect? Circuit weight training includes many arm exercises, and the energy expenditure for doing arm work compared with leg work is approximately 68 per cent at the same HR level.[142] With arm training, $\dot{V}O_2$ max for arm ergometry has been shown to increase from approximately 70 to 80 percent of $\dot{V}O_2$ max of treadmill work.[121] Wilmore et al.,[143] using circuit weight training, trained men at 74 per cent and women at 84 per cent of their maximum HR, but this corresponded only to 39 and 45 per cent, respectively, of their $\dot{V}O_2$ max. In addition, studies evaluating the energy cost of circuit weight training found it to correspond to a slow jog (11 to 12 minutes per mile pace).[143-145]

In a more positive note about circuit weight training, a recent study using circuit weight training with a 1-minute jog-run between each bout of exercise resulted in a 17 per cent improvement in aerobic capacity.[146] Another study showed that once aerobic fitness had been attained by a jog-run program, a subsequent 8-week circuit weight training program was enough to maintain aerobic capacity.[134] This latter study supports the results mentioned earlier concerning reduced training, i.e., it takes less effort to maintain fitness than it does to attain it.

INITIAL LEVEL OF FITNESS

The level of fitness at which participants begin a program will dictate their level of training and the rate of progression. These factors will be discussed further in Chapter 7. The amount of improvement expected from a training program is directly related to initial level of fitness, i.e., the higher the initial fitness level, the lower the expected change.[67,68,147] Muller[148] first reported this observation after conducting a series of experiments dealing with improvement in strength. He concluded that the percentage of improvement was directly related to initial strength and its relative distance from a possible endpoint of improvement. This concept has also been true with training studies dealing with cardiorespiratory fitness parameters.[67,68,147] Sharkey[68] noted that the magnitude of change was inversely related to the initial level of fitness ($r = -0.54$). He went on to say that the failure to account adequately for this factor in previous training studies may have resulted in erroneous conclusions or interpretations of results. To illustrate this point further, Saltin,[147] using the data of Rowell,[149] Ekblom et al.,[97] and Saltin et al.,[52] plotted the $\dot{V}o_2$ max data of subjects at the start of physical conditioning against percentage of improvement and found a moderately good relationship, excluding the older men. See Figure 3–16. The authors mentioned that the older men did not train as much as the

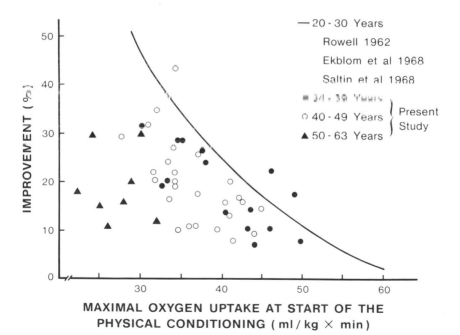

Figure 3–16. Improvement in $\dot{V}o_2$ max in young individuals (the line) and in middle-aged and older subjects in relation to initial level of $\dot{V}o_2$ max. (From Saltin, B., et al.: Physical training in sedentary middle-aged men, II. Scand. J. Clin. Lab. Invest. *24*:323–334, 1969, with permission from Blackwell Scientific Publications Limited.)

younger men, which would account for some of their lack of improvement.

As mentioned earlier, the average improvement in $\dot{V}O_2$ max with endurance training is between 15 and 25 per cent.[10] Other factors that tend to limit the amount of improvement include poor health status, which can limit the amount of training that a participant can handle, and programs conducted over too short a time span. Particularly for middle-aged and older adults, adaptation to training takes weeks and months; thus short-term experiments usually show only small-to-moderate improvements. Kavanagh et al.[150] showed that some cardiac patients continued to improve their $\dot{V}O_2$ max for up to 2 years. Young boys and young adults who are generally better fit early in life also may show more moderate improvements in aerobic capacity.[10] On the other hand, improvements may be inflated in individuals whose initial tests were stopped prematurely, i.e., true maximum tests were not initially performed[50] or large amounts of body weight were lost during the course of the program. The latter is particularly true if $\dot{V}O_2$ max is expressed in $ml \cdot kg^{-1} \cdot min^{-1}$. In addition, body weight is inversely related to treadmill performance time.[1,151]

AGE AND TRAINABILITY

In general, aerobic capacity can be improved at all ages.[8,10] Saltin et al.[147] mention that even though this training effect occurs as readily in middle-aged and older men as in young men, the absolute change is less, i.e., there appears to be an aging effect. For example, Pollock et al.[152] trained a group of sedentary men who were 49 to 65 years of age three times per week for 20 weeks. The training included a walk-jog regimen with mainly jogging occurring during the latter weeks. Figure 3–17 shows an 18 per cent improvement in $\dot{V}O_2$ max. The relative values were what would be expected for younger persons, but the absolute values were lower.

The results of earlier studies by DeVries,[153] which showed only an 8 per cent improvement in aerobic capacity, and by Benestad,[154] which showed no improvement, may be somewhat misleading. The latter program was of short duration, and the intensity and duration of training are considered minimal in relation to the criteria established by the American College of Sports Medicine.[27] DeVries' regimen was conducted over a much longer period of time, but the training intensity was minimal. The concern for protecting middle-aged and older subjects from overstress is important, and most investigators use much caution in their exercise prescription. As a result, sedentary groups need more time to adapt to training. This factor, as well as the confounding effects related to the previously discussed training stimuli, makes interpretation difficult. Additional information on rate of adaptation to training will be discussed in Chapter 7. More recent investigations[13,155] appear to support the findings of Saltin et al.[147] and Pollock et al.[152]

Can participants who continue to train their whole life or for periods

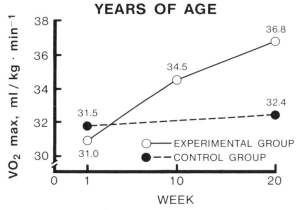

EFFECT OF TRAINING ON MAXIMUM OXYGEN UPTAKE OF MEN 49-65 YEARS OF AGE

Figure 3–17. Effects of training on $\dot{V}O_2$ max of men 49 to 65 years of age. (Data from Pollock, M. L., et al.: Physiologic responses of men 49 to 65 years of age to endurance training. J. Am. Geriatr. Soc. 24:97–104, 1976.)

of years maintain their aerobic capacity? Only a few longitudinal studies have been reported.[156–160] They generally show a rather linear reduction in $\dot{V}O_2$ max with age for both athletic and sedentary groups. The slopes of the curves tend to remain parallel, so that the athlete remains at a higher capacity at every age. The data of Robinson et al.,[156] who evaluated champion distance runners from 1936 to 1942 and subsequently in 1971 (25 to 43 years of follow-up), found different slopes, depending on whether the former champions continued to train. The two who continued to train had significantly less dropoff in aerobic capacity then their sedentary counterparts. Because longitudinal data are scarce, most research has focused on the cross sectional approach.

Cross-sectional data show trained athletes to be superior to their age-matched sedentary counterparts.[155,161–166] Their superior $\dot{V}O_2$ max is probably the result of both genetic endowment and physical training. The age decrement mentioned earlier also appears in the trained groups and becomes particularly evident after age 60. Can this decrement in $\dot{V}O_2$ max be explained by age itself, or are training factors also apparent? Current evidence supports both notions. Young endurance runners will train 100 to 200 miles per week (sometimes less if interval training is used), whereas middle-aged and older runners rarely accomplish this. In data collected from the 1971 National Master's AAU track and field meet and subsequent laboratory evaluations conducted by Pollock, Miller, and Wilmore,[163] the average number of miles trained per week was 40, 40, 30, and 20 for the fourth, fifth, sixth, and seventh decades, respectively. Another interesting fact was that most of these men were former college athletes who had not trained all their lives. Most of the older athletes had been sedentary for

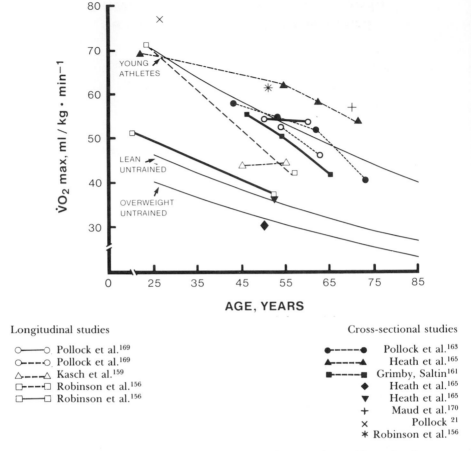

Figure 3–18. Maximum oxygen uptake of endurance athletes and nonathletes of various ages. See legend and text for group descriptions. (Data from Pollock, M. L., et al.: Ten year follow-up on aerobic capacity of champion master's track athletes [abstract]. Med. Sci. Sports Exer. *14:* 105, 1982.)

Longitudinal studies

○——○ Pollock et al.[169]
○---○ Pollock et al.[169]
△---△ Kasch et al.[159]
□---□ Robinson et al.[156]
□——□ Robinson et al.[156]

Cross-sectional studies

●-----● Pollock et al.[163]
▲-----▲ Heath et al.[165]
■-----■ Grimby, Saltin[161]
◆ Heath et al.[165]
▼ Heath et al.[165]
+ Maud et al.[170]
× Pollock[21]
∗ Robinson et al.[156]

many years and had been back in training for only 5 to 10 years. Grimby and Saltin's[161] data on middle-aged and older athletes who had trained all of their lives are comparable at the fourth decade but are lower for the fifth and sixth decades (Fig. 3–18). Other data of Pollock et al.[167] for men who had been training for 5.5 years are significantly higher than for men completing their first 6 months of training but are less than for the aforementioned athletic groups. Dill et al.[160] and Costill and Winrow's[168] data on competitive marathon runners agree. Thus, the conclusions from the above-mentioned studies and a review by Hodgson and Buskirk[164] showed a 9 per cent reduction per decade in $\dot{V}O_2$ max with age, ranging from 20 to 70 years. The athletic groups showed the same decrease as their sedentary counterparts and, therefore, remained significantly higher at all ages.

In an attempt to rule out the training and mileage differences found in the studies comparing younger and older runners, Heath et al.[165] investigated a group of younger and older runners matched for mileage and training characteristics. Their data suggest less difference between groups by age than had been found by previous studies (approximately 5 per cent per decade). See Figure 3–18.

In contrast to the above-mentioned findings, Kasch and Wallace[159] found no reduction in aerobic capacity after a 10-year follow-up of middle-aged noncompetitive runners. The subjects were 45 years of age initially and continued to run approximately 15 miles per week. Maximum oxygen uptake (43.7 versus 44.4 ml $\cdot$ kg^{-1} $\cdot$ min^{-1}), resting HR (63 versus 61 beats/min), and body weight (76.8 versus 76.0 kg) remained constant over the 10-year period. Only maximum HR decreased significantly (178 versus 171 beats/min). More recently, Pollock et al.[169] completed a 10-year follow-up study on champion master's runners. Important questions include the following: (1) Is the aging curve linear over a broad range of ages? (2) If a person continues to train at the same level, will a reduction in aerobic capacity occur? The cross-sectional results from this group's 1971 data showed the expected decrease in $\dot{V}O_2$ max up to approximately 65 years of age, with a more dramatic reduction occurring thereafter (see Fig 3–18). As a result of the small sample studied who were older than the age of 70 and the significant difference in the quantity and quality of training among the various age groups, conclusions were considered somewhat tenuous. Was the reduction in aerobic capacity a result of aging or the difference in training level? The follow-up data were collected on 25 men 50 to 82 years of age. All of the subjects had continued their training, but only 11 were training at approximately the same level and were still highly competitive. Training mileage remained unchanged for both groups, but the noncompetitors slowed their training pace by approximately 2 minutes per mile. Figure 3–18 shows the results in $\dot{V}O_2$ max. The competitive group showed no significant change in $\dot{V}O_2$ max (54.2 versus 53.3 ml $\cdot$ kg^{-1} $\cdot$ min^{-1}), whereas the noncompetitive group decreased significantly (52.5 versus 45.9 ml $\cdot$ kg^{-1} $\cdot$ min^{-1}). The results of this study help to confirm the hypothesis that the reduction in aerobic capacity found with age is affected by maintenance of training. This hypothesis is in agreement with the results of Kasch and Wallace.[159] The data also showed the aging curve for aerobic capacity to be curvilinear rather than linear, as reported by previous research.[164,165] The competitive group who continued to train at the same intensity level showed no reduction until after age 60 to 65 years. See Figure 3–19. After this age, a decrease was evident but not at the same rate as shown in the cross-sectional report. Although these longitudinal studies seem to answer important questions about how exercise may affect cardiorespiratory fitness, more data using larger numbers of subjects and longer follow-up periods are necessary before final conclusions can be drawn.

Although the above-mentioned studies of Kasch and Wallace,[159] Heath et al.,[165] and Pollock et al.[169] showed that the reduction in aerobic capacity with age is affected by training, there seemed to be no effect on maximum HR, i.e., HR$_{max}$ declines with age independent of training. See Figure 3–20. The explanation of this phenomenon is not clear.

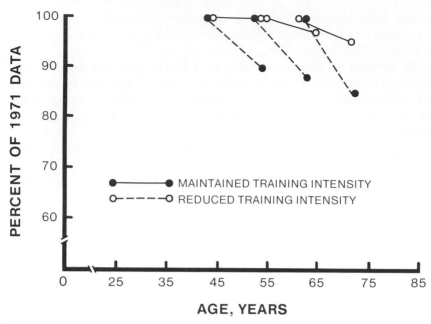

Figure 3–19. Reduction of maximum oxygen uptake after 10 years of follow-up for master's athletes who maintained or reduced their training intensity. (Data from Pollock, M. L., et al.: Ten year follow-up on aerobic capacity of champion master's track athletes [abstract]. Med. Sci. Sports Exer. *14:*105, 1982.)

Is the aerobic capacity of children and youth affected the same as that of adults? The $\dot{V}O_2$ max improvement with training in young boys is complicated somewhat by the maturation process, making interpretation more difficult. The data of Ekblom,[172] Sherman,[173] Larsson et al.,[174] and Lussier and Buskirk[175] show significant improvements with training, whereas those of Daniels and Oldridge[176] do not. Inspection of the results shows Daniels and Oldridge's initial values to be much higher than the others, thus again bringing up initial status of fitness and its relationship to possible improvement. The age-related average $\dot{V}O_2$ max values reported by Robinson[24] and Cumming[177] are in agreement with values found by Ekblom and Sherman, whereas those of Larsson et al. are lower. The 24 per cent improvement found by Larsson et al.[174] probably was related to the subjects' lower initial fitness. Thus, it appears that children and youth adapt to aerobic training about the same as adults.

Will training during youth give added benefits and advantages to aerobic performance capacity at maturity? Longitudinal studies conducted by Ekblom et al.,[97] Astrand et al.,[110] and Zauner and Benson[178] on young boys and girls showed higher than normal improvements in many physiological parameters with endurance training regimens, thus suggesting the probability of significant cardiopulmonary and anthropometric modifications occuring during the formative years. Although these results seem promising, further study is necessary before more definitive conclusions can be made.

Can aerobic training be harmful to younger children? Cureton and Barry[29] found that children adapt well to endurance training. In over 20 years of study with boys 7 to 14 years of age, no significant problems were noted. Whether a marathon type of training is detrimental for youngsters is not known. Possibly this type of activity creates more psychological problems—resulting from parental pressure, and so on, in children and youth—than physical ones.

HEREDITY

The effects of training have been well documented, with clear differences being established between sedentary, moderately trained, and highly trained athletes. Even with these differences, there are broad overlappings among these groups on most physiological variables. This fact, plus the

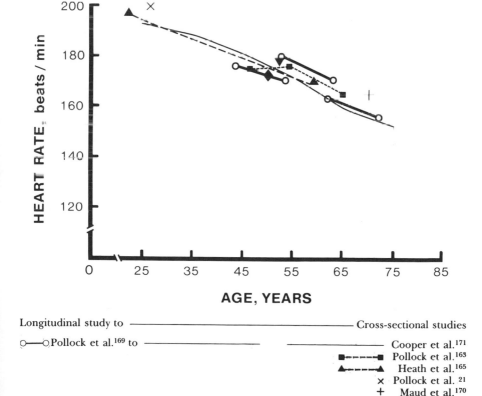

| Longitudinal study to | ————————————————— | Cross-sectional studies |

○—○ Pollock et al.[169] to ——————————   Cooper et al.[171]
■------■ Pollock et al.[163]
▲------▲ Heath et al.[165]
× Pollock et al. [21]
+ Maud et al.[170]

Figure 3–20. Maximum heart rate of groups of various ages. See legend and text for group description.

aging process, makes various standards awkward and somewhat misleading. That is, much of our ability is endowed by heredity.[1,179–181] Åstrand[182] stated that the best way to become a champion athlete is to be selective in the manner in which you pick your parents. Therefore, the fact of having a high $\dot{V}O_2$ max, must be interpreted with caution. It is certainly possible to have a high $\dot{V}O_2$ max and be considered in poor condition and to have a low one and be considered fit. The former would be true with a highly trained endurance athlete who has become inactive. Klissouras[180] has suggested, somewhat speculatively, that hereditary factors account for approximately 75 to 80 per cent of biological variability, leaving only 20 to 25 per cent that can be affected by training and detraining. Thus, it is recommended that physiological results also be interpreted with respect to genetic makeup as well as individual differences and variations.

TRAINING IN WOMEN

Treating the effects of aerobic training on women in a separate section should not be interpreted as a minimization of the subject's importance, but the fact is that only a limited number of investigations of this type are present in the literature. In fact, only a few training investigations dealing with women have been designed to quantify training regimens as described earlier.[10,17,18,27,87] Several studies have evaluated working capacity and anthropometric measurements[87,114,184,185,188,191] of young girls and women.[67,115,183,186,190,192,193] Some investigations have evaluated highly trained women athletes.[1,2,18,19,110,194] Others[67,87,106,113–115,135,183–193] have shown significant cardiovascular function and body composition changes with endurance training. The former data show significant differences between men and women, which become apparent after puberty.[1,2] These differences have been minimized in the last decade, since women have begun training at the same level as men.[2,195]

Most of the information concerning training has been conducted on men. Although information on women is lacking, the available evidence indicates that women tend to adapt to endurance training in the same manner as men.[184,189,190,192,193]

TRAINING WITH CARDIAC PATIENTS

Endurance training with cardiac patients has produced significant improvements in aerobic capacity.[196–203] Some relate this improvement to peripheral changes (A-$\dot{V}O_2$ *diff*) rather than central factors (cardiac output).[202–205] Although the mechanism for improvement is controversial, the answer may be related more to the status of ventricular dysfunction and to intensity and duration of training. Patients with low left ventricular function (ejection fraction < 50 per cent) can increase their working capacity, but they may have difficulty in increasing stroke volume.[205,206] In contrast, patients with normal left ventricular function may adapt to endurance training like nonpatients.[207] Previous studies often did not measure specific central and peripheral factors or did not measure left ventricular function; thus, inference for locus of improvement could not be made.

Improvement in rate pressure product (RPP) or myocardial blood supply with training has not been well documented in humans.[205,206] These studies with cardiac patients usually have been conducted 2 to 3 days per week for 2 to 6 months at a training intensity of 60 to 70 per cent of maximum HR reserve. Recently, Ehsani et al.[196] showed a significant improvement in RPP of cardiac patients who were trained for 1 year at approximately 85 per cent of maximum HR reserve. Their data also showed a significant reduction in angina pectoris and ST-segment depression at maximal exercise. Patients were jogging or running 4 to 5 miles for 4 or 5 days per week during the last 6 months of training. The authors speculate that their results differed from previous studies because of intensity of training and duration of the project period. Repeat studies of similar design are necessary to confirm these data.

Most investigators feel that ejection fraction and coronary blood supply (perfusion or increased capillarization) are not affected by endurance training. However, rate pressure product, angina pectoris, and ST-segment depression at standard submaximal work loads have been shown to be significantly reduced for cardiac patients participating in aerobic training.[200-205]

SUMMARY

The chronic effects of physical activity on cardiorespiratory functions were reviewed. Generally, $\dot{V}O_2$ max, cardiac output, stroke volume, A-V O_2 difference, and working capacity improved with endurance training. At submaximal work loads, $\dot{V}O_2$ and cardiac output remain fairly constant, with HR and systolic blood pressure decreasing and stroke volume increasing. Whether cardiac patients show both central and peripheral physiological adaptations to endurance training is not known. Central changes in cardiac patients may depend on increased intensity of training (85 per cent HR_{max} reserve) and normal left ventricular function.

Research findings showed that improvement in cardiorespiratory endurance was dependent on the intensity, duration, and frequency of the training program. Intensity and duration of training were found to be interrelated, and total kilocalorie expenditure was the important factor. Although there appears to be a minimum threshold for improving cardiorespiratory fitness (50 to 60 per cent of maximum), programs of 20 to 40 minutes of continuous activity, performed 3 to 5 days per week, generally produced significant improvement in cardiorespiratory fitness. Weight training resulted in increased muscular strength but showed little or no improvement in aerobic capacity. To help prevent musculoskeletal injuries and improve adherence to endurance training, moderate-intensity programs appear to be superior to high-intensity ones.

Although women have been shown to have a lower $\dot{V}O_2$ max compared with men, their adaptation to training is similar.

The aging curve for $\dot{V}O_2$ max may not be the same for active and sedentary populations. Middle-aged and elderly men who continued to train in a consistent fashion for 10 years showed no reduction in aerobic capacity.

REFERENCES

1. Åstrand, P. O., and Rodahl, K.: Textbook of Work Physiology. 2nd ed. New York, McGraw-Hill Book Co., 1977.
2. Wilmore, J. H.: Training for Sport and Activity: The Physiological Basis of the Conditioning Process. 2nd ed. Boston, Allyn and Bacon, 1982.
3. McArdle, W. D., Katch, F. I., and Katch, V. L.: Exercise Physiology, Energy, Nutrition and Human Performance. Philadelphia, Lea and Febiger, 1981.
4. Taylor, H. L., and Rowell, L. D.: Exercise and metabolism. In Johnson, W., and Buskirk, E. R., editors: Science and Medicine of Exercise and Sport. 2nd ed. New York, Harper and Row, 1974, pp. 84–111.
5. Mitchell, J. H., Sproule, B. J., and Chapman, C.: The physiological meaning of the maximal oxygen intake test. J. Clin. Invest. 37:538–547, 1958.
6. Åstrand, P. O.: Measurement of maximal aerobic capacity. Can. Med. Assoc. J. 96: 732–735, 1967.
7. Taylor, H. L., Buskirk, E. R., and Henschel, A.: Maximal oxygen intake as an objective measure of cardiorespiratory performance. J. Appl. Physiol. 8:73–78, 1955.
8. Pollock, M. L., Wilmore, J. H., and Fox, S. M.: Health and Fitness Through Physical Activity. New York, John Wiley and Sons, 1978.
9. Buskirk, E. R., and Taylor, H. L.: Maximal oxygen intake and its relation to body composition, with special reference to chronic physical activity and obesity. J. Appl. Physiol. 11:72–78, 1957.
10. Pollock, M. L.: The quantification of endurance training programs. In Wilmore, J. H., editor: Exercise and Sport Sciences Reviews, Vol. 1. New York, Academic Press, Inc., pp. 155–188, 1973.
11. Kitamura, K., Jorgenson, C. R., Gobel, F. L., Taylor, H. L., and Wang, Y.: Hemodynamic correlates of myocardial oxygen consumption during upright exercise. J. Appl. Physiol. 32:516–522, 1972.
12. Robinson, B. F.: Relationship of heart rate, and systolic blood pressure to the onset of pain in angina pectoris. Circulation 35:1073–1083, 1967.
13. Tzankoff, S. P., Robinson, S., Pyke, F. S., and Brawn, C. A.: Physiological adjustments to work in older men as affected by physical training. J. Appl. Physiol. 33:346–350, 1972.
14. Boyer, J., and Kasch, F.: Exercise therapy in hypertensive men. J.A.M.A. 211:1668–1671, 1970.
15. Choquette, G., and Ferguson, R. J.: Blood pressure reduction in borderline hypertensives following physical training. Can. Med. Assoc. J. 108:699–703, 1973.
16. Bjorntorp, P.: Hypertension and exercise. Hypertension 4(Suppl III):56–59, 1982.
17. Drinkwater, B. L.: Physiological responses of women to exercise. In Wilmore, J. H.: Exercise and Sports Sciences Reviews, Vol. 1. New York, Academic Press, pp. 126–154, 1973.
18. Wilmore, J. H., and Brown, C. H.: Physiological profiles of women distance runners. Med. Sci. Sports 6:178–181, 1974.
19. Saltin, B., and Åstrand, P. O.: Maximal oxygen uptake in athletes. J. Appl. Physiol. 23: 353–358, 1967.
20. Costill, D. L.: Physiology of marathon running. J.A.M.A.221:1024–1029, 1972.
21. Pollock, M. L.: Submaximal and maximal working capacity of elite distance runners. Ann. N.Y. Acad. Sci. 301:310–322, 1977.
22. Cooper, K. H.: The New Aerobics. New York, J. B. Lippincott, 1970.
23. Hurst, W.: The Heart. New York, McGraw Hill Book Co., 1982.

24. Robinson, S.: Experimental studies of physical fitness in relation to age. Arbeitsphysiol. *10:*251–323, 1938.
25. Asmussen, E., Fruensgaard, K., and Norgaard, S.: A follow-up longitudinal study of selected physiologic functions in former physical education students after forty years. J. Am. Geriatr. Soc. *23:*442–450, 1975.
26. Cureton, T. K.: The Physiological Effects of Exercise Programs upon Adults. Springfield, Ill., Charles C Thomas Co., 1969.
27. American College of Sports Medicine: Position statement on the recommended quantity and quality of exercise for developing and maintaining fitness in healthy adults. Med. Sci. Sports *10:*vii–x, 1978.
28. Costill, D. L.: A Scientific Approach to Distance Running. Los Altos, Calif., Track and Field News, 1979.
29. Cureton, T. K., and Barry, A. J.: Improving the Physical Fitness of Youth. Monograph of the Society of Research for Child Development, 1964.
30. Pollock, M. L., and Blair, S. N.: Action into analysis: exercise prescription. J. Phys. Educ. Rec. *52:*30–35, 1981.
31. The Perrier Study: Fitness in America. New York, Perrier, Great Waters of France, 1979.
32. Davies, C. T. M., and Knibbs, A. V.: The training stimulus, the effects of intensity, duration and frequency of effort on maximum aerobic power output. Int. Z. Angew. Physiol. *29:*299–305, 1971.
33. Shephard, R. J.: Intensity, duration, and frequency of exercise as determinants of the response to a training regime. Int. Z. Angew. Physiol. *26:*272–278, 1969.
34. Hill, J. S.: The effects of frequency of exercise on cardiorespiratory fitness of adult men. M.S. Thesis. London, University of Western Ontario, 1969.
35. Jackson, J. H., Sharkey, B. J., and Johnson, P. L.: Cardiorespiratory adaptations to training at specified frequencies. Res. Q., *39:*295–300, 1968.
36. Sidney, K. H., Eynon, R. B., and Cunningham, D. A.: Effect of frequency of exercise upon physical working performance and selected variables representative of cardiorespiratory fitness. *In* Taylor, A. W., and Howell, M. L., editors: Training: Scientific Basis and Application. Springfield, Ill., Charles C Thomas Co., pp. 144–148, 1972.
37. Pollock, M. L., Cureton, T. K., and Greninger, L.: Effects of frequency of training on working capacity, cardiovascular function, and body composition of adult men. Med. Sci. Sports *1:*70–74, 1969.
38. Pollock, M. L., Tiffany, J., Gettman, L., Janeway, R., and Lofland, H.: Effect of frequency of training on serum lipids, cardiovascular function, and body composition. *In* Franks, B. D., editor: Exercise and Fitness, Chicago, Athletic Institute, pp. 161–178, 1969.
39. Pollock, M. L., Miller, H. S., Linnerud, A. C., and Cooper, K. H.: Frequency of training as a determinant for improvement in cardiovascular function and body composition of middle-aged men. Arch. Phys. Med. Rehab. *58:*141–145, 1975.
40. Gettman, L. R., Pollock, M. L., Durstine, J. L., Ward, A., Ayres, J., and Linnerud, A. C.: Physiological responses of men to 1, 3, and 5 day per week training programs. Res. Q. *47:*638–646, 1976.
41. Fox, E. L., Bartels, R. L., Billings, C. E., O'Brien, R., Bason, R., and Mathews, D. K.: Frequency and duration of interval training programs and changes in aerobic power. J. Appl. Physiol. *38:*481–484, 1975.
42. Pollock, M. L. Broida, J., Kendrick, Z., Miller, H. S., Janeway, R., and Linnerud, A. C.: Effects of training two days per week at different intensities on middle-aged men. Med. Sci. Sports *4:*192–197, 1972.
43. Kilbom, A., Hartley, L., Saltin, B., Bjure, J., Grimby, G., and Åstrand, I.: Physical training in sedentary middle-aged and older men. Scand. J. Clin. Lab. Invest. *24:*315–322, 1969.
44. Pollock, M. L., Gettman, L. R., Mileses, C. A., Bah, M. D., Durstine, J. L., and Johnson, R. B.: Effects of frequency and duration of training on attrition and incidence of injury. Med. Sci. Sports *9:*31–36, 1977.
45. Pollock, M. L.: How much exercise is enough? Phys. Sportsmed. *6:*50–64, 1978.
46. Chaffin, B. D., and Park, K. S.: A longitudinal study of low-back pain as associated with occupational weight lifting factors. Am. Indust. Hyg. Assoc. J. *34:*513–525, 1973.
47. Fisher, A. G., and Ebisu, T.: Splitting the duration of exercise: effects on endurance and blood lipid levels. Med. Sci. Sports Exer. (Abstr.) *12:*90, 1980.
48. Moffatt, R. J., Stamford, B. A., and Neill, R. D.: Placement of tri-weekly training sessions: Importance regarding enhancement of aerobic capacity. Res. Q. *48:*583–591, 1977.
49. Roskamm, H.: Optimum patterns of exercise for healthy adults. Can. Med. Assoc. J. *96:*895–899, 1967.

50. Cureton, T. K., and Phillips, E. E.: Physical fitness changes in middle-aged men attributable to equal eight-week periods of training, non-training and retraining. J. Sports Med. Phys. Fitness 4:1–7, 1964.
51. Taylor, H. L., Henschel, A., Brozek, J., and Keys, A.: Effects of bed rest on cardiovascular function and work performance. J. Appl. Physiol. 2:233–239, 1949.
52. Saltin, B., Blomqvist, G., Mitchell, J., Johnson, R. L., Wildenthal, K., and Chapman, C. B.: Response to exercise after bed rest and after training. Circulation 37 and 38 (Suppl.)7:1–78, 1968.
53. Convertino, V., Hung, J., Goldwater, D., and DeBusk, R. F.: Cardiovascular responses to exercise in middle-aged men after 10 days of bed rest. Circulation 65:134–140, 1982.
54. Fringer, M. N., and Stull, A. G.: Changes in cardiorespiratory parameters during periods of training and detraining in young female adults. Med. Sci. Sports 6:20–25, 1974.
55. Knuttgen, H. G., Nordesjo, L. O., Ollander, B., and Saltin, B.: Physical conditioning through interval training with young male adults. Med. Sci. Sports 5:220–226, 1973.
56. Kendrick, Z. B., Pollock, M. L. Hickman, T. N., and Miller, H. S.: Effects of training and detraining on cardiovascular efficiency. Am. Corr. Ther. J. 25:79–83, 1971.
57. Brynteson, P., and Sinning, W. E.: The effects of training frequencies on the retention of cardiovascular fitness. Med. Sci. Sports 5:29–33, 1973.
58. Hickson, R. C., and Rosenkoetter, M. A.: Reduced training frequencies and maintenance of increased aerobic power. Med. Sci. Sports Exer. 13:13–16, 1981.
59. Siegel, W., Blomqvist, G., and Mitchell, J. H.: Effects of quantitated physical training program on middle-aged sedentary males. Circulation 41:19–29, 1970.
60. Karvonen, M., Kentala, K., and Musta, O.: The effects of training heart rate: a longitudinal study. Ann. Med. Exp. Biol. Fenn. 35:307–315, 1957.
61. Hollmann, W., and Venrath, H.: Experimentelle Untersuchungen zur bedentung aines Trainings unterhalb and oberhalb der dauerbeltz Stungsgranze. In Korbs, editor: Carl Diem Festschrift. W.U.A., Frankfurt/Wein, 1962.
62. Åstrand, I., Åstrand, P. O., Christensen, E. A., and Hedman, R.: Intermittent muscular work. Acta Physiol. Scand. 48:448–453, 1960.
63. Taylor, H. L., Haskell, W., Fox, S. M., and Blackburn, H.: Exercise tests: a summary of procedures and concepts of stress testing for cardiovascular diagnosis and function evaluation. In Blackburn, H., editor: Measurement in Exercise Electrocardiography. Springfield, Ill., Charles C Thomas, pp. 259–305, 1969.
64. Shephard, R. J.: Future research on the quantifying of endurance training. J. Hum. Ergol. 3:163–181, 1975.
65. Sidney, K. H., Shephard, R. J., and Harrison, H.: Endurance training and body composition of the elderly. Am. J. Clin. Nutr. 30:326–333, 1977.
66. Gledhill, N. and Eynon, R. B.: The intensity of training. In Taylor, A. W., and Howell, M. L., editors: Training: Scientific Basis and Application. Springfield, Ill., Charles C Thomas, pp. 97–102, 1972.
67. Kilbom, A.: Physical training in women. Scand. J. Clin. Lab. Invest. (Suppl.)119:1–34, 1971.
68. Sharkey, B. J., and Holleman, J. P.: Cardiorespiratory adaptations to training at specified intensities. Res. Q. 38:698–704, 1967.
69. Faria, I. E.: Cardiovascular response to exercise as influenced by training of various intensities. Res. Q. 41:44–50, 1970.
70. Olree, H. D., Corbin, B., Penrod, J., and Smith, C.: Methods of achieving and maintaining physical fitness for prolonged space flight. Final Progress Report to NASA, Grant No. NGR–04–002–004, 1969.
71. Sharkey, B. J.: Intensity and duration of training and the development of cardiorespiratory endurance. Med. Sci. Sports 2:197–202, 1970.
72. Pollock, M. L., Dimmick, J., Miller, H. S., Kendrick, Z., and Linnerud, A. C.: Effects of mode of training on cardiovascular function and body composition of middle-aged men. Med. Sci. Sports 7:139–145, 1975.
73. Pollock, M. L., Gettman, L. R., Raven, P. B., Ayres, J., Bah, M., and Ward, A.: Physiological comparisons of the effects of aerobic and anaerobic training. Presented to the American College of Sports Medicine. Washington, D.C., May 26, 1978.
74. Pollock, M. L., Miller, H., Janeway, R., Linnerud, A. C., Robertson, B., and Valentino, R.: Effects of walking on body composition and cardiovascular function of middle-aged men. J. Appl. Physiol. 30:126–130, 1971.
75. Hanson, J. S., Tabakin, B. S., Levy, A. M., and Nedde, W.: Long-term physical training and cardiovascular dynamics in middle-aged men. Circulation 38:783–799, 1968.
76. Hartley, L. H., Grimby, G., Kilbom, A., Nilsson, N. J., Åstrand, I., Bjure, J., Ekblom, B.,

and Saltin, B.: Physical training in sedentary middle-aged and older men. III Scand. J. Clin. Lab. Invest. 24:335–344, 1969.

77. Kilbom, A., Hartley, L., Saltin, B., Bjure, J., Grimby, G., and Åstrand, I.: Physical training in sedentary middle-aged and older men. I Scand. J. Clin. Lab. Invest. 24:315–322, 1969.

78. Oja, P., Teraslinna, P., Partaner, T., and Karava, R.: Feasibility of an 18 months' physical training program for middle-aged men and its effect on physical fitness. Am. J. Pub. Health 64:459–465, 1975.

79. Froelicher, V. F.: Exercise testing and training: clinical applications. J. Am. Coll. Cardiol. 1:114–125, 1983.

80. Hossack, K. F., and Hartwig, R.: Cardiac arrest associated with supervised cardiac rehabilitation. J. Card. Rehabil. 2:402–408, 1982.

81. Price, C., Pollock, M. L., Gettman, L. R., and Kent, D. A.: Physical fitness programs for law enforcement officers: a manual for police administrators. Washington, D.C., U.S. Government Printing Office, No. 027–000–00671–0, 1978.

82. Milesis, C. A., Pollock, M. L., Bah, M. D., Ayres, J. J., Ward, A., and Linnerud, A. C.: Effects of different durations of training on cardiorespiratory function, body composition and serum lipids. Res. Q. 47:716–725, 1976.

83. Terjung, R. L., Baldwin, K. M., Cooksey, J., Samson, B., and Sutter, R. A.: Cardiovascular adaptation to twelve minutes of mild daily exercise in middle-aged sedentary men. J. Am. Geriatr. Soc. 21:164–168, 1973.

84. Hartung, G. H., Smolensky, M. H., Harrist, R. B., and Runge, R.: Effects of varied durations of training on improvement in cardiorespiratory endurance. J. Hum. Ergol. 6:61–68, 1977.

85. Liang, M. T., Alexander, J. F., Taylor, H. L., Serfrass, R. C., Leon, A. S., and Stull, G. A.: Aerobic training threshold. Scand. J. Sports Sci. 4:5–8, 1982.

86. Wilmore, J. H., Royce, J., Girandola, R. N., Katch, F. I., and Katch, V. L.: Physiological alterations resulting from a 10-week jogging program. Med. Sci. Sports 2:7–14, 1970.

87. Yeager, S. A., and Brynteson, P.: Effects of varying training periods on the development of cardiovascular efficiency of college women. Res. Q. 41:589–592, 1970.

88. Blair, S. N., Chandler, J. V., Ellisor, D. B., and Langley, J.: Improving physical fitness by exercise training programs. South. Med. J. 73:1594–1596, 1980.

89. Knehr, C. A., Dill, D. B., and Neufeld, W.: Training and its effect on man at rest and at work. Am. J. Physiol. 136:148–156, 1942.

90. Saltin, B., Hartley, L., Kilbom, A., and Åstrand, I.: Physical training in sedentary middle-aged and older men. II Scand. J. Clin. Lab. Invest. 24:323–334, 1969.

91. Ismail, A. H., Corrigan, D., and McLeod, D. F.: Effect of an eight month exercise program on selected physiological, biochemical, and audiological variables in adult men. Br. J. Sports Med. 7:230–240, 1973.

92. Mann, G. V., Garrett, H., Farhi, A., Murray, H., Billings, T. F., Shute, F., and Schwarten, S. E.: Exercise to prevent coronary heart disease. Am. J. Med. 46:12–27, 1969.

93. Naughton, J., and Nagle, F.: Peak oxygen intake during physical fitness program for middle-aged men. J.A.M.A. 191:899–901, 1965.

94. Ribisl, P. M.: Effects of training upon the maximal oxygen uptake of middle-aged men. Int. Z. Angew. Physiol. 26:272–278, 1969.

95. Oscai, L. B., Williams, T., and Hertig, B.: Effects of exercise on blood volume. J. Appl. Physiol. 24:622–624, 1968.

96. Skinner, J., Holloszy, J., and Cureton, T.: Effects of a program of endurance exercise on physical work capacity and anthropometric measurements of fifteen middle-aged men. Am. J. Cardiol. 14:747–752, 1964.

97. Ekblom, B., Åstrand, P. O., Saltin, B., Sternberg, J., and Wallstrom, B.: Effect of training on circulatory response to exercise. J. Appl. Physiol. 24:518–528, 1968.

98. Hickson, R. C., Bomze, H. A., and Holloszy, J. O.: Linear increase in aerobic power induced by a strenuous program of endurance exercise. J. Appl. Physiol. 42:372–376, 1977.

99. Pechar, G. S., McArdle, W. D., Katch, F. I., Magel, J. R., and Deluca, J.: Specificity of cardiorespiratory adaptation to bicycle and treadmill training. J. Appl. Physiol. 36:753–756, 1974.

100. Golding, L.: Effects of physical training upon total serum cholesterol levels. Res. Q. 32:499–505, 1961.

101. Kasch, F. W., Phillips, W. H., Carter, J. E. L., and Boyer, J. L.: Cardiovascular changes in middle-aged men during two years of training. J. Appl. Physiol. 314:53–57, 1972.

102. Wood, P. D., Haskell, W. L., Blair, S. N., Williams, P. T., Krauss, R. M., Lindgren, F. T., Albers, J. J., Ho, P. H., and Farquhar, J. W.: Increased exercise level and plasma lipoprotein concentrations: a one-year, randomized, controlled study in sedentary, middle-age men. Metabolism. *32:*31–39, 1983.

103. Leon, A. S., Conrad, J., Hunninghake, D. B., and Serfass, R.: Effects of vigorous walking program on body composition, and carbohydrate and lipid metabolism of obese young men. Am. J. Clin. Nutr. *32:*1776–1787, 1979.

104. Miyashita, M., Hagg, S., and Mizuta, T.: Training and detraining effects on aerobic power in middle-aged and older men. J. Sports Med. *18:*131–137, 1978.

105. Burke, E. J., and Franks, B. D.: Changes in $\dot{V}o_2$ max resulting from bicycle training at different intensities holding total mechanical work constant. Res. Q. *46:*31–37, 1975.

106. Atomi, Y., Ito, K., Iwasaski, H., and Miyashita, M.: Effects of intensity and frequency of training on aerobic work capacity of young females. J. Sports Med. *18:*3–9, 1978.

107. Magle, J., Foglia, G. F., and McArdle, W. D., Gutin, B., Pechar, G. S., and Katch, F. I.: Specificity of swim training on maximum oxygen uptake. J. Appl. Physiol. *38:*151–155, 1975.

108. Stransky, A. W., Mickelson, R. J., Van Fleet, C., and Davis, R.: Effects of a swimming training regimen on hematological, cardiorespiratory and body composition changes in young females. J. Sports Med. *19:*347–354, 1979.

109. Cureton, T. K.: Improvement in physical fitness associated with a course of U.S. Navy underwater trainees, with and without dietary supplements. Res. Q. *34:*440–453, 1963.

110. Åstrand, P. O., Eriksson, B. O., Nylander, I., Engstrom, L., Karlberg, P., Saltin, B., and Thoren, C.: Girl swimmers with special reference to respiratory and circulatory adaptation and gynecological and psychiatric aspects. Acta Paediatr. (Suppl.) *147:*1–75, 1963.

111. Holmer, I.: Physiology of swimming man. Acta Physiol. Scand. (Suppl.) *407:*1–55, 1974.

112. Christensen, E. H., and Hogberg, P.: Physiology of skiing. Arbeitsphysiol. *14:*292–303, 1950.

113. Daniels, S., Pollock, M. L., and Startsman, T.: Effects of dancing training on cardiovascular efficiency and body composition of young obese women. Proceedings of the 37th Annual Convention of the Southern District American Association for Health, Physical Education, and Recreation, pp. 99–101, 1970.

114. Vaccaro, P., and Clinton, M.: The effects of aerobic dance conditioning on the body composition and maximal oxygen uptake of college women. J. Sports Med. *21:*291–294, 1981.

115. Rockefeller, K. A., and Burke, E. J.: Psycho-physiological analysis of an aerobic dance programme for women. Br. J. Sports Med. *13:*77–80, 1979.

116. Wilmore, J. H., Davis, J. A., O'Brien, R. S., Vodak, P. A., Walder, G. R., and Amsterdam, E. A.: Physiological alterations consequent to 20-week conditioning programs of bicycling, tennis, and jogging. Med. Sci. Sports Exer. *12:*1–8, 1980.

117. Jones, D. M., Squires, C., and Rodahl, K.: Effect of rope skipping on physical work capacity. Res. Q. *33:*236–238, 1962.

118. Baker, J. A.: Comparison of rope skipping and jogging as methods of improving cardiovascular efficiency of college men. Res. Q. *39:*240–243, 1968.

119. Fardy, P. S.: Effects of soccer training and detraining upon selected cardiac and metabolic measures. Res. Q. *40:*502–508, 1969.

120. Claussen, J. P., Trap-Jensen, T., and Lassen, N. A.: Effects of training on heart rate during arm and leg exercise. Scand. J. Clin. Lab. Invest. *26:*295–301, 1970.

121. Pollock, M. L., Miller, H. S., Linnerud, A. C., Laughridge, E., Coleman, E., and Alexander, E.: Arm pedaling as an endurance training regimen for the disabled. Arch. Phys. Med. Rehabil. *55:*418–424, 1974.

122. Gass, G. C., Watson, J., Camp, E. M., Court, H. J., McPherson, L. M., and Redhead, P.: The effects of physical training on high level spinal lesion patients. Scand. J. Rehabil. Med. *12:*61–65, 1980.

123. Miles, P. S., Sawka, M. N., Wilde, S. W., Durbin., R. J., Gotshall, R. W., and Glaser, R. M.: Pulmonary function changes in wheelchair athletes subsequent to exercise training. Ergonomics *25:*239–246, 1982.

124. Campney, H. K., and Wehr, R. W.: Effects of calisthenics on selected components of physical fitness. Res. Q. *36:*393–402, 1965.

125. Taddonio, D. A.: Effect of daily fifteen-minute periods of calisthenics upon the physical fitness of fifth grade boys and girls. Res. Q. *37:*276–281, 1966.

126. Getchell, L.: An analysis of the effects of a season of golf on selected cardiovascular,

metabolic, and muscular fitness measures on middle-age men. Ph.D. dissertation, University of Illinois, Urbana, Illinois, 1965.

127. Nagle, F., and Irwin, L.: Effects of two systems of weight training on circulorespiratory endurance and related physiological factors. Res. Q. 31:607–615, 1960.

128. Fahey, T. D., and Brown, C. H.: The effects of an anabolic steroid on the strength, body composition, and endurance of college males when accompanied by a weight training program. Med. Sci. Sports 5:272–276, 1973.

129. Gettman, L. R., and Pollock, M. L.: Circuit weight training: a critical review of its physiological benefits. Phys. Sportsmed. 9:44–60, 1981.

130. Allen, T. E., Byrd, R. J., and Smith, D. P.: Hemodynamic consequences of circuit weight training. Res. Q. 47:299–306, 1976.

131. Wilmore, J. H., Parr, R. B., Girandola, R. N., Ward, P., Vodak, P. A., Barstow, T. J., Pipes, T. V., Romero, G. T., and Leslie, P.: Physiological alterations consequent to circuit weight training. Med. Sci. Sports 10:79–84, 1978.

132. Gettman, L. R., Ayres, J. J., Pollock, M. L., and Jackson, A.: The effect of circuit weight training on strength, cardiorespiratory function, and body composition of adult men. Med. Sci. Sports 10:171–176, 1978.

133. Gettman, L. R., and Ayres, J. J.: Aerobic changes through 10 weeks of slow and fast speed isokinetic training (abstract). Med. Sci. Sports 10:47, 1978.

134. Gettman, L. R., Ayres, J. J., Pollock, M. L., Durstine, J. L., and Grantham, W.: Physiological effects on adult men of circuit strength training and jogging. Arch. Phys. Med. Rahabil. 60:115–120, 1979.

135. Garfield, D. S., Ward P., Cobb, R., Disch, J., and Southwick, D.: The Syracuse circuit weight training study report. Houston, Dynamics Health Equipment, 1979.

136. Gettman, L. R., Culter, L. A., and Strathman, T.: Physiologic changes after 20 weeks of isotonic vs. isokinetic circuit training. J. Sports Med. Phys. Fit. 20:265–274, 1980.

137. Kimura, Y., Itow, H., and Yamazakie, S.: The effects of circuit weight training on $\dot{V}_{O_2}$ max and body composition of trained and untrained college men. J. Physiol. Soc. Jpn. 43:593–596, 1981.

138. Hubbard, A. W.: Homokinetics: muscular function in human movement. In Johnson, W. R., and Buskirk, E. R., editors: Science and Medicine of Exercise and Sport. 2nd ed. New York, Harper and Row, pp. 5–23, 1974.

139. Brouha, L.: Training. In Johnson, W. R., and Buskirk, E. R., editors: Science and Medicine of Exercise and Sport. 2nd ed. New York, Harper and Row, pp. 276–286, 1980.

140. Saltin, B., Nazar, K., Costill, D. L., Stein, E., Jansson, E., Essen, B., and Gollnick, P. D.: The nature of the training response: peripheral and central adaptations to one legged exercise. Acta Physiol. Scand. 96:289–297, 1976.

141. Clausen, J. P.: Circulatory adjustments to dynamic exercise and effect of physical training in normal subjects and in patients with coronary disease. Progr. Cardiovasc. Dis. 18:459–493, 1976.

142. Åstrand, P. O., and Saltin, B.: Maximal oxygen uptake and heart rate in various types of muscular activity. J. Appl. Physiol. 16:977–981, 1961.

143. Wilmore, J. H., Parr, R. B., Ward, P., Vodak, P., Barstow, T. J., Pipes, T. V., Grimditch, G., and Leslie, P.: Energy cost of circuit weight training. Med. Sci. Sports 10:75–78, 1978.

144. Strathman, T., Gettman, L., and Culter, L.: The oxygen cost of an isotonic circuit strength program (abstract). American Alliance for Health, Physical Education, and Recreation Research Papers, 1979, p. 70.

145. Gettman, L. R., The aerobic cost of isokinetic slow- and fast-speed circuit training programs (abstract). American Alliance for Health, Physical Education, and Recreation Research Papers, 1979, p. 31.

146. Gettman, L. R., Ward, P., and Hagan, R. D.: A comparison of combined running and weight training with circuit weight training. Med. Sci. Sports Exer. 14:229–234, 1982.

147. Saltin, B., Hartley, L., Kilbom, A., and Åstrand, I.: Physical training in sedentary middle-aged men, II. Scand. J. Clin. Lab. Invest. 24:323–334, 1969.

148. Muller, E., and Rohmert, W.: Die Geschwindigkeit der Muskelkraft—Zunahme bei isometrischem Training. Arbeitsphysiol. 19:403–419, 1963.

149. Rowell, L. B.: Factors affecting the prediction of the maximal oxygen intake from measurements made during submaximal work. Ph.D. dissertation, University of Minnesota, Minneapolis, 1962.

150. Kavanagh, T., Shephard, R. J., Doney, H., and Pandit, V.: Intensive exercise in coronary rehabilitation. Med. Sci. Sports 5:34–39, 1973.
151. Cooper, K. H., Pollock, M. L., Martin, R., and White, S. R.: Levels of physical fitness versus selected coronary risk factors—a cross sectional study. J.A.M.A. 236:166–169, 1976.
152. Pollock, M. L., Dawson, G. A., Miller, H. S. Jr., Ward, A., Cooper, D., Headly, W., Linnerud, A. C., and Nomeir, M. M.: Physiologic responses of men 49 to 65 years of age to endurance training. J. Am. Geriatr. Soc. 24:97–104, 1976.
153. DeVries, H. A.: Physiological effects of an exercise training regimen upon men aged 52 to 88. J. Gerontol. 24:325–336, 1970.
154. Benestad, A. M.: Trainability of old men. Acta Med. Scand. 178:321–327, 1965.
155. Skinner, J.: The cardiovascular system with aging and exercise. In Brunner, D., and Jokl, E., editors: Physical Activity and Aging. Baltimore, University Park Press, pp. 100–108, 1970.
156. Robinson, S., Dill, D. B., Robinson, R. D., Tzankoff, S. P., and Wagner, J. A.: Physiological aging of champion runners. J. Appl. Physiol. 41:46–51, 1976.
157. Robinson, S., Dill., D. B., Ross, J. C., Robinson, R. D., Wagner, J. A., and Tzankoff, S. P.: Training and physiological aging in man. Fed. Proc. 32:1628–1634, 1973.
158. Asmussen, E., Fruensgaard, K., and Norgaard, S.: A follow-up longitudinal study of selected physiologic functions in former physical education students after forty years. J. Am. Geriatr. Soc. 23:442–450, 1975.
159. Kasch, F., and Wallace, J. P.: Physiological variables during 10 years of endurance exercise. Med. Sci. Sports 8:5–8, 1976.
160. Dill, D. B., Robinson, S., and Ross, J. C.: A longitudinal study of 16 champion runners. J. Sports Med. Phys. Fitness 7:1–27, 1967.
161. Grimby, G., and Saltin, B.: Physiological analysis of physically well-trained middle-aged and old athletes. Acta Med. Scand. 179:513–526, 1966.
162. Pollock, M. L., Miller, H. S., Linnerud, A. C., Royster, C. L., Smith, W. E., and Sonner, W. H.: Physiological findings in well-trained middle-aged American men. Br. Assoc. Sport Med. J. 7:222–229, 1973.
163. Pollock, M. L., Miller, H. S., and Wilmore, J.: Physiological characteristics of champion American track athletes 40 to 75 years of age. J. Gerontol. 29:645–649, 1974.
164. Hodgson, J. L., and Buskirk, E. R.: Physical fitness and age, with emphasis on cardiovascular function in the elderly. J. Am. Geriatr. Soc. 25:385–392, 1977.
165. Heath, G. W., Hagberg, J. M., Ehsani, A. A., and Holloszy, J. O.: A physiological comparison of young and older endurance athletes. J. Appl. Physiol. 51:634–640, 1981.
166. Drinkwater, B. L., Horvath, S. M., and Wells, C. L.: Aerobic power of females, ages 10 to 68. J. Gerontol. 30:385–394, 1975.
167. Pollock, M. L., Miller, H. S., and Ribisl, P. M.: Effect of fitness on aging. Phys. Sportsmed. 6:45–48, 1978.
168. Costill, D. L., and Winrow, E.: Maximal oxygen intake among marathon runners. Arch. Phys. Med. Rehabil. 51:317–320, 1970.
169. Pollock, M. L., Foster, C., Rod, J., Hare, J., and Schmidt, D. H.: Ten year follow-up on aerobic capacity of champion master's track athletes (abstract). Med. Sci. Sports Exer. 14:105, 1982.
170. Maud, P. J., Pollock, M. L., Foster, C., Anholm, J., Guten, G., Al-Nouri, M., Hellman, C., and Schmidt, D. H.: Fifty years of training and competition in the marathon: Wally Hayward aged 70—a physiological profile. S. Afr. Med. J. 59:153–157, 1981.
171. Cooper, K. H., Purdy, J. G., White, S. R., Pollock, M. L., and Linnerud, A. C.: Age-fitness adjusted maximal heart rates. In Brunner, D., and Jokl, E., editors: Medicine and Sport, Vol. 10, The Role of Exercise in Internal Medicine. Basel, S. Karger, pp. 78–88, 1977.
172. Ekblom, B.: Effect of physical training in adolescent boys. J. Appl. Physiol. 27:350–355, 1969.
173. Sherman, M.: Maximal oxygen intake changes of experimentally exercised junior high school boys. Ph.D. dissertation, University of Illinois, Urbana, Illinois, 1967.
174. Larsson, Y., Persson, B., Sterky, G., and Theren, C.: Functional adaptations to rigorous training and exercise in diabetic and non-diabetic adolescents. J. Appl. Physiol. 19:629–635, 1964.
175. Lussier, L., and Buskirk, E. R.: Effects of an endurance training regimen on assessment of work capacity in prepubertal children. Ann. N.Y. Acad. Sci. 301:734–747, 1977.

176. Daniels, J., and Oldridge, N.: Changes in oxygen consumption of young boys during growth and running training. Med. Sci. Sports 3:161–165, 1971.
177. Cumming, G. R.: Current levels of fitness. Can. Med. Assoc. J. 96:868–877, 1967.
178. Zauner, C. W., and Benson, N. Y.: Physiological alterations in young swimmers during three years of intensive training. J. Sports. Med. 21:179–185, 1981.
179. Gedda, L.: Sports and genetics: A Study on twins (351 pairs). In Larson, L. A., editor: Health and Fitness in the Modern World. Chicago, Athletic Institute, pp. 43–64, 1961.
180. Klissouras, V.: Heritability of adaptive variation. J. Appl. Physiol. 31:338–344, 1971.
181. Klissouras, V., Pirnay, F., and Petit, J.: Adaptation to maximal effort: genetics and age. J. Appl. Physiol. 35:288–293, 1973.
182. Astrand, P. O.: Do we need physical conditioning? J. Phys. Ed., Mar.-Apr., 1972, pp. 129–135.
183. Flint, M. M., Drinkwater, B. L., and Horvath, S. M.: Effects of training on women's response to submaximal exercise. Med. Sci. Sports 6:89–94, 1974.
184. Kearney, J. J., Stull, G. A., Ewing, J. L., and Strein, J. W.: Cardiorespiratory responses of sedentary college women as a function of training intensity. J. Appl. Physiol. 41: 822–825, 1976.
185. Smith, D. P., and Stransky, F. W.: The effects of jogging on body composition and cardiovascular response to submaximal work in young women. J. Sports Med. 15:26–32, 1975.
186. Cunningham, D. A., and Hill, J. S.: Effect of training on cardiovascular response to exercise in women. J. Appl. Physiol. 39:891–895, 1975.
187. Smith, D. P., and Stransky, F. W.: The effect of training and detraining on the body composition and cardiovascular response of young women to exercise. J. Sports Med. 16:112–120, 1976.
188. Marigold, E. A.: The effect of training at predetermined heart rate levels for sedentary college women. Med. Sci. Sports 6:14–19, 1974.
189. Burke, E. J.: Physiological effects of similar training programs in males and females. Res. Q. 48:510–517, 1977.
190. Getchell, L. H., and Moore, J. C.: Physical training: comparative responses of middle-aged adults. Arch. Phys. Med. Rehabil. 56:250–254, 1975.
191. Mayhew, J. L., and Gross, P. M.: Body composition changes in young women with high resistance weight training. Res. Q. 45:433–439, 1974.
192. Franklin, B., Buskirk, E., Hodgson, J., Gahagan, H., Kollias, J., and Mendez, J.: Effects of physical conditioning on cardiorespiratory function, body composition and serum lipids in relatively normal weight and obese middle-aged women. Int. J. Obesity 3: 97–109, 1979.
193. Hanson, J. S., and Nedde, W. H.: Long-term physical training effect in sedentary females. J. Appl. Physiol. 37:112–116, 1974.
194. Daniels, J., Krahenbuhl, G., Foster, C., Gilbert, J., and Daniels, S.: Aerobic responses of female distance runners to submaximal and maximal exercise. Ann. N.Y. Acad. Sci. 301:726–733, 1977.
195. Wilmore, J.: Inferiority of female athletes: myth or reality. J. Sports Med. 3:1–6, 1975.
196. Ehsani, A. A., Heath, G. H., Hagberg, J. M., Sobel, B. E., and Holloszy, J. O.: Effects of 12 months of intense exercise training on ischemic ST-segment depression in patients with coronary artery disease. Circulation 64:1116–1124, 1981.
197. Hellerstein, H. K.: Exercise therapy in coronary disease. Bull N.Y. Acad. Med. 44: 1028–1047, 1968.
198. Kavanagh, T., and Shephard, R. J.: Conditioning of postcoronary patients: comparison of continuous and interval training. Arch. Phys. Med. Rehabil. 56:72–76, 1975.
199. Naughton, J., Bruhn, J. G., and Lategola, M. T.: Effects of physical training on physiologic and behavioral characteristics of cardiac patients. Arch. Phys. Med. Rehabil. 49: 131–137, 1968.
200. Clausen, J. P.: Circulatory adjustments to dynamic exercise and effect of physical training in normal subjects and in patients with coronary disease. Progr. Cardiovasc. Dis. 18:459–495, 1976.
201. Ferguson, R. J. Petitclerc, R., Choquette, G., Chamiotis, L., Gauthier, P., Huot, R., Allard, C., Jankowski, L., and Campeau, L.: Effect of physical training on treadmill exercise capacity, collateral circulation, and progression of disease. Am. J. Cardiol. 34: 764–769, 1974.

202. Detry, J. M., and Bruce, R. A.: Effects of physical training on exertional ST-segment depression in coronary heart disease. Circulation *44:*390–396, 1971.
203. Clausen, J. P., and Trap-Jensen, J.: Effects of training on distribution of cardiac output in patients with coronary artery disease. Circulation *42:*611–624, 1970.
204. Haskell, W. L.: Mechanisms by which physical activity may enhance the clinical status of cardiac patients. *In* Pollock, M. L., and Schmidt, D. H., editors: Heart Disease and Rehabilitation. New York, J. Wiley and Sons, pp. 276–296, 1979.
205. Froelicher, V. F.: Exercise testing and training: clinical applications. J. Am. Coll. Cardiol. *1:*114–125, 1983.
206. Conn, E. H., Williams, R. S., and Wallace, A. G.: Exercise responses before and after physical conditioning in patients with severely depressed left ventricular function. Am. J. Cardiol. *49:*296–300, 1982.
207. Hagberg, J. M., Ehsani, A. A., and Holloszy, J. O.:Effect of 12 months of intense exercise training on stroke volume in patients with coronary artery disease. Circulation *67:* 1194–1199, 1983.

Chapter 4

BODY COMPOSITION ALTERATIONS WITH EXERCISE*

INTRODUCTION

What role does exercise play in the prevention, control, and treatment of obesity? For many years, it has been a common belief that exercise is of little or no value in programs of weight reduction and control. Many examples are given demonstrating the tremendous number of hours of vigorous exercise necessary to obtain even small losses in body weight. Compared with starvation or semi-starvation diets, exercise is not an efficient means of losing body fat. To complete a 26.2 mile marathon requires an energy expenditure of approximately 100 Kcal per mile, or 2,600 Kcal for the entire race. With 3,500 Kcal representing the energy equivalent of a single pound of fat, this race could be completed using less than a pound of fat, provided fat was the primary energy source! In reality, since carbohydrate is the predominant fuel source for such an activity, the total fat loss would be approximately one quarter of a pound or less. However, evidence shows that physical inactivity may be a major cause of obesity in the United States and may even be a more significant factor than overeating.[1] In addition, many studies to be reviewed in this chapter have shown that substantial changes in body composition do result from an exercise program, even when diet remains unchanged.

When weight is lost by diet alone, a substantial amount of the total weight loss comes from the lean tissue, primarily as a result of water loss. This was discussed in Chapter 2. Most of the recent fad diets have empha-

---

*Adapted in part from Jack H. Wilmore. Body composition in sport and exercise: Directions for future research. Med. Sci. Sports Exer. *15:* 21–31, 1983, with permission.

sized low carbohydrate intake, which results in a depletion of the body's carbohydrate stores. With the loss of 1 gram of carbohydrate from the body stores, there is a concomitant loss of approximately 3 g of water. With a total storage capacity of 400 to 500 g of carbohydrate, there is the potential for a water loss of 1.2 to 1.5 kg with depletion of the carbohydrate stores.[2] The ketosis resulting from these typical diets also promotes additional water loss. Thus, 1.5 to 2.5 kg (3 to 5 pounds) of weight loss per week can come from water loss associated with carbohydrate depletion and ketosis. Although the large decreases in scale weight resulting from this water loss are very rewarding on a day-to-day basis, the individual will eventually stop a particular diet when a target or goal weight is achieved. Typically, this individual will then revert to previous eating habits, and water storage will accompany the replenishment of the depleted carbohydrate stores. This initial water storage can approximate 2.0 to 2.5 kg (4 to 5 pounds) in the first 24 to 48 hours and is usually a devastating experience for the faithful dieter.

When exercise is used for weight loss or weight control purposes, there is usually a gain in lean body weight because of an increase in muscle mass, i.e., exercise-induced hypertrophy.[3] In addition, there is a substantial loss of body fat. Typically, body weight changes little, if at all, during the first 6 to 8 weeks of an exercise program, since gains in lean weight are compensating for losses in body fat.[3] This will frequently lead to frustration on the part of the individual attempting to lose weight, whose scale reads "no change" after weeks of hard work. It is important to alert those in exercise programs to this basic fact. Scale weight is not a good index of those changes in body composition that are taking place as a result of the exercise program. The tightness or looseness of clothing is probably a better index of the body composition changes.

When using exercise as a means of weight reduction and control, the total energy cost of the physical activity program is the most important consideration in program design. Activities that are continuous in nature and have a moderate-to-high rate of caloric expenditure are recommended, e.g., walking, jogging, running, cycling, swimming, and vigorous sports or games. By increasing caloric expenditure by 300 to 500 Kcal per exercise session through a properly prescribed physical activity program, it would be possible to lose a pound of fat in 7 to 12 exercise sessions, provided food intake remained constant. For most people, this would mean a moderate jog for 30 minutes per day or a brisk walk for 45 to 60 minutes. If a modest diet was also followed, weight and fat reduction would occur at an even faster rate. Reducing food intake by one buttered slice of bread or one glass of dry white wine per day (approximately 100 Kcal), combined with a 30-minute per day jogging program 3 days per week, would result in a fat weight loss of approximately 0.4 to 0.5 pound per week, or 20 to 25 pounds in a year.

The remainder of this chapter will investigate the role of exercise in weight control. First, the role of exercise in appetite regulation will be discussed. Second, studies that have investigated alterations in body composition with physical training will be reviewed. Finally, the body composition of athletic populations will be presented.

EXERCISE IN APPETITE REGULATION

A common myth that has been perpetuated for decades suggests that exercise is ineffective in weight loss programs owing to the stimulating effects of the exercise on one's appetite, i.e., the exercise will lead to a greater intake of kilocalories, negating the caloric expenditure of the exercise itself. Does exercise stimulate the appetite? The following review will be divided into those studies conducted on animals and those conducted on humans, for the data are not totally consistent.

ANIMAL STUDIES

Oscai,[4] in his review of the research literature up through 1972, concluded that exercise does tend to suppress the appetite in male animals, and the appetite suppression effect appears to be related to the intensity of the exercise. With long-duration, low-intensity exercise, animals that exercised and control animals had similar appetites. With high-intensity, short-term exercise, there was a distinct difference between the two groups, with the exercised groups consuming substantially fewer kilocalories. Katch et al.[5] investigated the effects of exercise intensity in two groups of male rats on subsequent food consumption and body weight changes. One group exercised at a considerably higher intensity, but the total caloric expenditure during exercise was equated between the two groups. The high-intensity group demonstrated a reduction in food consumption and a depression in body weight gain that exceeded that of the low-intensity group. However, both groups had depressed food consumption and rate of body weight gain compared with nonexercised control animals.

Studies using female animals have produced results that are not totally consistent with those for males as cited previously. In one of the first studies, Mayer et al.[6] investigated the role of exercise and food intake on body weight in normal rats and genetically obese mice. The results of this study are presented in Figure 4–1. Animals were exercised at each of the specified durations for a minimum of 14 days or until a steady state for weight had been achieved. The results indicated that exercise durations of 20, 40, and 60 minutes were not followed by increases in food intake over the amounts for total inactivity. In fact, a small decrease in food intake was observed at each of these exercise intervals. At durations of 2 or more hours, there was a linear increase in food intake through 6 hours, at which point the animals reached the stage of exhaustion. Body weight was reduced below control levels, i.e., physical inactivity, at each duration of exercise, with the weight stabilizing at durations of 1 to 6 hours per day.

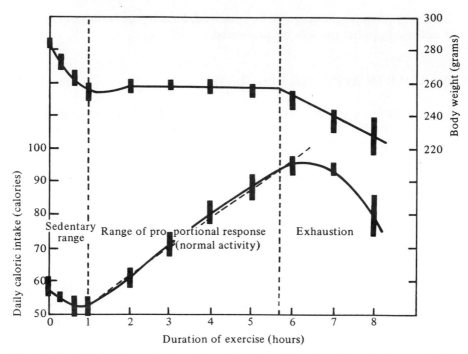

Figure 4–1. Food intake and body weight as functions of duration of exercise in normal adult rats. (From Mayer, J., et al.: Exercise, food intake and body weight in normal rats and genetically obese adult mice. Am. J. Physiol. *177:*544–548, 1954, with permission of The American Physiological Society.)

In Oscai's review,[4] several studies are cited that reported increased appetites in female animals exercised for long durations compared with sedentary controls. Oscai et at.[7] investigated the responses of both male and female rats to the same swimming program. The female rats that swam and were permitted unrestricted access to food took in an average of 75 Kcal per day compared with 61 Kcal per day for the sedentary female rats. In contrast, exercise had no effect on the voluntary intake of food in the male animals. The physiological basis for this sex-related paradox has not been elucidated.

What physiological mechanisms underlie the appetite suppression response to high-intensity exercise in animals, particularly male animals? Oscai concluded that the appetite suppression induced by exercise is possibly mediated through increased levels of catecholamines associated with the stress of exercise.[4] It is well recognized that catecholamine levels increase in direct response to exercise intensity, i.e., the higher the intensity, the greater the levels of the circulating catecholamines.[8] Thus, high-intensity exercise leading to marked increases in catecholamine levels would result in a greater suppression of appetite than would low-intensity exercise, during which catecholamine levels would only be moderately elevated. Brobek,[9] however, postulates that increased core temperature results in appetite suppression, which could also explain, at least in part, the appetite suppression effect of exercise. In addition, the increase in core temperature with exercise varies with the medium (swimming in water versus running through air) and the environmental conditions (heat, humidity, wind, and radiation). These factors must be considered when comparing studies conducted under different experimental conditions.

HUMAN STUDIES

With humans, does exercise increase or decrease the appetite, or does the appetite remain unchanged? Similarly, if the appetite is increased in response to exercise, is this increase in caloric intake equal to, greater than, or less than that which was expended directly as a result of that exercise? These are very difficult questions to answer owing to the inherent problems associated with accurately measuring both energy intake and energy expenditure. An increase or decrease in caloric intake of 100 Kcal per day above or below maintenance level would result in a 10-pound weight gain or loss, respectively, over the period of a year. To assess caloric intake to within 100 Kcal per day is extremely difficult, if not impossible, even when subjects are monitored directly and their food intake is measured very accurately with a balance scale.[10] Assessment of energy expenditure is even more difficult. Although direct calorimetry is a reasonably accurate method for measuring caloric expenditure, it is highly impractical, and more indirect techniques have been utilized. Activity diaries, mechanical activity monitors, and heart rate monitors all provide relative indices of activity, but the conversion of these indices to actual caloric expenditures is not precise.[10] Although the animal model for investigating the relationship between exercise and appetite suffers from the very basic fact that "man is not a rat"[10] and from the fact that applicability of data derived from studies on rats to humans is not well established, the human model suffers from its lack of control and precision. Thus, in reviewing the following data, these potential limitations must be recognized.

Mayer et al.[11] observed the relationship between caloric intake, body weight, and physical work in a group of 213 mill workers in West Bengal, India. The workers covered a wide range of physical activity, from sedentary to very hard work. They found that caloric intake increased with activity only within a certain zone, i.e., normal activity. With sedentary employees, the actual food intake was higher than that of the employees in the normal activity zone. For those employees in the medium–to–very heavy work zones, the caloric intake increased in proportion to the energy expenditure demands of the job. From this study and from his study on the food intake patterns of exercising rats, Mayer has concluded that when activity is reduced to below a minimum level, a corresponding decrease in food intake does not result and obesity develops.[12] This has led to the theory that a certain minimum level of physical activity is necessary before the body can precisely regulate food intake to balance energy expenditure. An appropriate analogy might be the television set in which a program can be selected by the use of both a channel selector and a fine tuner. The channel selector brings the viewer into the appropriate region, and the fine tuner allows for a precise regulation of the picture (M. Joyner, personal communication). It is possible that a certain level of physical activity is necessary before the body can exactly control food intake to match energy expenditure. Thus, a sedentary lifestyle may reduce the ability of the fine tuning device to control food intake precisely, resulting in a positive energy balance. This may amount to only a 10- to 100-Kcal, or a potato chip to a slice of buttered bread, imbalance per day, but this would produce a net yearly weight gain of from 1 to 10 pounds. Mayer et al.[6] have referred to the sedentary "nonresponsive" zone, in which a decrease in activity is *not* accompanied by a reduction in appetite and food intake. Mayer and Bullen[13] state that this has been known empirically to farmers for centuries and explains the practice of cooping up or penning up cattle, hogs, and geese for fattening.

Other studies have attempted to investigate experimentally the role of increased physical activity on appetite and food intake. Dempsey[14] studied a small group of obese and nonobese young men undergoing a program of vigorous physical exercise. Initially, overweight subjects experienced significant losses of body weight and subcutaneous and total body fat and increases in fat-free body weight and muscular mass. Daily caloric intake was unchanged over the 18-week program, when compared with a 3-week pretraining phase in which the subjects were relatively sedentary. These results could be interpreted in two ways. It would be logical to conclude that exercise had no effect on appetite; in fact, the trend was for a 100- to 200-Kcal increase in food intake, although this was not statistically significant. However, it must be remembered that the subjects were increasing their energy expenditures through 1 hour per day of vigorous exercise. Although the caloric equivalent of this exercise was not provided, walking 4 miles in 60 minutes (15 minutes per mile) or jogging 6 miles in 60 minutes (10 minutes per mile) would result in an average caloric expenditure of from 400 to 600 Kcal per day in addition to the normal caloric expenditure for 24 hours. Thus, the fact that the appetite did not increase implies a 400- to 600-Kcal deficit in intake over expenditure, provided the individual was in energy balance at the beginning of the study. The point to be made is that energy intake should not be expected to remain the same with increased caloric expenditure if caloric balance is to be maintained. It is therefore possible to interpret this study as showing a decrease in appetite even though kilocaloric intake did not change, since intake did not increase proportionally to expenditure.

Holloszy et al.[15] observed the effects of a 6-month program of endurance exercise on the serum lipids of middle-aged men. Skinner et al.[16] reported on the work capacity and anthropometric measurement changes in the same group of men. In these reports of this single study, the men who were placed on a 6-month exercise program participating in endurance calisthenics and distance running (2 to 4 miles per day) on the average of 3.3 times per week had no change in either body weight or average daily caloric intake, although there were changes in body composition, i.e., decreased body fat and increased lean weight. These results are in agreement with the study of Dempsey cited previously and could be interpreted to indicate that there was a net loss in appetite, since caloric intake did not increase with increasing caloric expenditure.

Jankowski and Foss[17] measured the postexercise changes in the 24-hour energy intake of 14 sedentary men after either a 440-yard or a 1-mile run on a treadmill. They found that the performance of these running tasks had no measurable effect on the 24-hour energy intake. This study can be criticized on the basis of the short period of the exercise bout, in which the energy expenditure would be 100 Kcal or less, and on the basis that it was an acute bout of exercise. Although the controls exerted in this study were excellent, the study would have been much more valuable if the observations would have been extended over a period of several weeks and the duration and intensity of the exercise bouts more substantive.

If exercise does act to suppress the appetite or to maintain food intake at a constant level while energy expenditure is increasing, how can this be explained physiologically? In the previous section on animal studies, Oscai[4] concluded that appetite suppression could be mediated through increases in plasma catecholamine levels. The possible influence of elevations in core temperature was also mentioned. Belbeck and Critz[18] have investigated the possibility of increased levels of a urinary anorexigenic substance with exercise as a contributing cause to appetite suppression. Stevenson et al.[19] first demonstrated this substance in 1964. Belbeck and Critz[18] found that 60 to 90 minutes after exhaustive treadmill exercise in seven healthy young men, there was a 21 per cent increase in the plasma concentration of this anorexigenic substance. The injection of this substance in amounts sufficient to cause a 50 per cent increase in its plasma concentration in rats had previously been shown to decrease food intake for 24 to 48 hours. They concluded that this substance may be responsible for the decreased appetite and food intake after exercise in humans. Unfortunately, no further studies have been conducted to determine more precisely the specific physiological mechanisms involved in appetite suppression with vigorous physical exercise.

BODY COMPOSITION ALTERATIONS WITH PHYSICAL TRAINING

To investigate those alterations in body composition that occur consequent to physical training, both the animal and the human models have been used. Although the animal model is much easier to control, the validity of drawing conclusions for humans from animal studies is still under debate.

Thus, there is a need for human research as well, recognizing the inherent limitations in exerting tight controls. The following review of the literature will be divided into two sections: animal studies and human studies. The animal studies will be reviewed briefly, with a much more comprehensive review of the human investigations.

ANIMAL STUDIES

Oscai,[4] in a general review of the role of exercise in weight control published in 1973, provides a comprehensive summary of the animal studies that had been conducted through 1972. He concluded that male animals subjected to programs of regularly performed treadmill running or swimming gain weight more slowly and have lower final body weights than comparable freely eating sedentary controls. The slower rate of weight gain was due to an increased caloric expenditure associated with the exercise and, in some cases, to a significant reduction in food intake. Female rats, in contrast, gain weight at approximately the same rate as sedentary, freely eating controls. This is due to an increase in food intake that apparently balances the increase in caloric expenditure associated with exercise.

Analysis of the body composition changes in these animals after physical training reveals that the male animals are much lighter, have considerably lower fat weights, and have lower lean body weights compared with the sedentary, freely eating controls. The female exercisers have similar body weights, greatly reduced total body fat weights, and increased lean body weights.[4]

To better understand the physiological mechanisms involved, several investigators have attempted to determine actual cellular changes consequent to physical training. Oscai and Holloszy[20] studied five groups of rats matched for weight under the following conditions: baseline group sacrificed at the beginning of the study; a freely eating, swimming group; a freely eating, sedentary group; and two paired-weight groups who were calorie-restricted to match the weight loss of the exercise group, with the protein intake of the one paired-weight group matched to the exercise group. With an initial mean weight of 706 g for all five groups, the exercising group lost 182 g over 18 weeks as a result of both an increase in caloric expenditure and a decrease in appetite. The sedentary, food-restricted animals lost an average of 182 g, and the sedentary, freely eating animals gained 118 g. The composition of the weight lost by the exercising animals was 78 per cent fat, 5 per cent protein, 1 per cent minerals, and 16 per cent water, compared with 62 per cent fat, 11 per cent protein, 1 per cent minerals, and 26 per cent water for the sedentary, food-restricted animals. Thus, exercise provided greater increases in fat loss and reduced the loss of the lean tissue.

Oscai et al.[21] divided young rats, 8 days of age, into one of three groups: swim-trained for 14 to 16 weeks; sedentary, paired-weight, with caloric

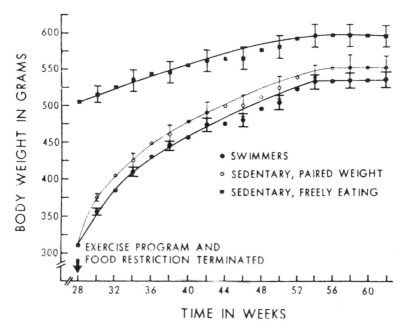

Figure 4–2. Influence of exercise and food restriction during the first 28 weeks of life on subsequent gains in body weight using male Wistar strain rats. (From Oscai, L. B., et al.: Exercise or food restriction: effect on adipose tissue cellularity. Am. J. Physiol. *227:*901–904, 1974, with permission of The American Physiological Society.)

intake regulated to match the weight gain of the exercising group; and sedentary, freely eating. At the conclusion of the study, the sedentary, freely eating rats weighed 418 g, compared with 260 g for the exercising rats and 266 g for the sedentary, paired-weight rats, with fat weights of 102 g, 26 g, and 45 g, respectively. The average caloric intake after weaning was 60 Kcal per day for the sedentary, freely eating rats, 59 Kcal per day for the exercising, freely eating rats, and 34 Kcal per day for the sedentary, paired-weight rats. Compared with the sedentary, freely eating control animals, the exercising and sedentary paired-weight animals had significantly lighter epididymal fat pads with fewer and smaller adipocytes. Compared with the food-restricted animals, the exercising animals had fewer and smaller adipocytes. They concluded that exercise in addition to food restriction early in life is effective in reducing the rate of adipocyte proliferation consequent to growth.

Oscai et al.[22] investigated the influence of both exercise and food restriction on adipose tissue cellularity in rats, starting at 5 days of age. The rats were divided into the following six groups: two groups of rats exercised by swimming 6 days per week, 360 minutes a day for 23 weeks; two groups of rats that were sedentary, but whose caloric intake was restricted to match the body weights of the exercised groups; and two groups of freely eating, sedentary rats. One group from each condition was sacrificed at the end of the 23-week exercise program, and the other group from each condition was followed through 62 weeks of age. During the final 34 weeks of the study, all three remaining groups were maintained sedentary without the opportunity to exercise and were allowed to eat freely. The body weight changes in these animals are illustrated in Figure 4–2. The average daily food intakes for the first 28 weeks were 19, 11, and 20 g for the exercising, sedentary, paired-weight, and sedentary, freely eating groups, respectively, and were 20, 19, and 20 g, respectively, from week 28 to week 62. The exercised animals, even following 34 weeks of a sedentary existence, had epididymal fat pads that were lighter and contained less fat than either of the sedentary groups. The lower fat content in the exercised group was the result of fewer adipocytes, as the cell diameters were similar among the three groups. The authors concluded that exercise in early life is effective in significantly reducing the rate of adipocyte proliferation, resulting in significantly lower body fat later in life.

Taylor et al.[23] observed the effects of fat pad removal in 54 exercised and control male Wistar rats. The animals were divided into three feeding pattern groups: freely eating, pair-fed, and pair-weight. The exercise program consisted of running on a motor-driven treadmill for a period of 16 weeks, 1 hour a day, 5 days per week. Animals had either one or both fat pads removed before starting the exercise program. Fat pad regeneration was noted in all animals. When one fat pad was removed, the regeneration was not as great per pad as after bilateral lipidectomy. Exercise further inhibited fat pad regeneration when both pads were removed. This inhibition was the result of a smaller cell diameter and cell number in the fat pads of the exercised rats.

Studies conducted on adult animals demonstrate a slightly different response to exercise training. Deb and Martin[24] investigated the effects of exercise and of food restriction on Zucker obese and lean rats. Zucker obese rats pair-fed to match their lean littermates gained more body fat on the same caloric intake, indicating greater efficiency of diet utilization. Exercise significantly reduced the fat pad weights and the body fat content of the obese rats. However, exercise had no effect on adipocyte number. Askew et al.[25] reported similar results, i.e., decreases in body weight, epididymal fat pad weight, and adipocyte size, with no change in adipocyte number, in a group of mature rats trained on a motor-driven treadmill for a period of 13 weeks. Taylor[26] also reported decreased fat cell diameter and lipid content, but no change in fat cell number after running or swimming programs in mature rats of 4 months' duration.

From the preceding studies, a fairly consistent pattern is apparent. In young, growing animals, physical training slows the rate of increase in body weight, total fat weight, and fat cell number. At maturity, the exercised animal has a lower body weight, lower total fat weight, and fewer adipocytes. The reduced number of adipocytes is the result of a decreased rate of proliferation, not a decrease in existing fat cell number. This latter point is an important one, for there appears to be no way, other than surgical removal, to decrease the number of adipocytes. When exercise is started later in life, after the attainment of maturity, there is a subsequent reduction or decreased rate of increase in total body weight, in total fat weight, and in adipocyte cell size, with no change in cell number. One additional factor, which is of considerable importance, concerns the alterations in lean tissue with weight loss. When weight is lost solely through caloric restriction, considerable losses in lean tissue of from 35 to 45 per cent of the total weight lost are common.[4] With exercise, or a combination of caloric restriction and exercise, there is a sparing of lean tissue and substantially greater losses in body fat.[20] Oscai[4] attributes the above alterations to the lipid-mobilizing effect of exercise, an effect that he feels is mediated, in part, by increased activity of the sympathetic nervous system. He states that the fat-mobilizing effect, which persists for a considerable time after the cessation of exercise, could play a role in the conservation of lean tissue by making available to the muscle and organ cells more of the energy stored as fat. It is clear that exercise training plays an important role in controlling the adipose tissue mass in animals both early in life and after attaining full maturity.

NORMAL HUMAN POPULATIONS

A number of studies have investigated body composition alterations with physical training. It would not be practical, nor serve any purpose, to review each of these studies. Thus, the following review includes only those studies that have made a unique contribution to this body of knowledge. There also appears to be a trend emerging from the existing literature that should be acknowledged. The response to physical training programs appears to be a function of the degree of obesity exhibited by the subjects at the start of the study. This is an inverse relationship, with those who are most obese receiving the least benefits and those who are only moderately obese receiving the greatest benefits.

Parizkova et al.[27] studied 18 obese boys and 15 obese girls with a mean age of 12.7 years, before and after 7 weeks of reducing treatment in a summer camp where they performed considerable physical activity and received a diet of 1,700 Kcal per day. The girls lost 12.8 per cent of their initial body weight compared with 11.1 per cent loss for the boys. The absolute lean body mass did not change; however, there were major increases in relative lean body mass and decreases in relative body fat. Parizkova and Poupa[28] conducted a longitudinal study of seven female gymnasts on the Czechoslovakian National Team and an additional group of female gymnasts attending a sports school for 3 to 4 years. Their observations were carried out over a period of several years. They found that there was a direct correlation between the intensity of training and alterations in body composition. With intense training, body density would increase, reflecting a loss in relative body fat, and skinfold thicknesses would decrease. During peri-

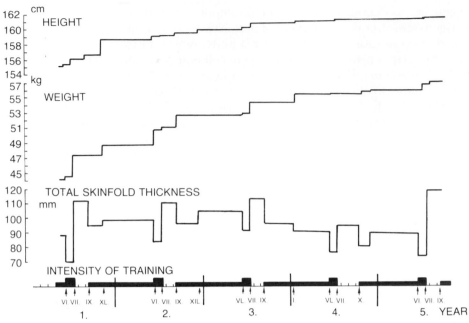

Figure 4–3. Changes in height, weight, and skinfold thickness in girl gymnasts during periods of various intensity of training. (From Parizkova, J.: Body composition and exercise during growth and development. *In* Rarick, G. L. [ed.]: Physical Activity Human Growth and Development. New York, Academic Press, 1973, p. 109, with permission.)

ods of rest or reduced activity, these changes were reversed. Interestingly, the caloric intake was highest during intense training when body fat levels were low and energy expenditure high and was lowest during rest periods when body fat levels were elevated. Parizkova's[29] study of 11 female gymnasts over a period of 5 years confirms these findings (Fig. 4–3).

Sprynarova and Parizkova[30] observed seven obese boys before and after a 7-week regimen of dietary restriction and regular exercise. All subjects experienced marked increases in body density and relative lean body weight and decreases in total body weight (mean loss of 6.6 kg, or 14.5 pounds) and in relative body fat. Wells et al.[31] found that after 4 weeks of intensive physical training, adolescent girls showed an increase in specific gravity of approximately 1.053 to 1.058, a decrease in the sum of 10 skinfolds from approximately 102 mm to 85 mm, and a slight increase in body weight of approximately 1.0 kg. These data were estimated from the original data that was presented in figure format. These changes reflect an increase in lean tissue and a decrease in the total body fat content.

Parizkova[32] studied a group of 143 boys from the age of 11 through 18 years. The group was divided into three subgroups on the basis of their habitual levels of activity. Relative lean body mass increased linearly with age, and relative body fat decreased linearly with age, with the more active groups exhibiting the more favorable body compositions. At each age, the most active group had lower absolute body fat and higher absolute lean body mass. Christakis et al.[33] studied the effect of a combined nutrition education and physical fitness program on the course of obesity in 55 randomly selected obese freshmen high school students. A control group of 35 obese boys was used for comparison. After an 18-month period of observation, the experimental group gained an average of 5.8 pounds and the control group, 13.5 pounds. With respect to percentage of overweight, there was a major shift toward normal weight in the experimental group compared with the control group.

Numerous studies have been conducted on the adult population. In one of the first studies to observe body composition changes with physical training, Thompson et al.[34] evaluated body weights and skinfold thicknesses on basketball and hockey players before and after a season of play in their respective sports. Although weight remained relatively stable, there were rather major decreases in subcutaneous skinfold fat measurements. In a similar study of football players, Thompson[35] reported no change in body weight, substantial decreases in skinfold thicknesses, and significant increases in estimated body density, indicating an overall decrease in total body fat and an increase in lean body weight.

Skinner et al.[16] used densitometry to determine longitudinal changes in body composition with training in a group of men who exercised a minimum of three times per week, approximately 40 minutes per session for a period of 6 months. Specific gravity increased from 1.058 to 1.063, and the sum of six skinfolds decreased from 107.7 to 99.3 mm. Oscai and Williams[36] studied five middle-aged men who ran three times per week, a minimum of 30 minutes per session for a total of 16 weeks. Compared with a group of five sedentary controls, the experimental group lost 4.5 kg of body weight, 3.6 kg of body fat, and 0.9 kg of lean body weight, as estimated from changes in skinfold thickness. Carter and Phillips[37] followed 13 subjects, 7 experimentals and 6 controls, for a 3-year period, with body composition evaluations occurring every 6 months. The experimental subjects participated in 1-hour sessions of calisthenics and jogging 3 days per week, with jogging mileage progressing from 1.5 to 7.5 miles per week. The experimental group made significant decreases in body weight, percentage of fat, skinfolds, girths, and the somatotype component of mesomorphy, while significantly increasing specific gravity, as estimated from underwater weighing. The majority of the change in each of these variables occurred during the first year of the program.

Pollock et al.[38] randomly assigned 19 middle-aged men to an exercise regimen of either 2 days per week or 4 days per week, with an additional 8 subjects serving as sedentary controls. The experimental subjects performed approximately 30 minutes of jog-run training per day for either 2 or 4 days per week, for a total of 20 weeks. The group training 2 days per week resulted in no significant changes in body composition, whereas the group that trained 4 days per week lost total body weight (79.7 to 76.8 kg), sum of six skinfold thicknesses (131.4 to 107.8 mm), and relative body fat estimated from skinfold thicknesses (19.6 to 18.6 per cent). Katch et al.[39] studied 10 members of the women's tennis team and 5 members of the women's swimming team at the University of California, Santa Barbara, before and after a season of competition. They found no significant alterations in body composition over 16 weeks of sports training.

Wilmore et al.[40] investigated body composition alterations in 55 men between the ages of 17 and 59 years after a 3-day per week, 10-week program of jogging. Small but significant decreases were found in total body weight, relative body fat, and in four of seven skinfold measurements, and a significant increase was found in body density. Boileau et al.[41] studied 23 college men who participated in a walking and running exercise program 60 minutes per day 5 days per week for 9 weeks. From the initial evaluations, 8 subjects were classified as obese (29 to 46 per cent fat) and the remaining 15 as normal (10 to 21 per cent fat). Total weight decreased by 3.2 kg in the obese and 1.0 kg in the normal groups, whereas fat-free, or lean weight increased by 2.7 and 1.4 kg, respectively. Relative fat decreased by 3.9 per cent in the obese and 3.0 per cent in the normal groups. In this study, as well as in the study of Wilmore et al.,[40] the actual fat loss was more than could be accounted for by the energy equivalent of the actual exercise performed.

Johnson et al.[42] followed 32 college women who participated in a 10-week cycle ergometer endurance training program 30 minutes per day, 5 days per week. Although body weight remained unchanged, four skinfold thicknesses were reduced substantially, and the relative body fat estimated from skinfolds decreased from an initial value of 24.9 per cent to 22.8 per cent. Mean caloric intake decreased from 1,751 Kcal per day to 1,584 Kcal per day from the beginning to the end of the exercise program. Pollock et al.[43] investigated the effects of a 20-week walking program, 40 minutes per day, 4 days per week, on the body composition of middle-aged men. Reductions were found in total body weight (−1.3 kg) and in relative body fat (−1.1 per cent). In a subsequent study, Pollock et al.[44] determined the physiological responses to training 2 days per week at different intensities, 45 minutes per day for 20 weeks. The group training at 90 per cent of maximum heart rate demonstrated small but significant decreases in the sum of seven skinfolds and in relative fat estimated from skinfolds. The group training at 80 per cent of maximum heart rate exhibited no change in body composition. In a third study by Pollock et al.,[45] the effects of mode of training on cardiovascular function and body composition were determined. Sedentary middle-aged men were assigned to one of four groups: running, walking, cycling, or control. All training groups exercised for 30 minutes per day 3 days per week for 20 weeks at 85 to 90 percent of maximal heart rate. The experimental groups had significant decreases in body weight, skinfold fat, and relative body fat estimated from skinfolds. The studies of Pollock et al. are summarized in Figures 4-4 to 4-6.

Kollias et al.[46] conducted a 15-week weight reduction study, with 19 women assigned to a volitional dieting, a volitional exercising, or a com-

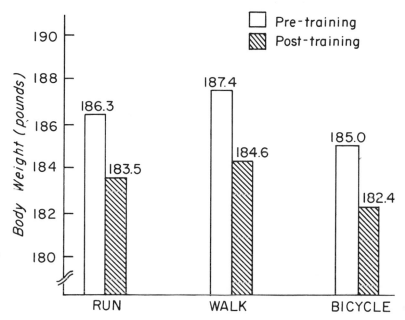

Effect of Mode of Training on Body Weight
Data from Pollock, M.L., Department of Physical Education,
Wake Forest University.

Figure 4–4. Alterations in body weight consequent to a 20-week training program of running, walking, or bicycling. (From Pollock, M. L., et al.: Effects of mode of training on cardiovascular functions and body composition of adult men. Med. Sci. Sports Exer. 7:139–145, 1975, with permission.)

bined dieting and exercising group. Body weight decreased by 5.3, 5.7, and 3.4 kg, and relative body fat decreased by 2.2, 2.5, and 1.7 per cent in the diet, exercise, and combined groups, respectively. Girandola and Katch[47] studied the effects of 9 weeks of physical training on aerobic capacity and body composition of college men. The exercise program consisted of calisthenics, running, and weight lifting, 2 days per week, in a circuit training format. Relative body fat decreased by 1.0 per cent, but total and lean body weights remained unchanged.

Getchell and Moore[48] studied the adaptations of middle-aged men and women to a 10-week physical training program, consisting of 30 minutes of walking and jogging 3 to 4 days per week. Both groups lost a negligible amount of body weight, –0.7 and –0.8 kg for men and women, respectively. However, the sum of six skinfolds decreased substantially, from a mean value of 144.6 to 115.4 mm in women and from 148.8 to 110.6 mm in men. These changes suggest that there were losses of total body fat and gains in lean body weight. Girandola[49] investigated the effects of high- and low-intensity exercise training on body composition changes in college women. Twenty women participated in a 10-week program three times per week,

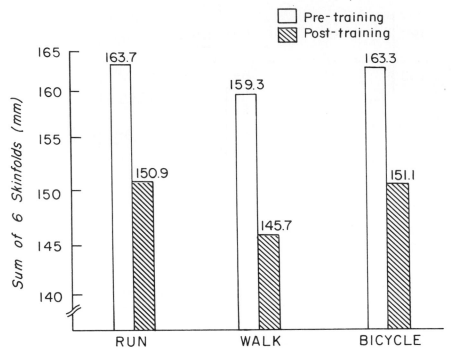

Effect of Mode of Training on the Sum of 6 Skinfold
Fat Measures.
Data from Pollock, M.L. and others, Department of
Physical Education, Wake Forest University.

Figure 4–5. Alterations in skinfold fat consequent to a 20-week training program of running, walking, or bicycling. (From Pollock, M. L., et al.: Effects of mode of training on cardiovascular functions and body composition of adult men. Med. Sci. Sports Exer. 7:139–145, 1975, with permission.)

which consisted of riding a cycle ergometer at either 840 and 420 kpm/ min for varying intervals of time. Body weight did not change over the course of the study; however, there was an increase in body density and a decrease in relative body fat in the low-intensity group (420 kpm/min). The high-intensity group exhibited no significant changes in body composition.

Wilmore et al.[50] observed changes in body composition after 20 weeks of bicycle, tennis, or jogging training. The subjects exercised for 30 minutes per day, 3 days per week at a prescribed training heart rate. The only alteration noted in body composition was an increase in the lean weight of members of the bicycle group. Although those in the jogging and bicycling group demonstrated rather major decreases in total body weight and relative and absolute body fat, these decreases were not statistically significant owing to similar unexplained changes in the control group.

EFFECTS OF FREQUENCY OF TRAINING
ON PERCENT BODY FAT

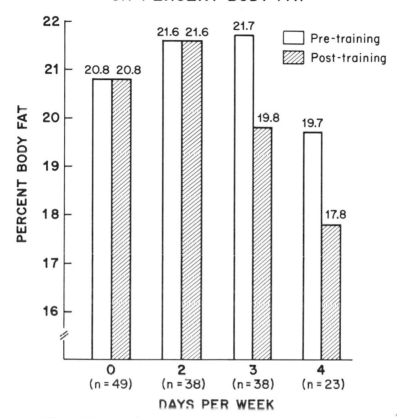

Figure 4–6. Effects of frequency of cardiorespiratory endurance training on percentage of body fat. (Data from Pollock, M. L., et al.: Frequency of training as a determinant for improvement in cardiovascular function and body composition of middle-aged men. Arch. Phys. Med. Rehab. 56:141 145, 1975, with permission.)

Most of the studies cited thus far have involved an aerobic type of exercise. There have been several studies that have evaluated the effects of weight training, in either a standard or a circuit format, on alterations in body composition. Fahey and Brown[51] investigated changes in strength, body composition, and endurance of college men performing a weight-training program 3 times per week for 9 weeks under placebo or steroid treatment. Body weight and lean body weight increased in both groups, whereas relative body fat decreased. Misner et al.[52] assigned 24 adult men to a weight-training, jogging, or control group, with the groups exercising 30 minutes per day, 3 days per week for 8 weeks. After the training period, the weight-training group gained body weight (1.0 kg) and fat-free, or lean body weight (3.1 kg) while losing absolute (–2.3 kg) and relative (–2.9 per cent) body fat. The jogging group lost body weight (–0.8 kg) and absolute (–2.3 kg) and relative (–2.5 per cent) body fat.

Wilmore conducted a 10-week weight-training program, 2 days per week for 40 minutes per day, involving 47 women and 26 men.[53] Neither group changed total body weight, but both groups decreased absolute body fat by 1.1 and 0.9 kg and relative body fat by 1.9 and 1.3 per cent and increased lean body weight by 1.1 and 1.2 kg in the women and men, respectively. Mayhew and Gross[54] conducted a similar study on 17 college women and reported nearly identical results. Brown and Wilmore[55] observed body composition changes in seven nationally ranked track and field throwing event athletes, 16 to 23 years of age, after 6 months of maximal resistance training for 3 days a week, 60 to 90 minutes per day. Body weight decreased slightly, as did relative and absolute body fat, and lean body weight increased.

Circuit weight training has also been shown to alter body composition. Wilmore et al.[56] circuit weight trained men and women subjects 3 days per week, approximately 30 minutes per day, for a period of 10 weeks. Although increases were found in lean body weight of 1.7 and 1.3 kg for men and women, respectively, there were no significant changes in body weight, and only the women exhibited a significant decrease in relative body fat (–1.8 per cent). Gettman and Pollock[57] have recently summarized the circuit weight training literature and found either small or no changes in body weight, increases in lean body weight, and decreases in relative body fat.

In a relatively recent series of studies, O'Hara et al.[58–61] have observed rather remarkable losses in fat mass and gains in lean mass after exercise in the cold. In one study,[58] 55 soldiers were observed over a vigorous 10-day sledding patrol in the Canadian arctic and subarctic. The authors claimed a fat loss of 3.9 kg and a gain in lean body weight of 3.9 kg in this relatively short exposure. In the second study,[59] 10 men spent 1 week in a cold climatic facility performing simulated arctic military exercises. The subjects lost an average of 2.6 kg of body weight and sustained a reduction in mean skinfold thickness of 2.6 mm. Body fat decreased by 2.35 kg, and lean body weight decreased by 0.25 kg. In the third study,[60] six obese men, 25 to 46 years of age, exercised vigorously in a cold chamber for 3.5 hours on 10 consecutive days. Lean body weight increased slightly, fat weight decreased by 3.1 kg, and body weight decreased by a mean of 3.2 kg. In their fourth study, O'Hara et al.[61] reported similar results for a group of 15 middle-aged, moderately obese men who exercised 2.5 hours per day for 2 weeks. Cold exposure and exercise led to reductions in skinfold thicknesses and body fat and to an increase in lean body weight. They felt that the observed fat loss in the cold can be explained by new protein synthesis, ketosis, and a small energy deficit. These studies certainly indicate a new area of research that could have major implications for the treatment of obesity.

To summarize this section, rather substantial alterations occur in body composition consequent to exercise training. Although body weight will usually decrease over long periods of time, i.e., 3 months or longer, it is not unusual for body weight to change very little during the initial few months of training. This lack of substantial change in the early phases on an exercise program is primarily the result of alterations in body composition, i.e., losses in body fat accompanied by similar gains in lean body weight. As the exercise program is extended beyond 3 months, lean weight changes very little, and decreases in body weight now start to reflect actual changes in body fat. The exercise program should be of an aerobic nature, although substantial alterations in body composition can occur with either traditional or circuit strength training. Pollock et al.[62] have established that frequency of training is important relative to body composition alterations; 3 and 4 day per week regimens provide significant changes, whereas no changes have been found with 2 day per week regimens. There may, in fact, be a threshold for the minimum number of kilocalories expended per exercise session or per week, in addition to a minimum duration and intensity, in order to achieve significant alterations in lean and fat weight.

OBESE AND LEAN POPULATIONS

The final part of this chapter is reserved for a review of those studies that have been conducted on obese or extremely lean populations. These studies were separated from the others, as there does appear to be a somewhat different response to physical training in these two subgroups. Moody et al.[63] placed 11 overweight college women on a physical activity program for 8 weeks, expending approximately 500 Kcal per day. Total body weight decreased by an average of 2.4 kg, and the skinfold thickness decreased by an average of 7.5 mm when comparing the mean of each 10 sites. Relative body fat, estimated from skinfolds, decreased from 38.6 to 28.5 per cent; fat weight decreased by 5.3 kg; and lean body weight increased by 2.9 kg. Moody et al.[64] measured body composition changes in 40 normal and obese high school girls after participation in a 15- or 29-week physical activity program of walking, jogging, and running 4 days per week, covering up to 3 to 3.5 miles per day. Total weight decreased by 1.15 kg, fat weight decreased by 2.66 kg, and relative body fat decreased by 3.1 per cent in the obese group after 29 weeks of activity. Kollias et al.[65] reported similar results for a group of eight obese college students after 9 weeks of physical conditioning for 5 days per week. Weight decreased by 3.2 kg, and relative body fat decreased from 38.5 to 34.6 per cent.

Gwinup[66] placed 11 obese women on a progressively increasing program of walking each day for 1 year or longer, with no dietary restriction imposed. No weight loss occurred until walking exceeded 30 minutes per day. Generally, the weight loss paralleled the length of time spent walking. Weight loss varied from 10 to 38 pounds, with an average of 22 pounds. The rate of weight loss seldom exceeded 0.5 pound per week. There was also a striking decrease in skinfold thickness, which could have indicated an even larger fat loss and a possible increase in lean body weight. Lewis et al.[67] evaluated the effects of physical activity on weight reduction in obese middle-aged women. They followed 22 obese women, ages 30 to 52 years, through a 17-week exercise program consisting of jog-walking 2.5 miles and 1 hour of calisthenics per week. Caloric restriction was also allowed on an individual basis and was felt to account for approximately 60 per cent of the total mean energy deficit. Relative body fat decreased by 5 per cent, absolute body fat decreased by 5.4 kg, and total body weight decreased by 4.2 kg.

Leon et al.[68] studied the effects of a vigorous walking program on the body composition of six sedentary obese men, ages 19 to 31 years. After 16 weeks of vigorous walking for 90 minutes a day 5 days per week on a treadmill at up to 3.2 mph on a 10 per cent grade, i.e., approximately 1,100 Kcal per session, lean body weight increased 0.2 kg, fat weight decreased 5.9 kg, and percentage of body fat decreased from 23.3 to 17.4 per cent. Monitored food intake initially increased and then progressively decreased below pretraining levels.

Franklin et al.[69] studied 36 sedentary women who participated in a 12-week physical conditioning program consisting of jogging 15 to 25 minutes per day for 4 days a week. Of the total group, 23 were classified as obese and 13 as normal. Although caloric intake remained unaltered throughout the training program, the obese subjects lost body weight and fat weight, whereas lean body weight was not significantly altered. Fifteen of the obese subjects were re-evaluated 18 months after termination of the training program and were found to have returned to their pretraining values.

Krotkiewski et al.[70] observed the effects of long-term physical training on adipose tissue cellularity and body composition in patients with either hypertrophic or hyperplastic obesity. The patients were trained as hard as possible for 45 minutes per session, 3 times per week, for a period of 6 months. Hypertrophic patients reduced body fat 6 kg after 3 months, which was the result of a decreased fat cell weight, as fat cell number was unchanged. In hyperplastic patients, there was no change in body fat. Thus, the form of obesity does appear to have an influence on the subsequent results from physical training programs. In a second study, Krotkiewski et al.[71] trained 27 women with varying degrees of obesity for a period of 6 months. Again, body fat changes were positively correlated with the number of fat cells in adipose tissue. Obese women with fewer fat cells decreased in weight during training, whereas women with severe obesity and an increased number of fat cells even gained weight. Warwick and Garrow[72] have found similar results with three obese women studied for periods of 12 to 13 weeks. Adding 2 hours per day of cycle ergometer exercise did not change the rate of weight loss in these women, who were on an 800-Kcal reducing diet. Judging from their weights, these women were most probably obese as a result of hypercellularity.

Few studies have been conducted on the body composition changes of the extremely lean or underweight individual. Dempsey[14] reported substantial gains in total weight, fat weight, and lean weight after an 18-week exercise program in one of his subjects who had an initial relative body fat of only 3 per cent. Wilmore[73] placed seven women, classified as being chronically underweight, on a 15-week exercise program consisting of walking-jogging for 30 minutes a day 5 days per week. Body weight and lean body weight increased slightly, and absolute and relative fat decreased slightly.

SPOT REDUCTION

Many individuals undertake an exercise program in an attempt to reduce fat in certain areas of the body, a practice that has been referred to as spot reduction. Many individuals, including athletes, believe that by exercising a specific area, the fat in that area will be selectively utilized, thus reducing the locally stored fat. Recent studies have shown the concept of spot reduction to be a myth, and they have revealed that exercise, even when localized, draws from all of the fat stores of the body, not just from the local deposits. A study by Gwinup et al.[74] demonstrated that the dominant arm of professional tennis players had greater muscular development than the nondominant arm because of the differences in activity levels of the two arms. However, no differences were found between the arms in localized fat stores, as assessed by multiple skinfold determinations. This study confirmed, in a rather interesting manner, previous studies that had concluded that spot reduction is a myth, not a reality.

DIET IN COMBINATION WITH EXERCISE

In this chapter, an attempt has been made to review selected studies that have investigated alterations in body composition with physical training. In all but one of the studies reviewed, diet was not manipulated as an experimental variable. In some studies, diet was monitored simply to observe spontaneous changes with training, but in most studies, diet was assumed to remain constant. Recognizing the important interaction between diet and exercise, Zuti and Golding[75] designed a study to investigate changes in body composition with diet, exercise, and a combination of diet and exercise. A caloric deficit of 500 Kcal per day was maintained by each of three groups of adult women during a 16-week period of weight loss. The diet group simply reduced their daily caloric intake by 500 Kcal. The exercise group increased their energy expenditure by 500 Kcal per day, exercising 5 days per week. The combination group reduced their caloric intake by 250 Kcal per day and increased their caloric expenditure by 250 Kcal per day. The results of this study are illustrated in Figure 4–7. Although all three groups lost the same amount of weight over 16 weeks, there was a substantial difference in the alterations in body composition. The exercise group and the exercise and diet group both increased their lean body weights, whereas the diet group lost lean body weight. In addition, the two exercise groups both lost substantially more body fat. These findings have particular

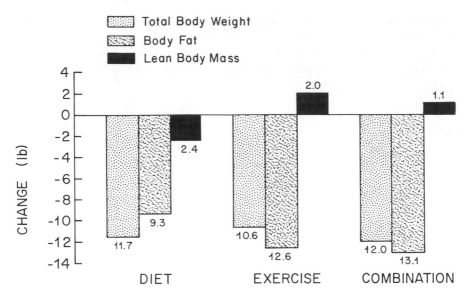

EFFECT OF DIET (n=8), EXERCISE (n=9), AND COMBINATION
OF DIET AND EXERCISE (n=8) ON LOSS OF BODY WEIGHT,
FAT, AND LEAN TISSUE

Data from Zuti and Golding

Figure 4–7. Changes in body weight, body fat, and lean body weight for diet, exercise, and combination groups. (From Zuti, W. B., and Golding, L. A.: Comparing diet and exercise as weight reduction tools. Phys. Sportsmed. *4:*49–53, 1976. Reproduced by permission of *The Physician and Sportsmedicine,* McGraw-Hill Publication.)

relevance for those individuals who are on a weight-reducing regimen with dietary intervention. Exercise does appear to protect the lean tissue, particularly when moderate dietary restriction is imposed upon the individual.

BODY COMPOSITION OF ATHLETIC POPULATIONS

Recent advances in sports physiology have led to an interest in the development of physiological profiles to describe the qualities and characteristics of elite athletes in their various sports. These profiles have considerable application in developing a better understanding of the sport and in providing data on elite athletes against which data from aspiring athletes can be compared. With respect to understanding the sport better, the profile of the elite athlete provides insights into those areas of training that should be emphasized and those areas that would need little, if any, attention.

With respect to body composition, those profiles reflect both the levels of training that are necessary for the sport and the genetic endowment of the athlete who finds success in that sport. Height, weight, and relative body fat for athletes in various sports are presented in Table 4–1. From this table,

TABLE 4–1. BODY COMPOSITION VALUES IN MALE AND FEMALE ATHLETES*

ATHLETIC GROUP OR SPORT	SEX	AGE (YR)	HEIGHT (CM)	WEIGHT (KG)	RELATIVE FAT (%)	REFERENCE
Baseball	male	20.8	182.7	83.3	14.2	Novak et al., 1968[76]
	male	—	—	—	11.8	Forsyth and Sinning, 1973[77]
Basketball	male	27.4	183.1	88.0	12.6	Wilmore, unpublished
	female	19.1	169.1	62.6	20.8	Sinning, 1973[78]
	female	19.4	167.0	63.9	26.9	Conger and Macnab, 1967[79]
Centers	male	27.7	214.0	109.2	7.1	Parr et al., 1978[80]
Forwards	male	25.3	200.6	96.9	9.0	Parr et al., 1978[80]
Guards	male	25.2	188.0	83.6	10.6	Parr et al., 1978[80]
Canoeing	male	23.7	182.0	79.6	12.4	Rusko et al., 1978[81]
Football	male	20.3	184.9	95.4	13.8	Novak et al., 1968[76]
	male	—	—	—	13.9	Forsyth and Sinning, 1973[77]
Defensive backs	male	17–23	178.3	77.3	11.5	Wickkiser and Kelly, 1975[82]
	male	24.5	182.5	84.8	9.6	Wilmore et al., 1976[83]
Offensive backs	male	17–23	179.7	79.8	12.4	Wickkiser and Kelly, 1975[82]
	male	24.7	183.8	90.7	9.4	Wilmore et al., 1976[83]
Linebackers	male	17–23	180.1	87.2	13.4	Wickkiser and Kelly, 1975[82]
	male	24.2	188.5	102.2	14.0	Wilmore et al., 1976[83]
Offensive linemen	male	17–23	186.0	99.2	19.1	Wickkiser and Kelly, 1975[82]
	male	24.7	193.0	112.6	15.6	Wilmore et al., 1976[83]
Defensive linemen	male	17–23	186.6	97.8	18.5	Wickkiser and Kelly, 1975[82]
	male	25.7	192.4	117.1	18.2	Wilmore et al., 1976[83]
Quarterbacks, kickers	male	24.1	185.0	90.1	14.4	Wilmore et al., 1976[83]
Gymnastics	male	20.3	178.5	69.2	4.6	Novak et al., 1968[76]
	female	19.4	163.0	57.9	23.8	Conger and Macnab, 1967[79]
	female	20.0	158.5	51.5	15.5	Sinning and Lindberg, 1972[84]
	female	14.0	—	—	17.0	Parízkova, 1973[85]
	female	23.0	—	—	11.0	Parízkova, 1973[85]
	female	23.0	—	—	9.6	Parízkova and Poupa, 1963[28]
Ice hockey	male	26.3	180.3	86.7	15.1	Wilmore, unpublished
	male	22.5	179.0	77.3	13.0	Rusko et al., 1978[81]
Jockeys	male	30.9	158.2	50.3	14.1	Wilmore, unpublished

TABLE 4-1. BODY COMPOSITION VALUES IN MALE AND FEMALE ATHLETES* (Continued)

ATHLETIC GROUP OR SPORT	SEX	AGE (YR)	HEIGHT (CM)	WEIGHT (KG)	RELATIVE FAT (%)	REFERENCE
Orienteering	male	31.2	—	72.2	16.3	Knowlton et al., 1980[86]
	female	29.0	—	58.1	18.7	Knowlton et al., 1980[86]
Pentathlon	female	21.5	175.4	65.4	11.0	Krahenbuhl et al., 1979[87]
Racketball	male	25.0	181.7	80.3	8.1	Pipes, 1978[88]
Rowing						
Heavyweight	male	23.0	192.0	88.0	11.0	Hagerman et al., 1979[89]
	male	21.0	186.0	71.0	8.5	Hagerman et al., 1979[89]
Lightweight	female	23.0	173.0	68.0	14.0	Hagerman et al., 1979[89]
	male†	25.9	176.6	74.8	7.4	Sprynarova and Parizkova, 1971[90]
Skiing						
Alpine	male	21.2	176.0	70.1	14.1	Rusko et al., 1978[81]
	male	21.8	177.8	75.5	10.2	Haymes and Dickinson, 1980[91]
	female	19.5	165.1	58.8	20.6	Haymes and Dickinson, 1980[91]
Cross-country	male	21.2	176.0	66.6	12.5	Niinimaa et al., 1978[92]
	male	25.6	174.0	69.3	10.2	Rusko et al., 1978[81]
	male	22.7	176.2	73.2	7.9	Haymes and Dickinson, 1980[91]
	female	24.3	163.0	59.1	21.8	Rusko et al., 1978[81]
	female	20.2	163.4	55.9	15.7	Haymes and Dickinson, 1980[91]
Nordic combination	male	22.9	176.0	70.4	11.2	Rusko et al., 1978[81]
	male	21.7	181.7	70.4	8.9	Haymes and Dickinson, 1980[91]
Skijumping	male	22.2	174.0	69.9	14.3	Rusko et al., 1978[81]
Soccer	male	26.0	175.0	75.5	9.6	Raven et al., 1976[93]
Speed skating	male	21.0	181.0	76.5	11.4	Rusko et al., 1978[81]
Swimming	male†	21.8	182.3	79.1	8.5	Sprynarova and Parizkova, 1971[90]
	male†	20.6	182.9	78.9	5.0	Novak et al., 1968[76]
	female†	19.4	168.0	63.8	26.3	Conger and Macnab, 1968[79]
Sprint	female	—	165.1	57.1	14.6	Wilmore et al., 1977[94]
Middle distance	female	—	166.6	66.8	24.1	Wilmore et al., 1977[94]
Distance	female	—	166.3	60.9	17.1	Wilmore et al., 1977[94]
Tennis	male	—	—	—	15.2	Forsyth and Sinning, 1973[77]
	male	42.0	179.6	77.1	16.3	Vodak et al., 1980[95]
	female	39.0	165.3	55.7	20.3	Vodak et al., 1980[95]
Track and field	male†	21.3	180.6	71.6	3.7	Novak et al., 1968[76]

Group	Sex					Reference
Runners						
Distance	male†	—	—	—	8.8	Forsyth and Sinning, 1973[77]
	male	22.5	177.4	64.5	6.3	Sprynarova and Parizkova, 1971[90]
	male	26.1	175.7	64.2	7.5	Costill et al., 1970[96]
	male	26.2	177.0	66.2	8.4	Rusko et al., 1978[81]
	male	40–49	180.7	71.6	11.2	Pollock et al., 1974[97]
	male	55.3	174.5	63.4	18.0	Barnard et al., 1974[98]
	male	50–59	174.7	67.2	10.9	Pollock et al., 1974[97]
	male	60–69	175.7	67.1	11.3	Pollock et al., 1974[97]
	male	70–75	175.6	66.8	13.6	Pollock et al., 1974[97]
	male	47.2	176.5	70.7	13.2	Lewis et al., 1975[99]
	female	19.9	161.3	52.9	19.2	Malina et al., 1971[100]
	female	32.4	159.4	57.2	15.2	Wilmore and Brown, 1974[101]
Middle distance	male	24.6	179.0	72.3	12.4	Rusko et al., 1978[81]
Sprint	female	20.1	164.9	56.7	19.3	Malina et al., 1971[100]
	male	46.5	177.0	74.1	16.5	Barnard et al., 1979[98]
Discus	male	28.3	186.1	104.7	16.4	Fahey et al., 1975[102]
	male	26.4	190.8	110.5	16.3	Wilmore, unpublished
Jumpers and hurdlers	female	21.1	168.1	71.0	25.0	Malina et al., 1971[100]
	female	20.3	165.9	59.0	20.7	Malina et al., 1971[100]
Shot put	male	27.0	188.2	112.5	16.5	Fahey et al., 1975[102]
	male	22.0	191.6	126.2	19.6	Behnke and Wilmore, 1974[3]
	female	21.5	167.6	78.1	28.0	Malina et al., 1971[100]
Volleyball	female	19.4	166.0	59.8	25.3	Conger and Macnab, 1968[79]
	female	19.9	172.2	64.1	21.3	Kovaleski et al., 1980[103]
Weight lifting	male	24.9	166.4	77.2	9.8	Sprynarova and Parizkova, 1971[90]
Power	male	26.3	176.1	92.0	15.6	Fahey et al., 1975[102]
Olympic	male	25.3	177.1	88.2	12.2	Fahey et al., 1975[102]
Body builders	male	29.0	172.4	83.1	8.4	Fahey et al., 1975[102]
	male	27.6	178.8	88.1	8.3	Pipes, 1979[104]
Wrestling	male	26.0	177.8	81.8	9.8	Fahey et al., 1975[102]
	male	27.0	176.0	75.7	10.7	Gale and Flynn, 1974[105]
	male	22.0	—	—	5.0	Parizkova, 1973[85]
	male	23.0	—	79.3	14.3	Taylor et al., 1979[106]
	male	19.6	174.6	74.8	8.8	Sinning, 1974[107]
	male	15–18	172.3	66.3	6.9	Katch and Michael, 1971[108]
	male	20.6	174.8	67.3	4.0	Stine et al., 1979[109]

* Adapted from Wilmore, J. H. et al: Body physique and composition of the female distance runner. Ann. N.Y. Acad. Sci. 301: 764–776, 1977.
† Specific events were not specified.

it is apparent that the female athlete is typically fatter than her male counterpart and that athletes who are involved in endurance activities or who must control their weight to meet a certain competitive weight classification have very low relative body fats. It is generally felt that a low relative body fat is desirable for successful competition in almost any sport. There is a high negative correlation between percentage of body fat and performance in those activities in which the body mass must be moved through space, either vertically, as in jumping, or horizontally, as in running.[83]

Figure 4–8 illustrates the relative body fat values for a number of national and international class track and field female athletes. This figure illustrates several very important points. First, although not obvious from the figure, the better runners generally had low relative body fat values, usually below 12 per cent body fat. However, one of the best runners, who held most of the American middle-distance records, had over 17 per cent body fat. She was training very intensely, with a great volume of both high-intensity training and long-distance running. It is unlikely that this athlete could have reduced her relative body fat to levels below 12 per cent without having a negative influence on her subsequent performance. This points to the importance of treating each athlete as an individual and not as a member of a group in which all athletes in the same sport, or even within an event, have to achieve the same level of body fat. It is appropriate to establish guidelines for a sport, but consideration must be given to the exceptions.

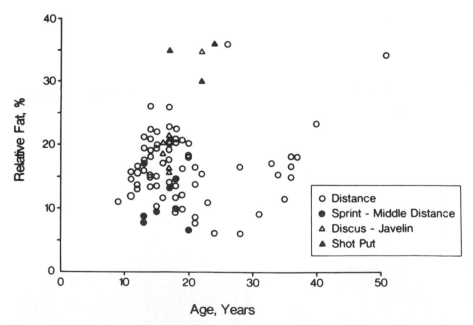

Figure 4–8. Relative body fat values for female track and field athletes. (From Wilmore, J. H., Brown, C. H., and Davis, J. A.: Body physique and composition of the female distance runner. Ann. N.Y. Acad. Sci. *301:*764–776, 1977, with permission.)

TABLE 4-2. ALTERATIONS IN TOTAL WEIGHT, FAT WEIGHT AND LEAN WEIGHT WITH PHYSICAL TRAINING IN ADULTS

PRINCIPAL INVESTIGATOR	AGE	SEX	Program Duration (weeks)	Session Duration (min)	Frequency (days/wk)	Mode*	Weight (kg) Pre	Weight (kg) Post	Lean Weight (kg) Pre	Lean Weight (kg) Post	Fat (%) Pre	Fat (%) Post
Carter[37]	39–59	M	104	60	2–3	a	80.3	77.0	64.4	62.7	19.8	18.6
Pollock[110]	55	M	20	30	3	a	79.1	77.9	62.2	62.5	21.4	19.8
Pollock[43]	49	M	20	40	4	a	77.6	76.3	60.5	60.4	22.0	20.9
Oscai[36]	35–46	M	16	30	3	a	88.1	83.6	64.5	63.6	26.8	23.9
Getchell[48]	42	M	10	30	3–4	a	83.2	82.4	—	—	—	—
Skinner[16]	42	M	26	40	6	a, d	79.6	79.7	63.7	65.7	20.0	17.5
Terjung[111]	40	M	6	6	7	a	87.5	88.0	—	—	—	—
Kilbom[112]	40	M	8–10	—	2–3	a, d	77.9	78.2	58.8	58.8	24.5	24.8
Ribisl[113]	40	M	12	35	3	a, d	84.4	81.9	66.3	64.9	21.4	20.7
Pollock[44]	39	M	20	45	2	a	81.3	80.4	62.4	62.0	23.3	22.9
Pollock[44]	39	M	20	45	2	a	79.4	78.7	61.2	61.3	22.9	22.1
Pollock[38]	28–39	M	20	30	2	a	80.2	80.3	65.8	65.1	18.0	18.9
Pollock[38]	28–39	M	20	30	4	a	79.7	76.8	64.1	62.5	19.6	18.6
Pollock[45]	38	M	20	30	3	a	84.7	83.4	66.3	66.4	21.7	20.4
Pollock[45]	38	M	20	30	3	a	85.2	83.9	66.1	67.6	22.4	19.4
Pollock[45]	38	M	20	30	3	c	84.1	82.9	66.4	66.5	21.0	19.8
Misner[52]	38	M	8	30	3	a	84.7	83.9	60.8	62.1	27.9	25.4
Misner[52]	38	M	8	30	3	e	86.2	87.2	63.7	66.8	25.9	23.1
Wilmore[50]	37	M	20	30	3	c	85.7	85.3	66.4	67.4	21.2	19.6
Oscai[14]	37	M	16	30	3	a	79.5	77.1	60.9	60.8	23.3	21.1
Pollock[115]	37	M	16	30	4	a	79.4	78.5	62.8	64.7	20.7	17.4
Pollock[115]	37	M	16	30	2	a	80.6	79.8	62.0	61.5	22.8	23.2
Wilmore[50]	36	M	20	30	3	a	79.8	77.9	63.6	63.5	19.8	17.8
Gettman[16]	21–35	M	20	45	3	e	85.4	85.9	64.6	66.4	24.4	22.7
Gettman[16]	21–35	M	20	45	3	a	82.1	81.6	64.3	66.0	21.7	19.1
Leon[68]	19–31	M	16	90	5	a	99.1	93.4	75.8	76.0	23.5	18.6
Wilmore[40]	33	M	10	20	3	a	79.6	78.6	64.2	64.4	18.9	17.8
Wilmore[50]	29	M	20	30	3	f_4	88.3	87.4	67.8	67.3	21.9	21.8

123

Study	Age	Sex				Mode						
Gettman[117]	29	M	16	25	3	a, e	80.5	80.1	64.1	65.0	20.2	18.7
Garfield[118]	23	M	12	15–33	3	e	77.6	76.9	66.8	68.0	13.5	11.6
Thompson[34]	21	M	—	—	—	f_1	81.1	80.2	73.6	74.0	9.2	7.7
Thompson[34]	21	M	—	—	—	f_2	71.6	71.2	65.6	66.3	8.4	6.9
Thompson[35]	21	M	9	—	2	f_3	88.8	87.3	81.5	81.6	8.2	6.5
Girandola[47]	21	M	10	40	2	e	77.2	76.9	63.5	64.2	16.9	15.9
Wilmore[53]	20	M	10	25	3	e	72.9	73.2	63.0	64.2	13.2	11.9
Wilmore[56]	20	M	9	—	5	e	71.9	71.9	59.8	59.6	16.8	16.4
Kollias[65]	18	M	9	—	5	a	67.7	67.0	58.0	59.3	14.4	11.5
Kollias[65]	18	M	9	60	5	a	122.4	119.2	75.3	77.9	38.5	34.6
Boileau[41]	18	M	9	60	5	a	122.4	119.2	74.6	77.3	38.5	34.6
Boileau[41]	18	M	9	—	5	a	67.6	66.6	57.3	58.7	15.1	12.1
Fahey[51]	—	M	9	—	3	e	76.6	77.1	64.8	66.2	15.1	14.1
Lewis[67]	44	F	17	60	2	a	76.2	72.0	45.2	46.3	40.4	35.4
Wilmore[73]	19–39	F	15	30	5	a	48.7	49.5	41.6	42.7	14.1	13.2
Getchell[48]	35	F	10	30	3–4	a	59.5	58.8	—	—	—	—
Brown[55]	16–23	F	26	60–90	3	e	79.0	78.6	58.0	58.4	24.7	23.9
Katch[39]	18–22	F	16	60	5	f_4	58.6	59.0	45.2	44.7	22.8	24.2
Katch[39]	18–22	F	16	120	5	f_5	60.1	60.3	48.0	46.3	20.1	23.2
Garfield[118]	22	F	12	15–33	3	e	57.9	56.2	43.4	42.7	25.0	24.0
Smith[119]	21	F	7	16	3	c	57.9	59.3	45.5	46.6	21.4	21.1
Mayhew[54]	21	F	9	40	3	e	58.1	58.5	40.1	41.6	30.8	28.7
Johnson[42]	21	F	10	30	5	c	61.4	61.3	46.1	47.3	24.9	22.8
Wilmore[56]	20	F	10	25	3	e	61.5	61.1	43.2	43.0	29.2	29.1
Wilmore[53]	20	F	10	40	2	e	57.9	57.9	43.6	44.6	24.5	22.7
Kollias[46]	20	F	15	60	3–5	a	83.4	77.7	56.9	54.2	31.8	30.2
Girandola[49]	19	F	10	—	3	c	54.0	54.8	39.5	39.9	26.7	26.9
Girandola[49]	19	F	10	—	3	c	55.6	55.4	40.1	40.5	27.1	26.0
Moody[63]	19	F	8	—	6	a	67.1	64.7	49.0	51.9	38.6	28.5
Moody[64]	16	F	29	—	4	a	71.5	70.3	43.5	45.0	39.1	36.8
Moody[64]	16	F	15	—	4	a	59.4	58.8	45.0	45.1	24.3	23.3
Zuti[75]	—	F	16	—	5	a						

* a = walk, jog, run; b = swim; c = bicycle, cycle ergometer; d = calisthenics; e = circuit training, circuit weight training, weight training; f = competitive sports and games, f_1 = basketball, f_2 = hockey, f_3 = football, f_4 = tennis, f_5 = swimming.

SUMMARY

It has been the purpose of this chapter to ascertain those alterations in body composition that occur consequent to physical training. From the literature on both humans and animals, exercise does appear to have an influence on appetite, with either a reduction in food intake after intensive exercise or an increase in caloric intake that is less than that expected on the basis of the caloric expenditure. With respect to body composition alterations with exercise, there do appear to be slight decreases in total body weight, increases in lean body weight, and decreases in fat weight. The magnitude of these changes will vary directly with the intensity and duration of the activity or with the total daily caloric expenditure. Table 4–2 summarizes those studies that have been cited earlier in this chapter, in addition to several other studies that were not presented. In conclusion, exercise appears to be a major factor in both the prevention and the treatment of obesity.

REFERENCES

1. Mayer, J.: Overweight: Causes, Cost, and Control. Englewood Cliffs, N.J., Prentice-Hall, 1968.
2. McArdle, W. D., Katch, F. I., and Katch, V. I.: Exercise Physiology: Energy, Nutrition, and Human Performance. Philadelphia, Lea and Febiger, 1981.
3. Behnke, A. R., and Wilmore, J. H.: Evaluation and Regulation of Body Build and Composition. Englewood Cliffs, N.J.; Prentice-Hall, 1974.
4. Oscai, L. B.: The role of exercise in weight control. In Wilmore, J. H., editor: Exercise and Sport Sciences Reviews, Vol I. New York, Academic Press, 1973, pp 103–123.
5. Katch, V. L., Martin, R., and Martin, J.: Effects of exercise intensity on food consumption in the male rat. Am. J. Clin. Nutr. 32:1401–1407, 1979.
6. Mayer, J., Marshall, N. B., Vitale, J. J., Christensen, J. H., Mashayekhi, M. B., and Stare, F. J.: Exercise, food intake and body weight in normal rats and genetically obese adult mice. Am. J. Physiol. 177:544–548, 1954
7. Oscai, L. B., Mole, P. A., and Holloszy, J. O.: Effects of exercise on cardiac weight and mitochondria in male and female rats. Am. J. Physiol. 220:1944–1948, 1971.
8. Terjung, R. L.: Endocrine response to exercise. In Hutton, R. S., and Miller, D. I., editors: Exercise and Sport Sciences Reviews, Vol. 7. Philadelphia, Franklin Institute Press, 1980, pp. 153–180.
9. Brobeck, J. R.: Food intake as a mechanism of temperature regulation. Yale J. Biol. Med. 20:545, 1948.
10. Garrow, J. S.: Energy Balance and Obesity in Man, 2nd ed. New York; Elsevier/North Holland Biomedical Press, 1978.
11. Mayer, J., Roy, P., and Mitra, K. P.; Relation between caloric intake, body weight, and physical work: studies in an industrial male population in West Bengal. Am. J. Clin. Nutr. 4:169–175, 1956.
12. Mayer, J.: Inactivity, and etiological factors in obesity and heart disease. In Blix, G., editor: Nutrition and Physical Activity. Symposium of the Swedish Nutrition Foundation V. Uppsala, Almqvist and Wiksells, 1967.
13. Mayer, J., and Bullen, B. A.: Nutrition, weight control, and exercise. In Johnson, W. R., and Buskirk, E. R., editors: Science and Medicine of Exercise and Sport, 2nd ed. New York, Harper and Row, 1974.
14. Dempsey, J. A.: Anthropometrical observations on obese and nonobese young men undergoing a program of vigorous physical exercise. Res. Q. 35:275–287. 1964.

15. Holloszy, J. O., Skinner, J. S., Toro, G., and Cureton, T. K.: Effects of a 6 month program of endurance exercise on the serum lipids of middle-aged men. Am. J. Cardiol. *14:* 753–760, 1964.
16. Skinner, J. S., Holloszy, J. O., and Cureton, T. K.: Effects of a program of endurance exercises on physical work: capacity and anthropometric measurements of 15 middle-aged men. Am. J. Cardiol. *14:*747–752, 1964.
17. Jankowski, L. W., and Foss, M. L.: The energy intake of sedentary men after moderate exercise. Med. Sci. Sports *4:*11–13, 1972.
18. Belbeck, L. W., and Critz, J. B.: Effect of exercise on the plasma concentration of anorexigenic substance in man. Proc. Soc. Exp. Biol. Med. *142:*19–21, 1973.
19. Stevenson, J. A. F., Fox, B. M., and Szlavko, A. J.: A fat mobilizing and anorectic substance in the urine of fasting rats. Proc. Soc. Exp. Biol. Med. *115:*424, 1964.
20. Oscai, L. B., and Holloszy, J. O.: Effects of weight changes produced by exercise, food restriction, or overeating on body composition. J. Clin. Invest. *48:*2124–2128, 1969.
21. Oscai, L. B., Spirakis, C. N., Wolff, C. A., and Beck, R. J.: Effects of exercise and of food restriction on adipose tissue cellularity, J. Lipid Res. *13:*588–592, 1972.
22. Oscai, L. B., Babirak, S. P., Dubach, F. B., McGarr, J. A., and Spirakis, C. N.: Exercise or food restriction: effect on adipose tissue cellularity. Am. J. Physiol. *227:*901–904, 1974.
23. Taylor, A. W., Garrod, J., McNulty, M. E., and Secord, D. C.: Regenerating epididymal fat pad cell size and number after exercise training and three different feeding patterns. Growth *37:*345–354, 1973.
24. Deb, S., and Martin, R. J.: Effects of exercise and of food restriction on the development of spontaneous obesity in rats. J. Nutr. *105:*543–549, 1975.
25. Askew, E. W., Barakat, H., Kuhl, G. L., and Dohm, G. L.: Response of lipogenesis and fatty acid synthetase to physical training and exhaustive exercise in rats. Lipids *10:* 491–496, 1975.
26. Taylor, A. W.: The effects of different feeding regimens and endurance exercise programs on carbohydrate and lipid metabolism. Can. J. Appl. Sport Sci. *4:*126–130, 1979.
27. Parizkova, J., Vaneckova, M., and Vamberova, M.: A study of changes in some functional indicators following reductions of excessive fat in obese children. Physiol. Bohemoslov. *11:*351–357, 1962.
28. Parizkova, J., and Poupa, O.: Some metabolic consequences of adaptation to muscular work. Br. J. Nutr. *17:*341–345, 1963.
29. Parizkova, J.: Impact of age, diet, and exercise on man's body composition. N.Y. Acad. Sci. *110:*661–674, 1963.
30. Sprynarova, S., and Parizkova, J.: Changes in aerobic capacity and body composition in obese boys after reduction. J. Appl. Physiol. *20:*934–937, 1965.
31. Wells, J. B., Parizkova, J., and Jokl, E.: Exercise, excess fat and body weight. Assoc. Phys. Med. Ment. Rehab. *16:*35–40, 58, 1962.
32. Parizkova, J.: Somatic development and body composition changes in adolescent boys differing in physical activity and fitness: a longitudinal study. Anthropologie *X:*3–36, 1972.
33. Christakis, G., Sajecki, S., Hillman, R. W., Miller, E., Blumenthal, S., and Archer, M.: Effect of a combined nutrition education and physical fitness program on the weight status of obese high school boys. Fed. Proc. *25:*15–19, 1966.
34. Thompson, C. W., Buskirk, E. R., and Goldman, R. F.: Changes in body fat, estimated from skinfold measurements of college basketball and hockey players during a season. Res. Q. *27:*418–430, 1956.
35. Thompson, C. W.: Changes in body fat, estimated from skinfold measurements of varsity college football players during a season. Res. Q. *30:*87–93, 1959.
36. Oscai, L. B., and Williams, B. T.: Effect of exercise on overweight middle-aged males. J. Am. Geriatr. Soc. *16:*794–797, 1968.
37. Carter, J. E. L., and Phillips, W. H.: Structural changes in exercising middle-aged males during a 2-year period. J. Appl. Physiol. *27:*787–794, 1969.
38. Pollock, M. L., Cureton, T. K., and Greninger, L.: Effects of frequency of training on working capacity, cardiovascular function, and body composition of adult men. Med. Sci. Sports. *1:*70–74, 1969.
39. Katch, F. I., Michael, E. D., and Jones, E. M.: Effects of physical training on the body composition and diet of females. Res. Q. *40:*99–104, 1969.

40. Wilmore, J. H., Royce, J., Girandola, R. N., Katch, F. I., and Katch, V. L.: Body composition changes with a 10-week program of jogging. Med. Sci. Sports. *2:*113–117, 1970.
41. Boileau, R. A., Buskirk, E. R., Horstman, D. H., Mendez, J. and Nicholas, W. C.: Body composition changes in obese and lean men during physical conditioning. Med. Sci. Sports. *3:*183–189, 1971.
42. Johnson, R. E., Mastropaolo, J. A., and Wharton, M. A.: Exercise, dietary intake, and body composition. J. Am. Diet. Assoc., *61:*399–403, 1972.
43. Pollock, M. L., Miller, H. S., Janeway, R., Linnerud, A. C., Robertson, B., and Valentino, R.: Effects of walking on body composition and cardiovascular function of middle-aged men. J. Appl. Physiol. *30:*126–130, 1971.
44. Pollock, M. L., Broida, J., Kendrick, Z., Miller, H. S., Janeway, R., and Linnerud, A. C.: Effects of training two days per week at different intensities on middle-aged men. Med. Sci. Sports *4:*192–197, 1972.
45. Pollock, M. L., Miller, H. S., Jr., Kendrick, Z., and Linnerud, A. C.: Effects of mode of training on cardiovascular functions and body composition of adult men. Med. Sci. Sports *7:*139–145, 1975.
46. Kollias, J., Skinner, J. S., Barlett, H. L., Bergsteinova, B. S., and Buskirk, E. R.: Cardiorespiratory responses of young overweight women to ergometry following modest weight reduction. Arch. Environ. Health *27:*61–64, 1973.
47. Girandola, R. N., and Katch, V.: Effects of nine weeks of physical training on aerobic capacity and body composition in college men. Arch. Phys. Med. Rehab *54:*521–524, 1973.
48. Getchell, L. H., and Moore, J. C.: Physical training: comparative responses of middle-aged adults. Arch. Phys. Med. Rehab. *56:*250–254, 1975.
49. Girandola, R. N.: Body composition changes in women: effects of high and low exercise intensity. Arch. Phys. Med. Rehab. *57:*297–300, 1976.
50. Wilmore, J. H., Davis, J. A., O'Brien, R. S., Vodak, P. A., Walder, G. R., and Amsterdam, E. A.: Physiological alterations consequent to 20-week conditioning programs of bicycling, tennis, and jogging. Med. Sci. Sports Exer. *12:*1–8, 1980.
51. Fahey, T. D., and Brown, C. H.: The effects of anabolic steroid on the strength, body composition, and endurance of college males when accompanied by a weight training program. Med. Sci. Sports *5:*272–276, 1973.
52. Misner, J. S., Boileau, R. A., Massey, B. H., and Mayhew, J. L.: Alterations in the body composition of adult men during selected physical training programs. J. Am. Geriatr. Soc. *22:*33–38, 1974.
53. Wilmore, J. H.: Alterations in strength, body composition and anthropometric measurements consequent to a 10 week weight training program. Med. Sci. Sports *6:*133–138, 1974.
54. Mayhew, J. L., and Gross, P. M.: Body composition changes in young women with high resistance weight training. Res. Q. *45:*433–440, 1974.
55. Brown, C. H., and Wilmore, J. H.: The effects of maximal resistance training on the strength and body composition of women athletes. Med. Sci. Sports *6:*174–177, 1974.
56. Wilmore, J. H., Parr, R. B., Girandola, R. N., Ward, P., Vodak, P. A., Barstow, T. J., Pipes, T. V., Romero, G. T., and Leslie, P.: Physiological alterations consequent to circuit weight training. Med. Sci. Sports *10:*79–84, 1978.
57. Gettman, L. R., and Pollock, M. L.: Circuit weight training: a critical review of its physiological benefits. Phys. Sportsmed. *9:*44–60, 1981.
58. O'Hara, W. J., Allen, C., and Shephard, R. J.: Loss of body fat during an arctic winter expedition. Can. J. Physiol. Pharm. *55:*1235–1241, 1977.
59. O'Hara, W. J., Allen, C., and Shephard, R. J.: Loss of body weight and fat during exercise in a cold chamber. Eur. J. Appl. Physiol. *37:*205–218, 1977.
60. O'Hara, W. J., Allen, C., and Shephard, R. J.: Treatment of obesity by exercise in the cold. Can. Med. Assoc. J. *117:*773–779, 1977.
61. O'Hara, W. J., Allen, C., Shephard, R. J., and Allen, G.: Fat loss in the cold—a controlled study. J. Appl. Physiol. *46:*872–877, 1979.
62. Pollock, M. L., Miller, H. S., Jr., Linnerud, A. C., and Cooper, K. H.: Frequency of training as a determinant for improvement in cardiovascular function and body composition of middle-aged men. Arch. Phys. Med. Rehab. *56:*141–145, 1975.
63. Moody, D. L., Kollias, J., and Buskirk, E. R.: The effect of a moderate exercise program on body weight and skinfold thickness in overweight college women. Med. Sci. Sports *1:*75–80, 1969.
64. Moody, D. L., Wilmore, J. H., Girandola, R. N., and Royce, J. P.: The effects of a jogging

program on the body composition of normal and obese high school girls. Med. Sci. Sports *4:*210–213, 1972.

65. Kollias, J., Boileau, R. A., Barlett, H. L., and Buskirk, E. R.: Pulmonary function and physical conditioning in lean and obese subjects. Arch. Environ. Health *25:*146–150, 1972.

66. Gwinup, G.: Effect of exercise alone on the weight of obese women. Arch. Int. Med. *135:* 676–680, 1975.

67. Lewis, S., Haskell, W. L., Wood, P. D., Manoogian, N., Bailey, J. E., and Pereira, M.: Effects of physical activity on weight reduction in obese middle-aged women. Am. J. Clin. Nutr. *29:*151–156, 1976.

68. Leon, A. S., Conrad, J., Hunninghake, D. B., and Serfass, R.: Effects of a vigorous walking program on body composition, and carbohydrate and lipid metabolism of obese young men. Am. J. Clin. Nutr. *33:*1776–1787, 1979.

69. Franklin, B. A., Mackeen, P. C., and Buskirk, E. R.: Body composition effects of a 12-week physical conditioning program for normal and obese middle-aged women, and status at 18-month follow-up. Int. J. Obesity *2:*394, 1978.

70. Krotkiewski, M., Sjostrom, L., and Sullivan, L.: Effects of long-term physical training on adipose tissue cellularity and body composition in hypertrophic and hyperplastic obesity. Int. J. Obesity *2:*395, 1978.

71. Krotkiewski, M., Mandroukas, K., Sjostrom, L., Sullivan, L., Wetterqvist, H., and Bjorntorp, P.: Effects of long-term training on body fat, metabolism, and blood pressure in obesity. Metabolism *28:*650–658, 1979.

72. Warwick, P. M., and Garrow, J. S.: The effect of addition of exercise to a regime of dietary restriction on weight loss, nitrogen balance, resting metabolic rate and spontaneous physical activity in three obese women in a metabolic ward. Int. J. Obesity *5:*25–32, 1981.

73. Wilmore, J. H.: Exercise-induced alterations in weight of underweight women. Arch. Phys. Med. Rehab. *54:*115–119, 1973.

74. Gwinup, G., Chelvam, R., and Steinberg, T.: Thickness of subcutaneous fat and activity of underlying muscles. Ann. Int. Med. *74:*408–411, 1971.

75. Zuti, W. B., and Golding, L. A.: Comparing diet and exercise as weight reduction tools. Phys. Sportsmed. *4:*49–53, 1976.

76. Novak, L. P., Hyatt, R. E., and Alexander, J. F.: Body composition and physiologic function of athletes. J.A.M.A. *205:*764–770, 1968.

77. Forsyth, H. L., and Sinning, W. E.: The anthropometric estimation of body density and lean body weight of male athletes. Med. Sci. Sports *5:*174–180, 1973.

78. Sinning, W. E.: Body composition, cardiovascular function, and rule changes in women's basketball. Res. Q. *44:*313–321, 1973.

79. Conger, P. R., and MacNab, R. B. J.: Strength, body composition and work capacity of participants and nonparticipants in women's intercollegiate sports. Res. Q. *38:*184–192, 1967.

80. Parr, R. B., Wilmore, J. H., Hoover, R., Bachman, D., and Kerlan, R.: Professional basketball players: athletic profiles. Phys. Sportsmed. *6:*77–84, 1978.

81. Rusko, H., Hara, M., and Karvonen, E.: Aerobic performance capacity in athletes. Eur. J. Appl. Physiol. *38:*151–159, 1978.

82. Wickkiser, J. D., and Kelly, J. M.: The body composition of a college football team. Med. Sci. Sports *7:*199–202, 1975.

83. Wilmore, J. H., Parr, R. B., Haskell, W. L., Costill, D. L., Milburn, L. J., and Kerlan, R. K.: Athletic profile of professional football players. Phys. Sportsmed. *4:*45–54, 1976.

84. Sinning, W. E., and Lindberg, G. D.: Physical characteristics of college age women gymnasts. Res. Q. *43:*226–234, 1972.

85. Parizkova, J.: Body composition and exercise during growth and development. *In* Rarick, G. L., editor: Physical Activity Human Growth and Development. New York, Academic Press, 1972, pp. 97–124.

86. Knowlton, R. G., Ackerman, K. J., Fitzgerald, P. I., Wilde, S. W., and Tahamont, M. V.: Physiological and performance characteristics of United States championship class orienteers. Med. Sci. Sports Exer. *12:*164–169, 1980.

87. Krahenbuhl, G. S., Wells, C. L., Brown, C. H., and Ward, P. E.: Characteristics of national and world class female pentathletes. Med. Sci. Sports *11:*20–23, 1979.

88. Pipes, T. V.: The racquetball pro: a physiological profile. Phys. Sportsmed. *7:*91–94, 1979.

89. Hagerman, F. C., Hagerman, G. R., and Mickelson, T. C.: Physiological profiles of elite rowers. Phys. Sportsmed. 7:74–83, 1979.
90. Sprynarova, S., and Parizkova, J.: Functional capacity and body composition in top weight-lifters, swimmers, runners and skiers. Int. Z. Angew. Physiol. 29:184–194, 1971.
91. Haymes, E. M., and Dickinson, A. L.: Characteristics of elite male and female ski racers. Med. Sci. Sports Exercise 12:153–158, 1980.
92. Niinimaa, V., Dyon, M., and Shepard, R. J.: Performance and efficiency of intercollegiate cross-country skiers. Med. Sci. Sports 10:91–93, 1978.
93. Raven, P. B., Gettman, L. R., Pollock, M. L., and Cooper, K. H.: A physiological evaluation of professional soccer players. Br. J. Sports Med. 10:209–216, 1976.
94. Wilmore, J. H., Brown, C. H., and Davis, J. A.: Body physique and composition of the female distance runner. Ann. N.Y. Acad. Sci. 301:764–776, 1977.
95. Vodak, P. A., Savin, W. M., Haskell, W. L., and Wood, P. D.: Physiological profile of middle-aged male and female tennis players. Med. Sci. Sports Exercise 12:159–163, 1980.
96. Costill, D. L., Bowers, R., and Kammer, W. F.: Skinfold estimates of body fat among marathon runners. Med. Sci. Sports 2:93–95, 1970.
97. Pollock, M. L., Miller, H. S., Jr., and Wilmore, J.: Physiological characteristics of champion American track athletes 40 to 75 years of age. J. Gerontol. 29:645–649, 1974.
98. Barnard, R. J., Grimditch, G. K., and Wilmore, J. H.: Physiological characteristics of sprint and endurance masters runners. Med. Sci. Sports 11:167–171, 1979.
99. Lewis, S., Haskell, W. L., Klein, H., Halpern, J., and Wood, P. D.: Prediction of body composition in habitually active middle-aged men. J. Appl. Physiol. 39:221–225, 1975.
100. Malina, R. M., Harper, A. B., Avent, H. H., and Campbell, D. E.: Physique of female track and field athletes. Med. Sci. Sports 3:32–38, 1971.
101. Wilmore, J. H., and Brown, C. H.: Physiological profiles of women distance runners. Med. Sci. Sports 6:178–181, 1974.
102. Fahey, T. D., Akka, L., and Rolph, R.: Body composition and $\dot{V}_{O_2}$ max of exceptional weight-trained athletes. J. Appl. Physiol. 39:559–561, 1975.
103. Kovaleski, J. E., Parr, R. B., Hornak, J. E., and Roitman, J. L.: Athletic profile of women college volleyball players. Phys. Sportsmed. 8:112–118, 1980.
104. Pipes, T. V.: Physiological characteristics of elite body builders. Phys. Sportsmed. 7:116–122, 1979.
105. Gale, J. B., and Flynn, K. W.: Maximal oxygen consumption and relative body fat of high-ability wrestlers. Med. Sci. Sports 6:232–234, 1974.
106. Taylor, A. W., Brassard, L., Proteu, L., and Robin, D.: A physiological profile of Canadian Greco-Roman wrestlers. Can. J. Appl. Sport Sci. 4:131–134, 1979.
107. Sinning, W. E.: Body composition assessment of college wrestlers. Med. Sci. Sports 6:139–145, 1974.
108. Katch, F. I., and Michael, E. D.: Body composition of high school wrestlers according to age and wrestling weight category. Med. Sci. Sports 3:190–194, 1971.
109. Stine, G., Ratliff, R., Shierman, G., and Grana, W. A.: Physical profile of the wrestlers at the 1977 NCAA championships. Phys. Sportsmed. 7:98–105, 1979.
110. Pollock, M. L., Dawson, G. A., Miller, H. S., Jr., Ward, A., Cooper, D., Headley, W., Linnerud, A. C., and Nomeir, M. M.: Physiologic responses of men 49 to 65 years of age to endurance training. J. Am. Geriatr. Soc. 24:97–104, 1976.
111. Terjung, R. L., Baldwin, K. M., Cooksey, J., Samson, B., and Sutter, R. A.: Cardiovascular adaptations to twelve minutes of mild daily exercise in middle-aged sedentary men. J. Am. Geriatr. Soc. 21:164–168, 1973.
112. Kilbom, A., Hartley, L. H., Saltin, B., Bjure, J., Grimby, G., and Åstrand, I.: Physical training in sedentary middle-aged and older men. Scand. J. Clin. Lab. Invest. 24:315–322, 1969.
113. Ribisl, R. M.: Effects of training upon the maximal oxygen uptake of middle-aged men. Int. Z. Angew. Physiol. 27:154–160, 1969.
114. Oscai, L. B., Williams, B. T., and Hertig, B.: Effect of exercise on blood volume. J. Appl. Physiol. 24:622–624, 1968.
115. Pollock, M. L., Tiffany, J., Gettman, L., Janeway, R., and Lofland, H.: Effects of frequency of training on serum lipids, cardiovascular function, and body composition. In Franks, B. D., editor: Exercise and Fitness. Chicago, Athletic Institute, 1969, pp. 161–178.
116. Gettman, L. R., Ayres, J. J., Pollock, M. L., and Jackson, A.: The effect of circuit weight

training on strength, cardiorespiratory function, and body composition of adult men. Med. Sci. Sports *10:*171–176, 1978.

117. Gettman, L. R., Ayres, J. J., Pollock, M. L., Durstine, J. L., and Grantham, W.: Physiological effects on adult men of circuit strength training and jogging. Arch. Phys. Med. Rehab. *60:*115–120, 1979.

118. Garfield, D. S., Ward, P., Cobb, R., Disch, J., and Southwick, D.: Circuit weight training. Houston, Dynamics Health Equipment, 1979.

119. Smith, D. P., and Stransky, F. W.: The effect of training and detraining on the body composition and cardiovascular response of young women to exercise. J. Sports Med. *16:*112–120, 1976.

Chapter 5

MUSCULOSKELETAL FUNCTION

INTRODUCTION

Sound musculoskeletal function is essential to optimal health and physiological function. Although it is true that very few people die from a lack of strength or poor flexibility, a number of otherwise healthy people suffer from chronic lower back problems, and decreases in muscle strength with aging are associated with decreases in muscle mass. As the body loses lean tissue, there is a concomitant reduction in its basal and resting metabolic rate. Frequently, food intake is not reduced in proportion to the decrease in metabolic rate, and increases in fat stores result. Finally, without proper stimulation, bones lose strength through loss of the bone matrix as well as bone mineral. Osteoporosis and hip and vertebral fractures are frequently the result of this process.

Back pain is a major malady of modern society. In 1971, insurance companies reported more claims for back disability than for any other cause.[1] Kraus and Raab have demonstrated that over 80 per cent of low back pain is due to muscular deficiency.[2] Further, in a 2- to 8-year follow-up study of 233 low back pain patients on a muscle strengthening and flexibility program, 82 per cent reported good, 15.5 per cent reported fair, and only 2.5 per cent reported poor responses to the exercise regimen.[2] It is now clearly recognized that inadequate muscular strength and flexibility can lead to serious musculoskeletal disorders that result in considerable pain and discomfort, losses in income, increased disability, and premature retirement.

Losses of lean tissue with aging have been associated with physical inactivity. Existing longitudinal data using both whole-body potassium-40 and densitometry indicate rates of loss ranging from 0.13 to 0.36 kg per year, with the higher rates of loss occurring later in life, when individuals are less active.[3] This decline in lean body mass has been associated with decreases in basal metabolic rate (BMR) with aging.[3] From cross-sectional

131

studies, Quenouille, et al.[4] have concluded that the BMR declines at a rate of 3 per cent per decade from the age of 3 to over 80 years. Keys, et al.[5] conducted both a cross-sectional and a longitudinal study of changes in BMR with aging. Comparing men 21.9 years of age with men 49.8 years of age indicated a 4.5 to 5.0 per cent decrease in BMR per decade. Of the original group of younger men, 63 were evaluated a second time 19.4 years later. There was an average decrease in BMR of 3.2 per cent per decade. A reduction in BMR with age without a concomitant reduction in energy intake will lead to increases in body fat stores. This is one of several mechanisms postulated for the increases in body fat identified with aging that was referred to in Chapter 2. Thus, maintaining one's lean body weight through a carefully designed exercise program should help in the prevention of obesity.

Bone also undergoes deterioration with aging, which is again related to reduced physical activity. Bed rest and immobilization are accompanied by calcium deficits. Birge and Whedon,[6] summarizing the research literature through 1967, concluded that disuse atrophy of bone has been observed to be clinically associated with varying degrees of immobilization, resulting largely from bone resorption. Vogel and Whittle,[7] in reviewing the changes in bone mineral content in the Skylab astronauts, concluded that mineral losses do occur from the bones of the lower extremities during missions of up to 84 days and that these mineral losses generally follow the loss patterns observed in the bed rest situation. Although the astronauts are mobile in space, they are working in a gravity-free environment, and the weight-bearing bones are not placed under the same degree of stress as they experience while in a normal 1-G environment. Thus, with reduced use, bone loses both structure and function, which will eventually lead to osteoporosis.[8] Aloia et al.[9] and Smith et al.[10] have recently demonstrated that exercise can prevent involutional bone loss in women with an average age of 52.3 and 81.0 years, respectively. In fact, exercise resulted in increases in bone mineral content[10] and in total body calcium,[9] whereas the nonexercising control groups demonstrated losses in both.

It is apparent that regular exercise is important for optimal musculoskeletal function. The remainder of this chapter will include a discussion of the physiology of strength and flexibility and procedures for the development of strength and flexibility.

PHYSIOLOGY OF STRENGTH AND FLEXIBILITY

DEFINITIONS

Before discussing the physiology of strength and flexibility, it is important to define several key words that are used frequently in the literature. Strength refers to the ability of the muscle or muscle group to apply force.[11] Typically, strength is defined relative to maximum force-producing capabilities. The individual who can maximally curl a barbell weighing 150 pounds is twice as strong as the individual who can lift only 75 pounds. When sophisticated laboratory equipment is unavailable for assessing strength, having the individual lift as much as he or she can just one time provides a simple but accurate estimate of strength. This is referred to as the one repetition maximum (1-RM). In many fitness programs, the 1-RM is assessed for both the bench press and the leg press, providing estimates of both upper and lower body strength.

Power is a term that refers to the maximum strength-producing capacity of the individual expressed relative to time,[11] i.e., force X distance X time^{-1}. An individual who can bench press 200 pounds a distance of 2 feet in 0.5 second would have a power output of 800 foot-pounds X second^{-1}. When training athletes, power is a most important component that is often ignored. The basketball player leaping for a rebound, the football player lunging across the line to block his opponent, and the tennis player serving to his or her opponent are all relying on power for peak performance.

Muscular endurance refers to the ability of the muscle or muscle group to sustain contractions of a given force over time.[11] A simple measure of muscular endurance involves determining the number of repetitions a person can complete while lifting a fixed percentage of his or her 1-RM. If two individuals had identical 1-RMs for the bench press of 200 pounds, the individual who could perform more repetitions at 75 per cent of that 1-RM, i.e., 150 pounds, would have the greater muscular endurance. More accurate estimates of endurance can be performed in the laboratory with specific dynamometers and strain gauges attached to recording devices.

Flexibility refers to the looseness or suppleness of the body or specific joints and involves the interrelationships between muscles, tendons, ligaments, and the joint itself.[11] Limited flexibility is usually the result of muscles and tendons that are too tight, restricting the range of motion; however, excessive fatness is also a contributing factor. Flexibility is not easy to measure, even in a laboratory setting. Several tests, such as the sit and reach test, have been devised, but they provide only estimates, not absolute measures of flexibility. Chapter 6 will provide more information concerning the testing for strength, muscular endurance, and flexibility.

Mechanisms of Strength Gains

When one gains strength through a planned program of strength training exercises, what physiological alterations occur to allow these gains? For many years, it was assumed that gains or losses in strength simply reflected changes in the size of the muscle or muscle group: As the muscles increased in size, or underwent hypertrophy, there was an increase in strength; and as the muscles decreased in size, or underwent atrophy, there was a decrease in strength. It is now recognized that changes in strength are not so simply explained. Wilmore[12] demonstrated substantial gains in strength in college-aged women after a 10-week strength training program with little or no change in muscle girth. In fact, some women were able to double their strength for certain weight-training exercises but experienced no perceptible hypertrophy.

It is important to recognize that in the intact human it is impossible to separate the muscle from its motor nerve. More specifically, a single motor nerve innervates a few to several thousand individual muscle fibers that compose the motor unit. When a motor nerve is activated by a simple reflex or by the higher brain centers, all of the muscle fibers innervated by that motor unit contract. The grading of a muscle's force production capabilities is accomplished by any one or a combination of the following: an increase in the number of motor units activated; rate of activation; and an increased synchronization of motor unit firing. Thus, strength and gains in strength must be discussed relative to neuromuscular integration, i.e., the muscle's ability to produce tension and the nervous system's ability to activate the muscle.

Examples of the neural component in the expression of strength are available from human experiences as well as from controlled laboratory studies. Periodically, newspapers provide detailed accounts of superhuman feats of strength, as illustrated by the small, middle-aged woman who lifts the automobile that has slipped off of its jack, freeing her son who was trapped beneath. In one of the first laboratory experiments to investigate this phenomenon, Ikai and Steinhaus[13] measured the strength of the right forearm flexors during normal testing conditions and after hypnosis, a gunshot, a loud shout, alcohol ingestion, an injection of epinephrine, and ingestion of an amphetamine. Compared with control conditions, strength was affected by +26.5 per cent to −31.0 per cent by the various interventions. This study pointed to the importance of specific inhibitory mechanisms employed by the body to protect the integrity of the muscles, tendons, ligaments, joints, and other tissues that might be subject to tear or injury consequent to the generation of high peak forces. Overcoming these inhibitory mechanisms appears to be an important adaptation in allowing the body to express greater levels of strength.

Moritani and deVries[14] proposed a model to differentiate the mechanisms for gains in strength into the components of "neural factors" and hypertrophy. If the gains in strength are attributed solely to neural factors, such as learning to disinhibit, then increases in maximal integrated electromyographic activation without any change in force per fiber or motor units innervated would be expected. If strength gains are attributable solely to muscular hypertrophy, increases in force production capabilities without increases in maximal integrated electromyographic activation would be expected. With this model, they demonstrated in seven young males and eight females that neural factors accounted for the larger proportion of the initial strength gains, with hypertrophy becoming the dominant factor after the first 3 to 5 weeks. Coyle et al.[15] identified a neural component explaining at least a portion of the gains in strength they observed after a program of maximal two-legged knee extensions performed at one of three different velocities.

Milner-Brown et al.[16] found strength increases after training to be associated with significantly greater levels of synchronization of the various motor units. Komi et al.[17] also suggest improved synchronization of motor units to explain increases in strength. Finally, Gerchman et al.[18] have identified enlargement of the nucleolus in motor neurons with training, providing morphological evidence of motor neuron involvement in training adaptations.

Thus, strength is the result of complex neuromuscular integrations. Strength is more than just a simple linear function of muscle size. Although size is possibly the most important determinant of strength, neurological and psychological factors must also be considered.

MUSCLE HYPERTROPHY AND ATROPHY

To understand how a muscle can undergo both hypertrophy with training and atrophy with disuse or immobilization, it is first necessary to review the basic morphology of muscle. For many years, muscle was assumed to be composed of two major types of fibers, red and white. Red fibers were considered to be oxidative or endurance fibers owing to their high concentration of myoglobin. White fibers were considered to be glycolytic fibers with high force-producing capabilities but low endurance. More recently, with the use of the muscle biopsy procedure (see Fig. 5–1) pioneered by Bergstom in 1962,[19] muscle fibers have been classified into three basic fiber types: (1) slow, or type I; (2) fast-oxidative-glycolytic, or type IIa; and (3) fast glycolytic, or type IIb (see Fig. 5–2). Endurance athletes typically have a preponderance of type I fibers, whereas sprint-type athletes have a preponderance of type II fibers.[20] In addition, it appears that fiber type is largely genetically determined and that the relative proportions of the type I and type II fibers do not change with training.[21]

Muscle hypertrophy represents a normal response to exercise training and is characterized by an increase in the size of the individual muscle fibers but could also involve an increase in the number of muscle fibers, the latter phenomenon being referred to as hyperplasia.[22,23] Goldberg et al.[22] concluded that hypertrophy is the result of both an increased protein synthesis and a decreased protein degradation.

Morpurgo,[24] in 1897, trained dogs on the treadmill after removal of the sartorious to induce a compensatory hypertrophy. He found muscle hypertrophy to be solely the result of increases in fiber size with no increase in fiber number. Goldspink[23] reported similar results and concluded that individual fiber enlargement was the result of myofibril proliferation. In the late 1960s and early 1970s, researchers began to report muscle fiber hyperplasia under certain exercise training conditions, and these increases in fiber number were attributed to longitudinal fiber splitting.[24] Gonyea,[25] in a series of studies in which cats were trained to lift weights with their right forelimb, reported a 20.5 per cent increase in muscle fiber number after training, with a maximum increase in fiber diameter of only about 11 per cent. This hyperplasia was attributed to muscle fiber splitting. Gollnick and associates[26] produced muscular hypertrophy in groups of rats by both surgical ablation of a synergist and the combination of synergist ablation and exercise. Counting each fiber of the hypertrophied muscles, they were unable to identify any evidence of hyperplasia and concluded that hypertrophy was the result of enlarged fiber size, not hyperplasia. With such conflicting evidence, it is impossible at this time to state the exact mechanisms of hypertrophy.

Atrophy, or the reduction in the size of a muscle or muscle group, represents a normal response to disuse or immobilization. When aging is accompanied by an increasingly sedentary lifestyle, and when a limb is immobilized in a cast consequent to a broken bone or surgery, muscle atrophy is almost always the result. Goldberg et al.[22] make the important observation that whereas hypertrophy of a muscle can help the organism improve physical performance, acquire new skills, or compensate for disease or injury to other body parts, atrophy of inactive muscle insures that the organism does not have to maintain structures that are metabolically expensive but physiologically unnecessary.

Larsson[27] has reported that the proportion and the cross-sectional area of type II muscle fibers decrease with aging, with no change in type I fibers.

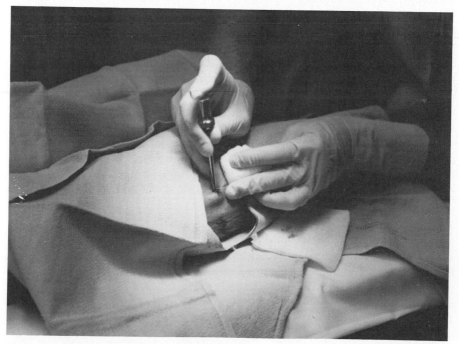

Figure 5–1. The muscle biopsy technique.

This decrease in the type II fibers correlates with decreases in strength observed with aging. Grimby et al.[28] reported a different aging pattern in their subjects. They did not find a decrease in type II fiber numbers, but they did confirm the decrease in type II fiber area with aging. Thus, it does appear that aging has a specific effect on the type II fiber, with decreased fiber area being associated with decreases in strength. Both are undoubtedly associated with decreased physical activity. Once the muscle undergoes atrophy with aging, it is difficult, if not impossible, to regain that muscle mass with strength training. Moritani and deVries[29] found that increases in strength with strength training, in 67- to 72-year-old men, was predominantly the result of neural factors, as described earlier in this chapter, with muscle hypertrophy accounting for less than 30 per cent of the strength gains.

Muscle atrophy has also been studied during periods of immobilization. Haggmark and Eriksson[30] studied 16 patients who had been placed in either standard cylinder casts or in a mobile cast brace after anterior cruciate ligament reconstruction surgery of the knee. Patients with the standard cast showed a significant atrophy of type I muscle fibers in the vastus lateralis, whereas those patients in the mobile brace demonstrated no significant changes in cross-sectional area of either type I or type II fibers. Evidently, the mobile brace, while maintaining the integrity of the surgical repair, still allowed sufficient movement of the involved muscles to prevent muscle

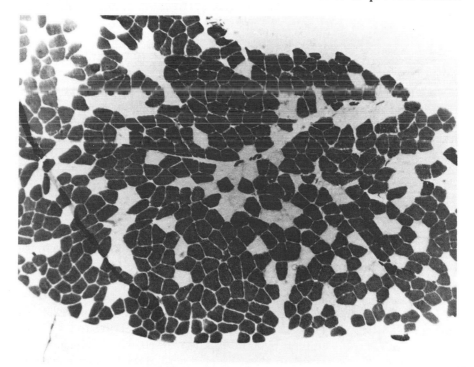

Figure 5–2. Illustration of muscle slow-twitch (dark) and fast-twitch (light) fiber types.

atrophy. Grimby et al.[31] reported somewhat lower fiber areas, particularly type II fibers, comparing the leg operated on with the leg not operated on in 30 subjects who had undergone surgery for knee ligament injuries. Sargeant et al.[32] studied seven patients who had suffered unilateral leg fractures after removal of their immobilizing plaster casts. After a mean casting period of 131 days, leg volume was reduced by 12 per cent in the injured leg, and this was accompanied by a reduction of 42 per cent in the cross-sectional area of the muscle fibers sampled from the vastus lateralis of the injured leg. Both type I and type II fibers were equally affected. MacDougall et al.[33] found decreases in fiber area of the triceps brachii of 33 per cent for the fast-twitch and 25 per cent for the slow-twitch fibers after 5 to 6 weeks of immobilization in elbow casts, coincident with a 41 per cent decrease in elbow extension strength.

Muscle atrophy has been shown to occur very rapidly. The studies of Booth et al.[34,35] have demonstrated that during the first 6 hours of hindlimb immobilization in rats, a significant decline of 37 per cent occurs in the fractional rate of protein synthesis. In addition, the position in which the limb is immobilized is extremely important. Atrophy exhibited a half-time response of 4 to 6 days, i.e., the time to reach one half of the final decrease, when the muscle was casted in a shortened position. When the muscle was fixed in a stretched position, i.e., greater than resting length, the onset of atrophy was delayed. In fact, in some cases, muscles hypertrophied when fixed in the stretched position. Wilmore et al.[36] casted a human subject for a period of 17 days and reported a net protein breakdown of 40 and 59 per cent on days 10 and 17 of casting, respectively.

STRENGTH TRAINING IN WOMEN

Women are generally considered to be the weaker sex. Is this stereotype justified? In a review article of nine separate studies, Laubach[37] compared basic strength differences between men and women. He reported the following: (1) upper extremity strength measurements in women were found to range from 35 to 79 per cent of men's, averaging 55.8 per cent; (2) lower extremity strength measurements in women ranged from 57 to 86 per cent of men's, averaging 71.9 per cent; and (3) trunk strength for women ranged from 37 to 70 per cent of men's, averaging 63.8 per cent. Wilmore[12] compared the absolute strength of college-age men and women for both the upper and the lower body, finding the women to have only 36.9 per cent of the bench press strength and 73.4 per cent of the leg press strength of men. When strength was expressed relative to body weight, the women had only 46.2 per cent of the bench press strength, but 92.4 per cent of the leg press strength of men. When expressed relative to lean body weight, removing the influence of body fat, women were only 53.4 per cent of the bench press strength, but 106.0 per cent of the leg press strength of the men. In other words, relative to the lean body weight, women were as strong as men when equated for lean weight, but only with respect to leg strength. Hosler and Morrow[38] reported similar findings in young women and men for leg and arm isokinetic strength. They found that once body composition and size were controlled, gender accounted for only 2 per cent of the variance in leg strength and 1 per cent in arm strength. Thus, it would appear that the quality of the muscle is similar for men and women, but the larger size of the man will always be a distinct advantage relative to absolute strength.

There is also evidence that women respond in a manner similar to men when placed in a strength training program. Brown and Wilmore[39] trained seven women throwing event athletes for a period of 6 months using a heavy resistance strength training program. After 6 months, bench press strength increased 15 to 44 per cent and half-squat strength increased by 16 to 53 per cent. In a study of nonathletic young women, Wilmore[12] observed a 29.5 per cent increase in leg press strength and a 28.6 per cent increase in bench press strength after a 10-week strength training program. A comparison group of men exhibited increases of 26.0 per cent and 16.5 per cent, respectively. In both of these studies, strength gains were accompanied by little or no change in muscle girth, indicating that hypertrophy is not a necessary concomitant to gains in strength. This may not be true with higher intensity programs. Mayhew and Gross[40] reported similar results for a group of college women who strength trained for a period of 9 weeks. Thus, it appears that women can gain benefits from strength training similar to men and that these benefits do not necessitate major increases in muscle bulk.

MUSCLE SORENESS

Muscle soreness may be present during the latter stages of an exercise, during immediate recovery, between 12 and 48 hours after a strenuous bout of exercise, or at each of these times. The pain that is felt during and immediately after exercise is probably due to the accumulation of the end products of exercise and tissue edema caused by the high hydrostatic pressure that forces fluid to shift from the blood plasma into the tissue. This pain and soreness is usually of short duration, disappearing within an hour after cessation of exercise.[41]

The muscle soreness that is felt a day or two after a heavy bout of exercise has been explained by several recent theories, but there is not total agreement about which of these most adequately explains the soreness phenomenon. DeVries[42] has developed the spasm theory to explain muscle soreness. According to this theory, exercise brings about localized muscle ischemia, the ischemia causes pain, the pain generates increased reflex motor activity, and greater motor activity creates even greater local muscle tension, which results in even greater degrees of ischemia. His research supports this theory, and he has also found that static stretching procedures help to prevent soreness, as well as to relieve soreness when it is present. More recently, Abraham[43,44] has provided data supporting Hough's torn tissue hypothesis, which was originally formulated in 1902.[45] Abraham found muscle soreness to correlate with the appearance of myoglobin in the urine, with myoglobin being a marker of muscle fiber trauma. Since myoglobin in the urine is associated with all strenuous work, independent of muscle soreness, he also looked at hydroxyproline excretion, indicative of connective tissue breakdown. He found a significant correlation between the day of maximum hydroxyproline excretion and the day when the subjects experienced their greatest soreness.

There are several interesting characteristics of muscle soreness that may eventually be important considerations when attempting to identify potential contributing mechanisms. First, muscle soreness is usually a transient phenomenon. The individual will typically experience extreme muscle soreness only during the first few weeks of a new exercise program. After this initial training period, there is relatively little soreness, even with substantially higher levels of exercise, provided the form of exercise is the same. Second, muscle soreness appears to be associated with only the eccentric phase of muscle contraction, i.e., the lengthening of a muscle as when a weight is gradually lowered back to its starting position after the completion of a lift. With eccentric contraction, the force of gravity brings the weight down, and the muscles execute a controlled lengthening to reduce the speed of this downward movement. Talag[46] investigated the relationship of muscle soreness to eccentric, concentric, and isometric contractions and found that the group that trained solely with eccentric contractions experienced extreme muscle soreness, whereas the isometric and concentric contraction groups experienced little muscle soreness. Assmussen[47] and Komi et al.[48,49] suggest that eccentric work overloads and overstretches the muscle's elastic components and that this insult results in muscle soreness. From the work of Abraham,[43,44] Assmussen,[47] and Komi et al.,[48,49] it would appear that muscle soreness is related to connective tissue irritation and is associated primarily with eccentric muscle contraction.

FLEXIBILITY

Flexibility is limited in some joints by either the bony structure or the bulk of the surrounding muscle or both. These mechanical factors cannot be greatly modified. However, for most joints, the limitation of movement through the range of movement is imposed by the soft tissues, including (1) the muscle and its fascial sheaths (2) the connective tissue, with tendons, ligaments, and joint capsules; and (3) the skin.[50] Johns and Wright,[51] studying wrist flexion and extension in the cat, found the muscles, the joint capsule, and the tendons to be the most important factors limiting free movement about the joint.

DeVries[50] has cited a number of factors other than those listed previously that influence the flexibility of joints. First, the more active the individual, generally the more flexible he or she is. It appears that this activity must be performed through the full range of motion of each specific joint in order to gain benefits. Most long distance runners who do little or no stretching before or after their workouts have limited or poor flexibility. The mechanics of the running movement are such that the runner does not utilize the full range of movement while running. Thus, even those who are very active must evaluate the nature of their activity to determine if that activity is promoting or reducing general body flexibility. Second, there appears to be a gender difference in flexibility, with girls and women being much more flexible than men. Third, flexibility is age-related, with flexibility decreasing to the age of 10 to 12 years and then increasing into adulthood. With aging, flexibility begins a progressive decline. Finally, flexibility is greatly influenced by temperature. Local warming of a joint will increase the flexibility of that joint, whereas local cooling will bring about the opposite effect.

STRENGTH AND FLEXIBILITY TRAINING PROCEDURES

Strength, power, muscular endurance, and flexibility can be altered through muscle and flexibility training programs. Although the intent of this chapter is to provide a basic overview of the physiological foundations of strength and flexibility, it is also important to understand basic procedural concepts in order to prescribe strength and flexibility training programs most effectively. The remainder of this chapter will give a brief overview of training procedures specific to strength and flexibility training programs.

STRENGTH TRAINING PROCEDURES

Strength training procedures can be classified according to whether the contraction is static or dynamic and whether the contraction is concentric, i.e., shortening, or eccentric, i.e., lengthening. In a static, or isometric, contraction, the muscle contracts, but there is no visible movement about the joint. With dynamic contraction, there is movement about the joint, and this movement can take one of several forms. With isotonic contraction, there is movement of a specific weight through the full range of motion, as illustrated by the two-arm curl, in which the barbell is lifted from a position with the elbows fully extended to a position of complete flexion. When curling a weight of 105 pounds, there is a constant resistance of 105 pounds that must be overcome by the application of a force in excess of 105 pounds. Owing to the mechanics of the elbow joint, however, the force of 105 pounds represents different fractions of the maximal potential at each angle in the range of motion. Strength is the result of the contractile force and the mechanics of movement about a joint, as illustrated in Figure 5–3. Thus, the 105 pounds in the biceps curl may represent maximal strength at the angle of 60 degrees and 180 degrees, but only 75 per cent of maximal strength at 100 degrees when the contractile force and joint mechanics are optimal.

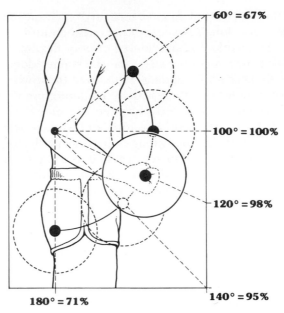

Figure 5–3. Variation in force relative to the angle of contraction, with 100 per cent representing the angle at which force is optimal. (From Wilmore, J.: Training for Sport and Activity, 2nd ed. Boston, Allyn and Bacon, 1982, with permission.)

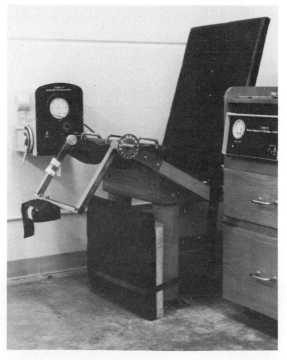

Figure 5–4. The Cybex II isokinetic muscle testing device.

In isotonic movements, therefore, the muscle is not contracting at its capacity or at a constant percentage of its capacity throughout the entire range of motion.

Isokinetic contraction is a form of dynamic contraction in which the speed of limb movement is constant. Typically, the muscle applies force against a resistance that is moving at a constant speed. Figure 5–4 illustrates a Cybex II isokinetic testing device. The lever arm, against which the subject is applying force, moves at a fixed rate of movement. The rate of movement can be adjusted to any speed between an isometric contraction at 0 degrees per second to a relatively fast speed of 300 degrees per second. Theoretically, if properly motivated, the individual can apply maximum force throughout the entire range of motion. This would be an apparent advantage over isotonic procedures, in which the muscle is taxed to its capacity only in the weakest portion of its range of motion. Isokinetic training has also been referred to as accommodating resistance training.

Variable resistance is an additional form of dynamic contraction in which the resistance is altered throughout the range of motion in an attempt to match the strength-producing potential of the muscle or muscle group. This is illustrated in Figure 5–5.

Isometric training procedures are based on the theory that strength can

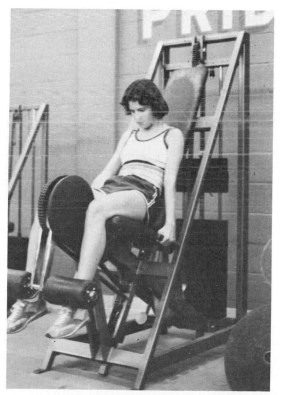

Figure 5–5. A Nautilus variable resistance weight training device.

be efficiently gained by training the muscle or muscle group against a fixed, immovable resistance. Although isometric training has been practiced for many years, it was popularized in the mid 1950s by the research of Hettinger and Muller[52] in Germany. Their initial studies indicated that strength gains of 5 per cent of the original strength value could be obtained each week as a result of only one 6-second contraction per day at only 67 per cent of maximum effort. Little additional improvement resulted with maximum effort or with repeated contractions totaling 45 seconds. Subsequent research has been unable to confirm this original work.[53] Clarke,[53] in reviewing the research literature through 1972, concluded that the best results from isometric training appear to be obtained by using maximum contractions, held for a period of 6 seconds, repeated 5 to 10 times per day. In a more recent review, Atha[54] concluded that isometric contractions, to have their greatest effect, should probably be performed at nearly maximum effort, should last long enough for all fibers in a muscle group to be fully recruited, and should be repeated several times daily.

Isotonic strength training typically involves the use of weights in the form of dumbbells, barbells, and pulleys. Two important principles govern isotonic strength training and, in fact, all forms of dynamic strength training. The principle of overload refers to the well-known fact that to gain strength through muscle training procedures, it is necessary to load the muscle beyond the point at which it is normally loaded. Closely related, the principle of progressive resistance exercise refers to the fact that as the muscle becomes stronger, it must work against a progressively greater resistance in order to continue to achieve gains in strength. To illustrate, an individual who can perform only 10 repetitions of a bench press using 150 pounds of weight will, as he weight trains and gets stronger, be able to increase his repetitions for the same weight, e.g., 14 or 15 repetitions. By adding 5 pounds of weight to the bar for a total of 155 pounds, he will reduce the maximum number of repetitions he can perform to 8 to 10. As he continues to train, his maximum number of repetitions for this new weight will continue to increase until it is time to add an additional 5 pounds of weight. Thus, there is a progressive increase in the amount of resistance, or weight, lifted.[11]

With isotonic procedures, what is the most effective procedure for training? DeLorme[55] and later DeLorme and Watkins[56] are credited with the initial efforts to systematize isotonic training procedures. They emphasized the use of heavy resistance and a low number of repetitions to develop muscular strength, as opposed to light resistance and a high number of repetitions to develop muscular endurance. Originally working with 100 repetitions divided into 7 to 10 sets, they modified this to 3 sets of 10 repetitions each. In 1951, Zinovieff[57] proposed the Oxford technique, in which 100 repetitions were performed over 10 sets, with the resistance decreasing with each progressive set as the individual fatigued.

Subsequent research has attempted to identify the best possible combination of sets, repetitions, and resistance to maximize strength gains.

Clarke,[58] in the January 1974 issue of the *Physical Fitness Research Digest,* summarized the research literature through 1973, and Atha[54] has recently conducted a review that was published in 1981. From these two reviews, it would appear that weight training should be performed at five to seven repetitions per set, with three sets of each exercise executed per training session, to maximize gains in muscle strength. The weight used for each set should be sufficient to tax the muscle maximally to fatigue by the last repetition of the set. Training frequency should be three times per week, although this can be increased to five times per week if the muscles have been preconditioned.

Isokinetic training procedures are relatively new in concept and in practice. This concept, which was introduced by Perrine in 1968,[59] is rather unique in that it does allow maximum force production throughout the full range of movement, provided the subject is properly motivated. Most isokinetic training devices also provide variation in the speed of the movement, allowing the subject to train at different velocities. Traditional weight training is performed at very slow velocities, whereas most human movement, particularly with respect to sport, is performed at relatively fast velocities. This raises the following question: Would the athlete be better off to train at faster velocities that more closely approximate the speeds at which he or she performs? Preliminary research suggests that fast speed training may, in fact, be more beneficial.[11,15] Thus, isokinetic training would seem to have at least two definite advantages over static or other dynamic forms of training: opportunity for maximum force production throughout the full range of motion and variable speed training.

Actual training procedures for isokinetic training are similar to those listed earlier for isotonic training. Typically, three sets are performed for each exercise, with five to seven repetitions at maximum force production. There may be some advantage to mixing slow and fast speed training, but this has yet to be confirmed by experimental research. As mentioned previously, accommodating resistance training is considered to be similar to isokinetic training, in that the resistance can be matched to the force-producing capabilities of the muscles at all points in the range of motion. However, with several of the commercial devices, although the resistance accommodates to the force production capabilities of the muscle, the movements are not truly isokinetic, since the speed of movement is not absolutely constant. The Hydra-Gym and the Cam II strength training devices are examples of accommodating resistance devices using hydraulics and air, respectively, to provide the accommodating resistance.

Variable resistance devices typically use several different means to alter the mechanical advantage of the lever arm, thus altering the resistance to the subject through the range of motion, even though the weight on the weight stack remains constant. The variable resistance cam used by Nautilus was illustrated in Figure 5–5. This is an ingenious device that attempts to alter the resistance of the weight stack to match the force-producing capabilities of the muscles throughout the full range of motion. The Universal Gym Centurion reduces the length of the lever arm as the subject progresses through the range of motion, decreasing the mechanical advantage and increasing the resistance.

Two additional training procedures that do not fit within the definitions of the training procedures noted previously are eccentric training and plyometric training. Eccentric training has received much interest, since a muscle can be loaded with considerably more weight eccentrically than concentrically. The research literature indicates that eccentric training is effective for increasing strength, but no more effective than concentric training.[54] Plyometric training was described by Wilt in 1975[60] but is considered to be an extension of the work of Verkhoshanski in 1966.[61] Verkhoshanski advocated a rebound jump after dropping from a fixed height. The muscle is loaded so suddenly that it is forced to yield and stretch before developing sufficient tension to arrest the motion of the load and to reverse the direction of movement.[54] Atha has described plyometric loading as a rhythmical hybrid of eccentric plus concentric activity, loading the elastic as well as the contractile components of the muscle.[54] Although the theory of plyometrics appears sound, there has not been sufficient research conducted to demonstrate its effectiveness relative to other training procedures.[54]

Which of the previously named training procedures provides the greatest gains in strength? Much early work compared isometric with isotonic training procedures and found that both procedures led to substantial increases in strength, with the isotonic procedures providing slightly greater gains in strength and substantially greater gains in muscular endurance and in muscular hypertrophy.[62] Few studies have compared isokinetic with isotonic and isometric training procedures. Atha[54] concludes that at the present time, isokinetic procedures have not been demonstrated to have superiority over other training procedures, but this may be due to an inadequate number of well-designed and controlled investigations. With respect to accommodating resistance devices, despite the claims of the manufacturers, no experimental evidence exists to demonstrate the superiority of one system over another or of accommodating resistance training procedures over other procedures.

SPECIFICITY OF STRENGTH TRAINING PROCEDURES

Over the years, the scientific community has become much more aware of the specificity of different training procedures. It is obvious that strength training will do very little to improve one's time in the marathon or that distance running will have little effect on improving the strength of the competitive weight lifter. Strength training improves strength, and distance running improves cardiorespiratory endurance capacity. This does not mean that the distance runner should not lift weights or that the weight lifter should not run, but simply that training is very specific in what it accomplishes.

With respect to strength training, there are currently two conflicting theories regarding training to improve sports performance. One theory states that the training should simulate the sport movement as closely as possible relative to anatomical movement pattern, velocity, contraction type, and contraction force.[63] The opposing theory holds that it is necessary to train only the appropriate muscle groups, i.e., there is no need to have movement-specific exercises. Sale and MacDougall,[63] in a review of research in this area, conclude that the scientific evidence to date strongly favors specificity in training. The pattern of movement has been shown to be very important relative to increases in strength with training. Thorstensson et al.[64] demonstrated this very clearly in a study in which they trained their subjects by having them perform barbell squats. The subjects were tested before and after training by performing 1-RM barbell squats and by performing an isometric leg press, both using the same muscle groups in approximately the same position. Strength gains after 8 weeks of training approached 75 per cent for the barbell squat test but averaged less than 30 per cent for the isometric leg press. Velocity of training is also highly specific, as illustrated by Coyle et al.[15] Training subjects at either a fast speed of 300 degrees per second or a relatively slow speed of 60 degrees per second, or a combination of fast and slow speeds, for maximal two-legged isokinetic knee extensions three times per week for 6 weeks, they found the improvements in strength, i.e., peak torque, to be highly specific to the speed of training. The group that trained at the high speed improved most when tested at high speeds, the group that trained at the slow speed demonstrated improvement only at the slow speed, and the combination group demonstrated intermediate changes.

Since specificity is a factor in strength development, is it also a factor when training to develop muscle power? Since most athletic events depend on power, should training be structured to emphasize power movements? Although this question has not yet been answered, the evidence previously presented relative to the specificity of training for strength would suggest that there is probably a high degree of specificity associated with training to maximize gains in power. Assuming that specificity does exist, how would one train to maximize power development? McLario[65] investigated the relative contribution of force and velocity to the development of peak power output in the bench press. Figures 5–6 and 5–7 represent the force-velocity and power-velocity relationships established in this study, respectively. Peak power was achieved at approximately 50 per cent of the 1-RM for the bench press. This would suggest that at least part of an individual's training should be performed at these low relative force outputs, emphasizing both speed and explosiveness of movement when executing the lift.

CIRCUIT WEIGHT TRAINING

Circuit training is a relatively new and innovative type of conditioning program that was developed by R. E. Morgan and G. T. Adamson in 1953 at the University of Leeds in London.[66] Circuit training can be designed to develop strength, power, muscular endurance, speed, agility, flexibility, and cardiovascular endurance. With circuit training, the individual proceeds through a series of selected exercises or activities that are performed in sequence or in a circuit. There are usually 6 to 10 stations in a circuit, which can be located inside gymnasiums, exercise rooms, or hallways or outside on courts, fields, or roof tops. The individual performs a specific exercise at each station and then proceeds to the next station. The idea is to progress

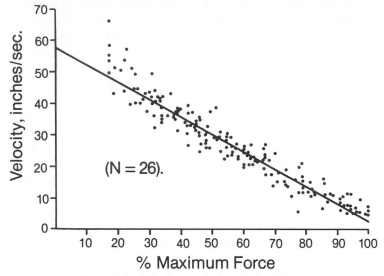

Figure 5–6. The force-velocity relationship.

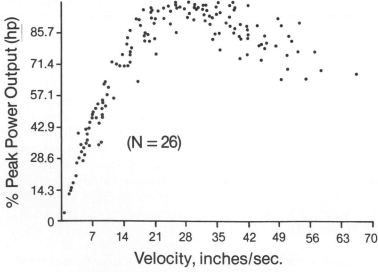

Figure 5–7. The power-velocity relationship.

through the circuit as rapidly as possible, attempting to improve either by decreasing the total time to complete the circuit or by increasing the amount of work accomplished at each station, or both.

Allen et al.[67] investigated the possibility of placing traditional weight training into a circuit training format. Traditional weight training is usually performed in a slow, methodical manner, with very short work periods and very long rest intervals. With circuit weight training, individuals work at approximately 40 to 60 per cent of their 1-RM for periods of approximately 30 seconds, with 15-second rest intervals interspersed between work periods. They start at the first station, completing as many repetitions as possible in 30 seconds, take a 15-second rest, during which they move to the next station, and then begin their second 30-second work period. This continues until they complete the six to eight stations in the circuit, and then they start their second set. The work and rest intervals can be varied to match the needs of the individual or group.

Gettman and Pollock[68] have published an excellent review of all research that has been conducted on circuit weight training since the original study of Allen et al.[67] Circuit weight training has been shown to provide modest increases in maximal oxygen uptake (see Chapter 3); major increases in strength, muscular endurance, and flexibility; and substantial alterations in body composition, i.e., increases in lean body weight and decreases in body fat.

FLEXIBILITY TRAINING PROCEDURES

Flexibility training is not difficult, requires little time and effort, and can be accomplished during either or both the warm-up and cool-down phases of the daily workout. In the performance of stretching exercises, the movement can be either static or dynamic. Dynamic stretching involves rapid or ballistic movements, e.g., bobbing or jerking, whereas static stretching involves a slow positioning of the body followed by a static stretch. As an example, with the hip flexion movement, the ballistic approach would have the individual bending forward at the waist in attempting to touch his or her toes with the fingers and hands extended downward using five or six rapid jerking or bouncing motions. In the static stretch, the individual grabs his or her ankles with the hands and slowly stretches forward, attempting to place the head on the knees. Research has shown both methods to be effective. However, it is believed that there is less danger of injury and soreness with static stretching. If a muscle contracts quickly or in a jerky motion, it will stretch the antagonist muscles, causing them to contract, thus limiting the range of dynamic motion. A firm static stretch involves the inverse myotatic reflex, which results in an inhibition of the antagonist group of muscles, allowing them to relax and enhancing the range of motion.[50]

SUMMARY

Attention must be given to maintaining optimal functioning of the musculoskeletal system. Prevention of poor posture, lower back complaints, lean tissue loss, and osteoporosis is dependent on the incorporation of a comprehensive strength and flexibility program into the daily workout. This chapter has presented the physiological foundations of both strength and flexibility and has attempted to review the most current thoughts relative to training procedures. Specific strength and flexibility exercises are presented in Chapters 7 and 8.

REFERENCES

1. Massachusetts Mutual Insurance Company: Disability income protection approved claims, 1974. World Supplement, June 1975.
2. Kraus, H., and Raab, W.: Hypokinetic Disease. Springfield, Ill, Charles C Thomas, 1961.
3. Forbes, G. B.: The adult decline in lean body mass. Hum. Biol. *48:*161–173, 1976.
4. Quenouille, M. H., Boyn, A. W., Fisher, W. B., and Leitch, I.: Statistical studies of recorded energy expenditure in man. Part 1. Basal metabolism related to sex, stature, age, climate and race. Commonwealth Agric. Bur. Tech. Comm. No. 17. Farnham Royal, Bucks, England, 1951.
5. Keys, A., Taylor, H. L., and Grande, F.: Basal metabolism and age of adult man. Metabolism *22:*579–587, 1973.
6. Birge, S. J., Jr., and Whedon, G. D.: Bone. *In* McCally, M., editor: Hypodynamics and Hypogravics. New York, Academic Press, 1968.
7. Vogel, J. M., and Whittle, M. W.: The Proceedings of the Skylab Life Sciences Symposium (NASA Technical Memorandum JSC-09275), Washington, D.C., 1974.
8. Bortz, W. M.: Disuse and aging. J.A.M.A. *248:*1203–1208, 1982.
9. Aloia, J. F., Cohn, S. H., Ostuni, J. A., Cane, R., and Ellis, K.: Prevention of involutional bone loss by exercise. Ann. Intern Med. *89:*356–358, 1978.
10. Smith, E. L., Reddan, W., and Smith, P. E.: Physical activity and calcium modalities for bone mineral increase in aged women. Med. Sci. Sports Exer. *13:*60–64, 1981.
11. Wilmore, J. H.: Training for Sport and Activity, 2nd ed. Boston, Allyn and Bacon, 1982.
12. Wilmore, J. H.: Alterations in strength, body composition and anthropometric measurements consequent to a 10-week weight training program. Med. Sci. Sports *6:*133–138, 1974.
13. Ikai, M., and Steinhaus, A. H.: Some factors modifying the expression of human strength. J. Appl. Physiol. *16:*157–163, 1961.
14. Moritani, T., and deVries, H. A.: Neural factors versus hypertrophy in the time course of muscle strength gain. Am. J. Phys. Med. *58:*115–130, 1979.
15. Coyle, E. F., Feiring, D. C., Rotkis, T. C., Cote, R. W., III, Roby, F. B., Lee, W., and Wilmore, J. H.: Specificity of power improvements through slow and fast isokinetic training. J. Appl. Physiol. *51:*1437–1442, 1981.
16. Milner-Brown, H. S., Stein, R. B., and Lee, R. G.: Synchronization of human motor units: possible roles of exercise and supraspinal reflexes. Electroencephalogr. Clin. Neurophysiol. *38:*245–254, 1975.
17. Komi, P. V., Viitasalo, J. T., Rauramaa, R., and Vihko, V.: Effect of isometric strength training on mechanical, electrical and metabolic aspects of muscle function. Eur. J. Appl. Physiol. *40:*45–55, 1978.
18. Gerchman, L., Edgerton, V. R., and Carrow, R.: Effects of physical training on the histochemistry and morphology of the ventral motor neurons. Exp. Neurol. *49:*790–801, 1975.
19. Bergstom, J.: Muscle electrolytes in man. Scand. J. Clin. Lab. Invest. *68:*11–13, 1962.
20. Costill, D. L.: A Scientific Approach to Distance Running. Los Altos, CA: Track and Field News, 1979.

21. Komi, P. V., and Karlsson, J.: Physical performance, skeletal muscle enzyme activities, and fibre types in monozygous and dizygous twins of both sexes. Acta Physiol. Scand. Suppl. 462, 1979.
22. Goldberg, A. L., Etlinger, J. D., Goldspink, D. F., and Jablecki, C.: Mechanism of work-induced hypertrophy of skeletal muscle. Med. Sci. Sports 7:248–261, 1975.
23. Goldspink, G.: The proliferation of myofibrils during muscle fibre growth, J. Cell Sci. 6: 593–604, 1970.
24. Edgerton, V. R.: Exercise and the growth and development of muscle tissue. In Rarick, G. L., editor: Physical Activity Human Growth and Development. New York, Academic Press, 1973.
25. Gonyea, W. J.: Role of exercise in inducing increases in skeletal muscle fiber number. J. Appl. Physiol. 48:421–426, 1980.
26. Gollnick, P. D., Timson, B. F., Moore, R. L., and Riedy, M.: Muscular enlargement and number of fibers in skeletal muscles of rats. J. Appl. Physiol. 5:936–943, 1981.
27. Larsson, L.: Morphological and functional characteristics of the aging skeletal muscle in man: a cross-sectional study. Acta Physiol. Scand. Suppl. 457, 1978.
28. Grimby, G., Danneskiold-Samsoe, B., Hvid, K., and Saltin, B.: Morphology and enzymatic capacity in arm and leg muscles in 78–81 year old men and women. Acta Physiol. Scand. 115:125–134, 1982.
29. Moritani, T., and deVries, H. A.: Potential for gross muscle hypertrophy in older men. J. Gerontol. 35:672–682, 1980.
30. Haggmark, T., and Eriksson, E.: Cylinder or mobile cast brace after knee ligament surgery. Am. J. Sports Med. 7:48–56, 1979.
31. Grimby, G., Gustafsson, E., Peterson, L., and Renstrom, P.: Quadriceps function and training after knee ligament surgery. Med. Sci. Sports Exer. 12:70–75, 1980.
32. Sargeant, A. J., Davies, C. T. M., Edwards, R. H. T., Maunder, C., and Young, A.: Functional and structural changes after disuse of human muscle. Clin. Sci. Molec. Med. 52:337–342, 1977.
33. MacDougall, J. D., Elder, G. C. B., Sale, D. G., Moroz, J. R., and Sutton, J. R.: Effects of strength training and immobilization on human muscle fibers. Eur. J. Appl. Physiol. 43: 25–34, 1980.
34. Booth, F. W.: Time course of muscular atrophy during immobilization of hindlimbs in rats. J. Appl. Physiol. 43:656–661, 1977.
35. Booth, F. W., and Seider, M. J.: Early change in skeletal muscle protein synthesis after limb immobilization of rats. J. Appl. Physiol. 47:974–977, 1979.
36. Wilmore, J. H., Tischler, M. E., Percy, E. C., Rotkis, T. C., Roby, F. B., Stanforth, P. R., Constable, S. H., Buono, M. J., Maxwell, B. D., and Sather, T. M.: Alterations in cardiovascular, metabolic and muscle function consequent to 17 days of single-leg casting. Int. J. Sports Med. 4:142, 1983.
37. Laubach, L. L.: Comparative muscular strength of men and women: a review of the literature. Aviat. Space Environ. Med. 47:534–542, 1976.
38. Hosler, W. W., and Morrow, J. R.: Arm and leg strength compared between young women and men after allowing for differences in body size and composition. Ergonomics 25: 309–313, 1982.
39. Brown, C. H., and Wilmore, J. H.: The effects of maximal resistance training on the strength and body composition of women athletes. Med. Sci. Sports 6:174–177, 1974.
40. Mayhew, J. L., and Gross, P. M.: Body composition changes in young women with high resistance weight training. Res. Q. 45:433–440, 1974.
41. Fox, E. L., and Mathews, D. K.: The Physiological Basis of Physical Education and Athletics, 3rd ed. Philadelphia, Saunders College Publishing, 1981.
42. deVries, H. A.: Quantitative electromyographic investigation of the spasm theory of muscle pain. Am. J. Phys. Med. 45:119–134, 1966.
43. Abraham, W. M.: Factors in delayed muscle soreness. Med. Sci. Sports 9:11–20, 1977.
44. Abraham, W. M.: Exercise-induced muscle soreness. Phys. Sportsmed. 7:57–60, 1979.
45. Hough, T.: Ergographic studies in muscular soreness. Am. J. Physiol. 7:76–92, 1902.
46. Talag, T. S.: Residual muscular soreness as influenced by concentric, eccentric and static contractions. Res. Q. 44:458–469, 1973.
47. Assmussen, E.: Observations on experimental muscle soreness. Acta Rheumatol. Scand. 1:19–116, 1956.
48. Komi, P. V., and Buskirk, E. R.: The effect of eccentric and concentric muscle activity on tension and electrical activity of human muscle. Ergonomics 15:417–434, 1972.

49. Komi, P. V., and Rusko, H.: Quantitative evaluation of mechanical and electrical changes during fatigue loading of eccentric and concentric work. Scand. J. Rehab. Med. (Suppl.) *3*:121–126, 1974.
50. deVries, H. A.: Physiology of Exercise for Physical Education and Athletics, 3rd ed. Dubuque, Iowa, Wm. C. Brown, 1980.
51. Johns, R. J., and Wright, V.: Relative importance of various tissues in joint stiffness. J. Appl. Physiol. *17*:824–828, 1962.
52. Hettinger, T., and Muller, E. A.: Muskelleistung und Muskel Training. Arbeitsphysiol. *15*:111–126, 1953.
53. Clarke, D. H.: Adaptations in strength and muscular endurance resulting from exercise. *In* Wilmore, J. H., editor: Exercise and Sport Sciences Reviews, Vol. 1. New York, Academic Press, 1973.
54. Atha, J.: Strengthening muscle. *In* Miller, D. I., editor: Exercise and Sport Sciences Reviews, Vol. 9. Philadelphia, The Franklin Institute Press, 1982.
55. DeLorme, T. L.: Restoration of muscle power by heavy resistance exercise. J. Bone Joint Surg. *27*:645–667, 1945.
56. DeLorme, T. L., and Watkins, A. L.: Technics of progressive resistance exercise. Arch. Phys. Med. *29*:263–273, 1948.
57. Zinovieff, A. N.: Heavy resistance exercises: the Oxford technique. Br. J. Phys. Med. *14*: 129–132, 1951.
58. Clarke, H. H.: Development of muscular strength and endurance. Physical Fitness Research Digest, Series 4, No. 1, January 1974.
59. Perrine, J. J.: Isokinetic exercise and the mechanical energy potentials of muscle. J. Health Phys. Ed. Rec. *39*:40–44, 1968.
60. Wilt, F.: Plyometrics: what it is—how it works. Athlet. J. *55*:89–90, 1975.
61. Verkhoshanski, Y.: Perspectives in the improvement of speed-strength preparation of jumpers. Track and Field *9*:11–12, 1966.
62. Clarke, H. H: Strength development and motor-sports improvement. Physical Fitness Research Digest, Series 4, No. 4, October, 1974.
63. Sale, D., and MacDougall, D.: Specificity in strength training; a review for the coach and athlete. Science Periodical on Research and Technology in Sport. Ottawa, The Coaching Association of Canada, March 1981.
64. Thorstensson, A., Karlsson, J., Viitasalo, J.T., Luhtanen, P., and Komi, P.V.: Effect of strength training on EMG of human skeletal muscle. Acta Physiol. Scand. *94*: 313–318, 1975
65. McLario, D. J.: The Contribution of Force and Velocity in the Development of Peak Power Output. M.S. thesis, University of Arizona, 1981.
66. Morgan, R. E., and Adamson, G. T.: Circuit Weight Training. London, G. Bell and Sons, 1961.
67. Allen, T. E., Byrd, R. J., and Smith, D. P.: Hemodynamic consequences of circuit weight training. Res. Q. *47*:299–306, 1976.
68. Gettman, L. R., and Pollock, M. L.: Circuit weight training: a critical review of its physiological benefits. Phys. Sportsmed. *9*:44–60, 1981.

PRESCRIPTION FOR PROGRAMS OF PREVENTION AND REHABILITATION

Chapter 6

MEDICAL SCREENING AND EVALUATION PROCEDURES

PRELIMINARY CONSIDERATIONS

This chapter will focus on the medical screening and evaluation procedures necessary for participants to enter an exercise program safely. These procedures should be helpful in giving participants advice about their health and behavior as related to physical fitness and risk for the development of coronary artery disease (CAD), an exercise prescription, and monitoring the progress of their health maintenance and exercise program. Information and test procedures usually include a medical history, CAD risk factor analysis, and physical fitness assessment. The physical fitness assessment will include test items in the following areas: cardiorespiratory (functional capacity), body composition, muscular strength and endurance, and flexibility. The diagnosis and medical treatment of CAD is discussed in detail in other texts;[1,2] thus this chapter will emphasize the use of tests as they relate to participants entering a health maintenance and rehabilitation exercise program.

Preliminary information should include such items as a physical examination or consultation with the family physician or both, completion of a medical history questionnaire and its discussion, explanation and signing of an informed consent form, and, if possible, a symptom-limited graded exercise test (SL-GXT). The SL-GXT is used to determine functional capacity and to monitor the electrocardiogram (ECG) and blood pressure as well as other signs of exercise intolerance.

MEDICAL HISTORY QUESTIONNAIRE

The medical history form should include a record of personal and family history of CAD and the associated risk factors, present medication and treatment, eating habits and diet analysis, smoking history, and current physical activity pattern. In addition, any other pertinent medical problems and physical disabilities should be listed. Thus, the information obtained in the preliminary evaluation should help to identify in advance the person who might be classified at high risk for testing and program participation. Data from Bruce et al.[3] show the importance of a medical history in differentiating high- and low-risk patients. As will be discussed later in this chapter, knowledge of risk for CAD has importance in the diagnostic and prognostic interpretation of the exercise test. See Appendix A, Figure A–1, for an example of a medical history questionnaire. For mass screening to determine who needs a more extensive medical follow-up before entering an exercise program, a less complex, briefer medical questionnaire (PAR Q) has been used successfully in the Canadian Province of British Columbia.[4]

INFORMED CONSENT

The informed consent form should provide the participant with an adequate explanation and understanding of the tests and program and the potential risk and discomforts that may be involved. In this way, an individual should know exactly what is involved before testing and participating in an exercise program. All testing information should be held in strict confidence and not be released to anyone without permission. In addition, participants should not be coerced or inadequately advised with the objective of obtaining a better performance on a test or increasing adherence to a program. Such procedures are unethical, violate human rights, and are against policy established by the federal government and most professional organizations.[5] If the consent form is being used for research purposes, a statement concerning withdrawal without prejudice of future care is appropriate. See Appendix A, Figures A–2 and A–3, for examples of informed consent forms. In addition, refer to publications provided by the American College of Sports Medicine,[6] the American Heart Association,[7] and others.[8-11] The informed consent form shown in Appendix A, Figure A–2, is used when the main purpose of the GXT is for diagnostic purposes and the form in Figure A–3 is used for the purpose of entering an exercise program. An example of a form used for an outpatient cardiac rehabilitation program is shown in Appendix B, Figure B–7. In general, the informed consent form should contain certain basic components but should be individualized for each laboratory or program.

MEDICAL EVALUATION AND SUPERVISION

Is it important to have a physical examination and undergo tests before starting an exercise program? Ideally, the answer is yes, although there should be some flexibility in the requirements, depending upon the participant's age, health status, family history, and current fitness level. It is desirable for all persons to have a complete physical examination, including a 12-lead resting and exercise ECG before their physical fitness evaluation. As mentioned earlier, the more information known about a participant before testing and training, the safer and more accurate the exercise prescription. In reality, the ideal situation is not always practical. In addition, the risk for a major coronary event for young, low-risk persons is extremely low (see Chapter 8 for more details on risk for major coronary events for cardiac and noncardiac patients). The impracticality and considerable cost to the medical system or individual for doing mass medical testing (GXT) have been discussed by Shephard.[12] Thus, it does not appear to be realistic to recommend comprehensive medical evaluations for the total population. Mass nonmedical fitness evaluations have been successfully used in Canada for years.[12, 13]

If a GXT is for a diagnostic purpose or is performed on persons with known CAD or who are at high risk for such disease, direct medical supervision is necessary. Nondiagnostic tests on apparently healthy individuals can be safely administered without direct physician supervision. An example of the nondiagnostic test would be the physical fitness test used and administered by the YMCA.[14] For years, thousands of assessments of cardiorespiratory fitness for the purpose of entering an exercise program have been safely administered by allied health (nonphysician) personnel.

What is meant by low- and high-risk individuals? The term "at risk" is usually associated with a person's risk for having CAD. A low-risk person might be asymptomatic (no chest discomfort, shortness of breath, and so on) with no previous history of CAD and no known primary risk factors for CAD (see Chapter 1 for CAD risk factors). Therefore, for persons who are symptomatic of CAD, or who have known significant risk factors for CAD, a medical examination, including a resting and exercise ECG, is strongly recommended.

Is age alone a criterion for having a medical examination and diagnostic GXT before entering an exercise program? There is no set answer to this question. When the guidelines for exercise testing and exercise prescription were developed by the American College of Sports Medicine,[6] there was a wide variation of opinion: Some recommended that everyone (young and old) should have a GXT, and some favored a minimum age of 45 to 50. Most felt that a GXT was important or necessary for men between 30 and 45 years of age. The final agreed-upon recommendation was age 35. A recent publication by the National Heart, Lung, and Blood Institute recommends that asymptomatic, low-risk individuals over age 60 should see their doctor before starting an exercise program.[15] The recent popular application of the old theory developed by Bayes[16,17] would suggest that the recommendation by the American College of Sports Medicine is too conservative. The significance of a GXT to predict future events in an asymptomatic population is not significant until after age 40 for men and 50 for women.[16,17] In summary, in the absence of symptoms and primary risk factors, age in itself does not seem to be a strong indicator for requiring a physical examination or diagnostic GXT before age 40 to 45 for men and 50 to 55 for women.

RISK FACTOR ANALYSIS

Several risk factor profile charts are available for use. The problem with most charts is their lack of validity. That is, they have been developed on the basis that risk factors for CAD are important predictors, with cutoff points (high-low) and weighting factors (relative strength of predictor) arbitrarily determined. The general cardiovascular risk profile developed from the Framingham Study[18] is one of the few validated profiles. It uses age, sex, serum cholesterol, cigarette smoking, systolic blood pressure, glucose intolerance, and left ventricular hypertrophy by ECG criteria for calculating risk. From these data, a *Coronary Risk Handbook* was published by the American Heart Association.[19]

TABLE 6-1. RISK OF DEVELOPING CORONARY HEART DISEASE

	RELATIVE LEVEL OF RISK				
RISK FACTOR	*Very Low*	*Low*	*Moderate*	*High*	*Very High*
Blood pressure (mmHg)					
Systolic	<110	120	130–140	150–160	>170
Diastolic	<70	76	82–88	94–100	>106
Cigarettes (per day)	Never or none in 1 yr	5	10–20	30–40	>50
Cholesterol (mg/dl)	180	200	200–240	260–280	>300
Cholesterol (mg/dl) ÷ HDL* (mg/dl)	<3.0	<4.0	<4.5	5.2	>7.0
Triglycerides (mg/dl)	<50	<100	130	200	>300
Glucose (mg/dl)	<80	90	100–110	120–130	>140
Body fat (%)					
Men	12	16	20	25	>30
Women	16	20	25	32	>40
Stress-tension	Never	Almost	Occasional	Frequent	Nearly constant
Physical activity (minutes/week) above 6 Kcal/min (5 METs)† or	240	180–120	100	80–60	<30
above 60% HR max reserve	120	90	30	0	0
ECG abnormality (ST depression-mv)‡	0	0	0.05	0.10	0.20
Family history of premature heart attack (blood relative) §	0	0	1	2	3+
Age	<30	35	40	50	>60

* HDL = high density lipoprotein.

† A MET is equal to the oxygen cost at rest. One MET is generally equal to 3.5 ml/kg·min^{-1} of oxygen uptake or 1.2 Kcal/min.

‡ Other ECG abnormalities are also potentially dangerous and are not listed here.

§ Premature heart attack refers to those occurring in persons younger than 60 years of age.

(Adapted with permission from Pollock, M.L., Wilmore, J.H., and Fox, S.M.: Health and Fitness Through Physical Activity. New York, John Wiley and Sons, 1978.)

Does this mean that nonvalidated risk factor profile charts should not be used? No, not necessarily. As mentioned in Chapter 1, many significant risk factors have been identified, and an increased number of risk factors dramatically increases the risk for premature manifestations of CAD. As teaching tools for identifying risk factors and planning for their modification, some of these can be useful. Problems lie in their application to the prediction of future events.

How accurately can future events be predicted from coronary risk profiles? The Framingham Study cardiovascular risk profile was developed from 5,209 men and women who had clinical evaluations every 2 years and continuous surveillance for morbidity and mortality.[18] The 10 per cent of persons (ninetieth percentile) identified as at the highest risk accounted for 20 per cent of the 8-year incidence of CAD and 33 per cent of the 8-year incidence of atherothrombotic brain infarction, hypertensive heart disease, and intermittent claudication. These data show that the profile is significant in predicting high- and low-risk persons but is less than perfect. Thus, it is suggested that risk factor analyses (profiles) be used with caution and their predictability not overstated.

Table 6–1 is a risk factor profile chart recommended for use with participants entering a health maintenance and exercise program. In addition, see Appendix A, Tables A–1 to A–10, for age- and sex-adjusted norms for many of these variables. For variables listed in Table 6–1, the relative risk scale has not been validated but is estimated from published data. Additional years of inquiry will be necessary before more definitive results can be presented. As mentioned earlier, the chart should be used only for educational and descriptive purposes. In interpreting the risk factor profile for others, one should tell people that being at high risk in more than one factor greatly increases their chance of developing CAD. For example, the chances of developing CAD jumps from onefold to nearly fourfold when a person proceeds from having one to three primary risk factors.

For the purpose of rating potential risk, whether a patient has primary or secondary risk factors is important. As mentioned in Chapter 1, cigarette smoking, hypercholesterolemia, and hypertension are the three primary risk factors for the development of CAD. Having one primary risk factor would place a person at moderate risk, and two to three factors would mean high risk. Having one or two secondary factors puts one in a low-risk category, and having three to four factors or more puts one in the moderate- and high-risk categories, respectively.

Although most people with risk factors can be safely evaluated and started on an exercise program, under certain conditions it might be recommended that individuals not exercise. Conditions contraindicating exercise would include congestive heart failure, acute myocardial infarction, acute infectious diseases, severe valvular heart disease, dangerous dysrhythmias, severe angina pectoris with and without effort, and active myocarditis. Chapter 8 lists absolute and relative contraindications to exercise that can also be used for GXT. It also names other medical conditions that are considered of a less serious nature but still require special precautions during exercise testing and prescription.

PHYSICAL FITNESS EVALUATION

Thus far, we have discussed the desirability of having certain preliminary information and a medical examination before entering an exercise program. In addition to medical screening, a thorough physical fitness evaluation is also recommended. Although there is some duplication in classifying tests, the main differences between medical screening tests and physical fitness tests are as follows: (1) medical tests classify a person's status relative to health and disease and can provide an estimation of risk for developing disease, and (2) physical fitness evaluations classify a person relative to status of fitness. The results from both the medical and the fitness tests are used as a basis for an exercise prescription and as a baseline for future comparison. Like the medical examination, there can be some flexibility in the fitness testing program, depending upon individual health status, age, current fitness and activity level, as well as the presence of CAD and other risks. Table 6–2 lists the major categories of fitness and the test items that will be discussed. Although the physical fitness evaluation can be thought of in broader terms, we feel that these categories and test items are sufficient for the basic needs of the adult population entering an exercise program.

With the knowledge that the needs of patients and nonpatients often differ and that the amount of equipment and of technical and medical expertise varies with laboratories, three plans for testing are suggested. The test items listed in Table 6–2 become less complex and expensive from plan A to plan C. In some cases, the level of accuracy and diagnostic capability of the tests are also less between plans. For example, exercise tests listed under plan C, cardiorespiratory, should not be used as diagnostic tests. The maximal field type of test, which include a 1- to 2-mile run, are not recommended for patients with CAD or at high risk for CAD or for those without recent jogging-running experience. Medical advisors and program directors, as well as the participants, should take the cost, risk, and feasibility aspects of testing into consideration before setting up a test battery. Except for the blood sample measures, each aspect of testing listed in Table 6–2 will be discussed in the following sections.

SPECIAL CONSIDERATIONS IN THE SELECTION OF TESTS AND PERSONNEL

Often the type of test battery administered to participants depends on four major factors: time, expense, qualifications of personnel, and the population to be tested. If large numbers of individuals have to be tested in a short time, the test items may be limited to a less sophisticated test battery.

TABLE 6-2. RECOMMENDED TESTING PROGRAM FOR ADULTS

FITNESS COMPONENT	PLAN A*	PLAN B†	PLAN C‡
Cardiorespiratory Rest	Heart rate, blood pressure, ECG	Same as Plan A	Heart rate, blood pressure
Exercise	Symptom-limited GXT with heart rate, blood pressure and ECG monitoring and actual assessment of aerobic capacity	Symptom-limited GXT test with heart rate, blood pressure and ECG monitoring (aerobic capacity estimated)	Submaximal test without ECG and blood pressure monitoring and maximal field type of test (aerobic capacity estimated)
Body composition	Per cent fat by underwater weighing or equivalent (should include determination of residual volume), anthropometry (skinfold and girth measures, height and weight)	Per cent fat by skinfold and/or girth measures, height and weight	Same as Plan B
	Determine ideal weight	Same as Plan A	Same as Plan A
Blood measures	Serum cholesterol, triglycerides, glucose, high density lipoprotein (HDL-C)	Serum cholesterol, triglycerides and glucose	Serum cholesterol
Strength§	One-repetition maximum bench press	Same as Plan A	Same as Plan A
Muscular§ endurance	All-out push-ups, bent leg Sit-ups for 1 minute	Same as Plan A Same as Plan A	Same as Plan A Same as Plan A
Flexibility	Sit and reach	Same as Plan A	Same as Plan A

* Most preferred plan of testing physical fitness and risk factors for coronary heart disease.
† Next most preferred plan of testing.
‡ Least preferred plan of testing; cardiorespiratory tests not used for diagnostic purposes.
§ May not be appropriate for hypertensive and high-risk individuals.
(Adapted with permission from Pollock, M.L., Wilmore, J.H., and Fox, S.M.: Health and Fitness Through Physical Activity. New York, John Wiley and Sons, 1978.)

161

If high-risk patients are involved, the GXT with ECG and blood pressure monitoring should always be used.

With sedentary persons older than 40 years of age or with high-risk individuals, a physician should be present during exercise testing. Although for this same group, field tests for determination of cardiorespiratory fitness —e.g., a 1- to 2-mile run—should not be attempted, they are acceptable for use with young persons or middle-aged individuals who have been carefully screened and have had recent experience in jogging or running. A more definitive statement concerning subject safety has been established by the American Heart Association's Committee on Exercise.[20] It states the following:

> **Emergency equipment and qualified personnel should be available for exercise testing of all patients. Patients with known or suspected heart disease or dysfunction should not be tested without a qualified physician at the site or in the immediate area (within 30 seconds) in order to provide life saving emergency care. In the case of younger individuals (under age 35), free of clinical abnormalities or increased risk factors, the untoward responses to exercise are extremely uncommon. Direct physician presence is not considered necessary provided the health care personnel directing the sessions are trained to the satisfaction of the responsible physician in cardiopulmonary resuscitation (CPR) and emergency cardiac care (ECC) according to standards set by the American Heart Association and the Committee on Emergency Medical Services of the National Academy of Sciences–National Research Council, Division of Medical Sciences.**

The expense often dictates the kind of equipment that will be available for testing. If funds are limited, the most important pieces of equipment for GXT would be an ergometer, ECG recorder, and blood pressure apparatus. For diagnostic testing, the availability of emergency supplies and equipment (crash cart, defibrillator) is mandatory. Next, an oscilloscope and possibly a cardiotachometer could be purchased. The oscilloscope would allow the tester to observe the ECG at all times, and the cardiotachometer provides an instant visual readout of heart rate (HR). Multiple channel recorders have become the standard for diagnostic ECG evaluation, with many having computer averaging capabilities.

As mentioned in earlier chapters, $\dot{V}O_2$ max is considered one of the best measures of cardiorespiratory fitness. If so, why has not anything been mentioned about the purchase of equipment to be used for this procedure? In general, $\dot{V}O_2$ max can be estimated accurately from performance time on a treadmill, cycle ergometer, or field tests (running); thus actual measurement may not be necessary (see Tables 6–3 to 6–5).[20–24] Although this is true, methodological problems have been shown potentially to cause gross errors in estimation.[24–28] More details concerning the issue of predicting $\dot{V}O_2$ max rather than its actual measurement will be discussed in more detail later in this chapter. Other equipment—e.g., skinfold fat calipers, hydrostatic weighing tanks, and so on—will be discussed later.

Having the right personnel available for various phases of a physical

TABLE 6–3. ESTIMATION OF MAXIMUM OXYGEN UPTAKE—METs* FOR VARIOUS PROTOCOLS AND FITNESS CLASSIFICATIONS FOR EXERCISE PRESCRIPTION FOR DIFFERENT LEVELS OF CARDIORESPIRATORY FITNESS

FITNESS CLASSIFICATION	MAXIMUM O$_2$ UPTAKE ml/kg·min⁻¹	METs	TREADMILL PROTOCOLS					Åstrand (mph)	1.5-MILE RUN (min:sec)
			Bruce†	Ellestad†	Balke†,‡ (3.3 mph)	Balke†,§ (3.0 mph)	Naughton†,‖		
1	7	2	—	—	—	—	2:07	—	—
	10.5	3	—	—	1:00	3:00	4:17	—	—
	14	4	2:30	2:00	2:00	4:00	6:28	—	—
2	17.5	5	4:00	3:00	3:00	7:30	8:38	—	—
	21.0	6	6:00	4:45	6:00	10:30	10:49	—	—
	24.5	7	7:20	5:00	8:00	13:30	12:59	—	—
3	28.0	8	8:20	5:45	9:45	17:00	15:10	5.00	18:45
	31.5	9	9:15	6:40	12:00	19:30	17:20	5.25	16:30
	35.0	10	10:10	7:30	14:30	22:00	19:30	5.50	15:00
4	38.5	11	11:00	8:20	17:00	24:00	21:40	5.75	13:00
	42.0	12	12:00	9:10	19:00	27:00	23:51	6.25	12:00
5	45.5	13	12:45	10:15	21:30	30:00	26:01	6.50	11:00
	49.0	14	13:40	11:15	24:15	33:00	28:12	7.00	10:00
6	52.5	15	14:30	—	26:15	36:00	30:22	7.50	9:30
	56.0	16	15:15	—	27:45	—	32:33	8.00	9:00
7	59.5	17	16:10	—	29:00	—	—	8.50	8:15
	63.0	18	17:00	—	30:00	—	—	9.00	7:45
	66.5	19	18:00	—	31:15	—	—	9.25	7:15
8	70.0	20	19:20	—	32:00	—	—	9.75	6:52
	73.5	21	21:00	—	33:45	—	—	10.50	6:30
	77.0	22	22:30	—	35:45	—	—	11.00	6:10

* MET refers to metabolic equivalent above the resting metabolic level. Value at rest is approximately 3.5 ml/kg·min⁻¹.

† Data expressed in minutes and seconds of test protocol (duration completed).

‡ Balke protocol, 3.3 mph, at 1 per cent grade increase in work level per minute (Fig. 6–1).

§ Balke protocol, 3.0 mph, at 2.5 per cent grade increase in work level every 3 minutes.

‖ Naughton protocol, modified to use 2-minute rather than 3-minute stages.

(Adapted with permission from Pollock, M.L., Wilmore, J.H., and Fox, S.M.: Health and Fitness Through Physical Activity. New York, John Wiley and Sons, 1978.)

fitness program is important. Although the physician and the program director have overall control of the program, they must have qualified exercise leaders (specialists) and laboratory technicians to help them conduct the program. Exercise leaders should have a background in functional anatomy, exercise physiology, behavioral psychology and group dynamics, emergency procedures, and exercise prescription. The laboratory technician should have expertise in the mechanics of individual test procedures, screening a participant before exercise testing, administration of tests, emergency procedures, and data analysis. Programs for training personnel for such positions are becoming readily available in many universities. A certification program for program directors, exercise specialists, fitness instructors, and exercise test technologists is now available through the auspices of the American College of Sports Medicine.[6]

EVALUATION PROCEDURE

In general, if the medical history form is filled out at home before the testing session, the testing procedures can be completed in approximately 2 to 3 hours. If possible, a 15- to 30-minute orientation to the laboratory and various procedures may be helpful before the test day. The orientation may relieve apprehensions associated with testing and improve performance on the GXT.[11,27–30] The orientation should include an explanation of all tests, familiarization with laboratory facilities, and, if possible, practice in treadmill walking (or other ergometer) and with head gear apparatus (mouthpiece) and so on used in determining aerobic capacity.

Precise instructions should be given to the participant before reporting

TABLE 6–4. ENERGY EXPENDITURE IN METS DURING BICYCLE ERGOMETRY*

BODY WEIGHT		WORK RATE ON BICYCLE ERGOMETER (KPM/MIN AND WATTS)												
		75	150	300	450	600	750	900	1050	1200	1350	1500	1650	1800 (Kpm/min)
(kg)	(lb)	12	25	50	75	100	125	150	175	200	225	250	275	300 (watts)
20	44	4.0	6.0	10.0	14.0	18.0	22.0							
30	66	3.4	4.7	7.3	10.0	12.7	15.3	17.9	20.7	23.3				
40	88	3.0	4.0	6.0	8.0	10.0	12.0	14.0	16.0	18.0	20.0	22.0		
50	110	2.8	3.6	5.2	6.8	8.4	10.0	11.5	13.2	14.8	16.3	18.0	19.6	21.1
60	132	2.7	3.3	4.7	6.0	7.3	8.7	10.0	11.3	12.7	14.0	15.3	16.7	18.0
70	154	2.6	3.1	4.3	5.4	6.6	7.7	8.8	10.0	11.1	12.2	13.4	14.0	15.7
80	176	2.5	3.0	4.0	5.0	6.0	7.0	8.0	9.0	10.0	11.0	12.0	13.0	14.0
90	198	2.4	2.9	3.8	4.7	5.6	6.4	7.3	8.2	9.1	10.0	10.9	11.8	12.6
100	220	2.4	2.8	3.6	4.4	5.2	6.0	6.8	7.6	8.4	9.2	10.0	10.8	11.6
110	242	2.4	2.7	3.4	4.2	4.9	5.6	6.3	7.1	7.8	8.5	9.3	10.0	10.7
120	264	2.3	2.7	3.3	4.0	4.7	5.3	6.0	6.7	7.3	8.0	8.7	9.3	10.0

*Oxygen uptake $(ml/kg \cdot min^{-1})$ may be determined by multiplying the MET value by 3.5. These data are based on steady-state exercise; thus, caution should be taken in extrapolating to $\dot{V}O_2$ max. Data may overpredict $\dot{V}O_2$ max by 1 to 2 METs. See section on prediction of $\dot{V}O_2$ max for details.
(Reprinted with permission from American College of Sports Medicine: Guidelines for Graded Exercise Testing and Exercise Prescription, 2nd ed. Philadelphia, Lea and Febiger, 1980.)

to the laboratory. These instructions should include date and time of test; shoes and clothing requirements; and information concerning eating, drinking of alcohol or stimulants (coffee and so forth), taking medications, and prior exercise. If testing is in the morning, avoidance of fluids (except water), smoking, and breakfast may be appropriate. Most laboratories require a minimum of 2 to 3 hours of abstention from eating, drinking, and smoking before reporting for testing.[11,28-30] If serum lipids are to be determined, refraining from alcohol consumption and vigorous exercise for 24 hours and having, at minimum, a 12-hour fast is recommended.[31, 32] Vigorous exercise within 24 hours may also affect serum glucose.[32] Diabetics should be allowed to keep their dietary habits and injections of insulin as regular as possible. Extremes in hydration or dehydration should be avoided, since they can affect endurance performance, body weight, and results from hydrostatic weighing (body composition).[33,34] The 24-hour history questionnaire shown in Appendix A, Figure A-4, may be helpful for use in standardizing and keeping a record of the participant's condition when reporting to the laboratory.

For standardization purposes, the organization of the testing session is important. The testing session should begin with quiet (resting) tests. Under plan A, Table 6-2, this would include resting HR, blood pressure, ECG, and blood drawing. Depending on the standardized length of time used for relaxation before determining HR and blood pressure and the time taken for drawing a blood sample, the quiet tests should take approximately 20

TABLE 6-5. ENERGY EXPENDITURE IN METS DURING STEPPING AT DIFFERENT RATES ON STEPS OF DIFFERENT HEIGHTS*

STEP HEIGHT		STEPS/MIN			
(cm)	(in)	12	18	24	30
0	0	1.2	1.8	2.0	2.4
4	1.6	2.1	2.5	2.9	3.7
8	3.2	2.4	3.0	3.5	4.5
12	4.7	2.8	3.5	4.1	5.3
16	6.3	3.1	4.0	4.7	6.1
20	7.9	3.4	4.5	5.4	7.0
24	9.4	3.8	5.0	6.0	7.8
28	11.0	4.1	5.5	6.7	8.6
32	12.6	4.4	6.0	7.3	9.4
36	14.2	4.8	6.5	8.0	10.3
40	15.8	5.1	7.0	8.7	11.7

*Oxygen uptake $(ml/kg \cdot min^{-1})$ may be determined by multiplying the MET value by 3.5. These data are based on steady-state exercise; thus, caution should be taken in extrapolating to $\dot{V}O_2$ max. Data may overpredict $\dot{V}O_2$ max by 1 to 2 METs. See section on prediction of $\dot{V}O_2$ max for details.

(Reprinted with permission from American College of Sports Medicine: Guidelines for Graded Exercise Testing and Exercise Prescription, 2nd ed. Philadelphia, Lea and Febiger, 1980.)

to 30 minutes. Before quiet testing, usually a 5- to 15-minute rest period is recommended.

Body composition measures should be administered next. If both anthropometric and underwater weighing measures are taken, allow 30 to 45 minutes for testing. Anthropometric measures take approximately 5 minutes. Body composition measures are followed by the determination of strength, muscular endurance, and flexibility (30 minutes) and then by the GXT (45 minutes).

Once the testing has been completed, time should be scheduled to go over test results and give recommendations.

INITIAL EVALUATION. The medical and fitness evaluations are used as a basis for exercise prescription. The results of the initial tests are also used as a baseline for future comparisons. With respect to the latter, tests are excellent motivators for the participants in that they provide objective evidence about their initial status (health and fitness), as well as the progress and benefits attained from a regular exercise program. In contrast, if one is irregular in attendance or not devoting sufficient time and effort to training, testing may give added motivation to improve adherence or change the exercise prescription.

For the first evaluation, many persons are apprehensive and thus may not do as well on some test items. Apprehension will adversely affect most of the resting and submaximal cardiorespiratory tests. Heart rate, blood pressure, and metabolic measures are elevated under these conditions.[28] Many tests are sensitive to time of day and to the effects of eating or smoking before testing.[28,35] These factors adversely affect resting and submaximal cardiorespiratory tests. Individuals usually improve their performance on a GXT with some practice. If a tester cannot use ideal conditions (fasting, time of day) for testing, then the conditions in which the tests are administered should be noted and standardized for future comparisons.

Heart rate and blood pressure are particularly susceptible to time of day, smoking, apprehension, coffee and other stimulants, food, tension, temperature, and so on. Therefore, it is particularly important to standardize conditions for resting and submaximal HR tests. Maximal HR, $\dot{V}O_2$ max, performance, and other related variables are usually not significantly affected by time of day, moderate amounts of food or drink, tension, or anxiety. Most cardiorespiratory tests should allow a minimum of 2 to 3 hours of controlled conditions before testing. For more details on the standardization and interpretation of submaximal and maximal tests, refer to the work of Taylor et al.[28]

FOLLOW-UP EVALUATIONS. How often should follow-up examinations be administered? Unless something unusual is found in one's initial tests or unless a participant is considered at high risk or has had a change in health status, a regular medical examination may not be necessary. There is varied opinion on this subject. Many recommend a physical examination every 2 to 3 years for persons older than 40 years of age and yearly after 50 years of age. Under usual circumstances, a physical fitness test battery should be administered after approximately 3 to 6 months and again after 1 year of training. Yearly fitness evaluations are recommended after the first year.

Although fitness takes many months to attain, a progress check at 3 to 6 months is important for evaluating the participant's progress. With this information, the participant's exercise prescription can be verified and modified as necessary. Not only does the progress check give the physician and program director vital information about how the participant is responding to the program but also it acts as a motivational tool to the participant. Many times interest wanes about 10 to 15 weeks after beginning training; therefore, a motivational lift can help at this stage.

RESTING EVALUATION. The resting, or quiet test, will vary between plans A, B, and C but could include the determination of resting HR, blood pressure, serum lipids and glucose, and a standard 12-lead ECG. Standards for HR and blood pressure, serum cholesterol, triglycerides, and glucose, subdivided by age and sex, are shown in Appendix A, Tables A–1 to A–10. A comfortable armchair should be used for determining sitting HR and blood pressure, and a stretcher bed or table should be used for the resting ECG. Blood drawing should occur after the HR and blood pressure check, for minor discomfort may produce an "alarm reaction."

For persons who have a family history of heart disease, are over 40 years of age, or at a high risk for CAD, a preliminary cardiovascular examination is important. The medical history will be reviewed, and the physician will listen for specific heart and blood vessel abnormalities (auscultation). This is considered an important part of the physical examination, since many dangerous valve or vessel dysfunctions are found in this way. If the physical fitness evaluation is for nondiagnostic purposes, this part of the examination is usually omitted (nonphysician evaluations).

The HR is usually counted for 15 or 30 seconds and then multiplied appropriately to obtain beats per minute. To help insure accuracy and stablization of blood pressure, two to three readings may be necessary. For best results in taking blood pressure, do the following:

1. Take the measurement in a quiet room with a temperature approximately 70 to 74°F (21 to 23°C).

2. Have both men and women dressed in a T-shirt or sleeveless blouse (this makes it easier to adjust the pressure cuff properly).

3. Have the person sit in a comfortable chair with arm at midchest level.

4. Take the blood pressure from both the left and the right arms (because of arterial obstructions, sometimes the pressure in one arm is different from the other). In subsequent evaluations, the arm found to have the higher pressure initially should be used.

5. Use the proper-sized cuff (a large cuff on a small arm will cause the readings to be lower and vice versa). The three most frequently used cuff sizes are child (13 to 20 cm), adult (17 to 26 cm), and large adult (32 to 42 cm). The measurement shown in parentheses refers to the arm circumfer-

ence at midpoint. Refer to the American Heart Association standard booklet for more details on cuff size.[36]

6. Take the measure fairly rapidly and leave the pressure cuff deflated for approximately 30 seconds to 1 minute between determinations (this will allow normal circulation to return to the arm).

The width of the inflatable bladder should be 40 per cent of the circumference of the arm on which it is used; the length should be 80 per cent of the circumference. The bladder should be applied directly over the compressible artery approximately 2.5 cm above the antecubital space. With the stethoscope in place, the pressure cuff should be inflated rapidly to approximately 30 mm Hg above the point at which the pulse disappears and then deflated at a rate of 2 to 4 mm Hg per second. Usually just the systolic and fifth phase diastolic pressures are recorded at rest. During exercise and recovery from exercise, the fifth phase diastolic blood pressure is often heard all the way to zero; thus both fourth and fifth phase should be noted. Sphygmomanometers should be calibrated at least once a year. More detailed information concerning the methods of taking blood pressure and calibration of sphygmomanometers is found in American Heart Association Standards booklets.[36,37]

Persons with a resting systolic blood pressure more than 180 mm Hg or a diastolic blood pressure higher than 100 mm Hg may need to be referred to a physician before further testing or training. In these extreme cases, it would be wiser to have persons achieve a reduction in blood pressure (by drugs or dietary control program or both) before letting them begin a training program. If someone is hypertensive, the initial program should be of a low intensity. The hypertensive person should also avoid static holds and moderate-to-heavy lifting or pushing exercises. These types of exercises have a dramatic effect on elevating the blood pressure.[38, 39]

The blood serum measures listed in Table 6–2 are standard procedures and can be determined rather easily and economically by most medical laboratories. The determination of high density lipoprotein–cholesterol (HDL-C) gives a more accurate assessment of the serum cholesterol but is significantly more expensive. To complete the risk factor profile shown in Table 6–1, the determination of serum cholesterol, triglycerides, HDL-C, and glucose is necessary. In general, if serum cholesterol is above 300 mg/dl or below 150 mg/dl, the measurement of HDL-C becomes less important. At these levels, the pure cholesterol fraction of serum cholesterol measure would be already considered clinically high or low, respectively.

CARDIORESPIRATORY FITNESS

Maximum oxygen uptake is measured in the laboratory setting and can be directly assessed as part of a diagnostic GXT. Consolazio, Johnson, and Pecora[40] give a detailed description of the principles and methodology involved in the measurement of $\dot{V}O_2$ max. More recently, reliable semiauto-mated and automated systems to measure aerobic capacity have become commercially available.[41,42] Although the automated systems make it com-paratively easy to measure $\dot{V}O_2$ max directly, the equipment and supplies needed for its measurement, as well as the added technical assistance re-quired during testing and analysis, add to the expense of the GXT proce-dure. In addition, regular technical assistance is required to keep equipment calibrated and in good working condition. When research is involved and when evaluating pulmonary patients, the actual measurement of $\dot{V}O_2$ max is advisable.

The estimation of $\dot{V}O_2$ max can be made with relative accuracy from HR response at submaximal work loads and from performance time or distance on a standardized test protocol. Thus, because of time, expense, and the ease of estimating $\dot{V}O_2$ max indirectly, the direct measurement of $\dot{V}O_2$ max may not be practical for use in the general clinical setting.

There is no question that by not actually measuring $\dot{V}O_2$ max, large potential errors in its estimation are possible. Methodology problems—e.g., holding onto the handrails during treadmill walking—can cause overestima-tion of the $\dot{V}O_2$ max by as much as 30 per cent.[43,44] Average standard errors of estimate range from 2 to 5 percent ($r = 0.8$ to 0.9) for tests listed under plan B (Table 6–2) and 5 to 10 per cent ($r = 0.7$ to 0.9) under plan C.[23,27,45,46] The section on test interpretation will further discuss errors of estimation and suggestions that generally help decrease them.

In reference to the testing plans suggested in Table 6–2, the protocols shown under plans A and B are identical, except that $\dot{V}O_2$ max is directly measured under plan A and is estimated from performance under plan B. Tests under plan C are not diagnostic tests, but rather are tests to measure functional capacity. Most of the tests listed under plan C are submaximal tests and use HR and work load to predict $\dot{V}O_2$ max. The 1- to 2-mile run tests require a maximum effort but are generally used for mass testing in the schools, for police, and in the military.[27,47–49]

When deciding whether to use direct or indirect measurements of $\dot{V}O_2$ max, the purpose of the test should be considered, as well as the impact the error may have on test interpretation. In general, $\dot{V}O_2$ max is used mainly for identifying status of fitness and showing serial results; thus, a consistent (under- or overprediction) 5 to 10 per cent error may not be crucial. When procedures are carefully standardized, errors have been shown to be consis-tent on repeated tests.[27,50] Thus, results from serial testing should not be greatly affected.

As will be discussed later in this chapter, knowledge of functional capac-ity can have certain diagnostic implications and is important for designing the initial exercise prescription. Even so, the actual exercise prescription is usually based on HR and on signs and symptoms.

Going to a physician's office or other establishments (universities, YMCAs) to obtain a sophisticated GXT is impractical for many persons. Even so, the diagnostic test should be mandatory for high-risk persons and strongly recommended for sedentary persons who are more than 40 years of age and who are going to participate in moderate- to high-intensity activities. Once the status is determined and the participant begins his or her program, less sophisticated tests can often be used for future evaluations. If one has any difficulty deciding what to do, a physician should be consulted and, if available in the community, an expert in evaluation and fitness. Along with medical centers and clinics, many local YMCAs, Jewish community centers, and colleges and universities have experts in adult fitness who can give the participant good advice.

TESTING PROTOCOLS FOR DETERMINING CARDIORESPIRATORY FITNESS

Maximum oxygen uptake is generally estimated from standardized tests administered on a treadmill, cycle ergometer, or steps.[6,8,11,29,30,51-56] A national survey of 1,400 exercise testing facilities showed that the treadmill was the most used mode of testing (71 per cent), followed by the cycle ergometer (17 per cent), and steps (12 per cent).[57] Of the treadmill protocols, the Bruce (65.5 per cent),[23] Balke (9.7 per cent),[53] Naughton (6 per cent),[58] and Ellestad (3.1 per cent)[30] protocols were the most widely used.

TREADMILL PROTOCOLS. As mentioned above, several protocols can be used for diagnostic purposes and for the determination of $\dot{V}O_2$ max. Figure 6–1 describes the most commonly used treadmill protocols. The modified Åstrand protocol includes a 5-minute warm-up walk (3.5 mph, 2.5 per cent grade for nonathletes and 5-minute jog for athletes) followed by a continuous, multistage run to exhaustion.[46,51] The speed of the run is adjusted to exhaust each participant in 7 to 10 minutes; this time period is considered adequate for maximal physiological adjustments to occur.[51] The proper starting speed for the modified Åstrand test can be estimated from an initial screening test or from knowledge of the participant's current status of fitness. Usually sedentary, middle-aged participants who are starting an exercise program will run at 5 to 6 mph, moderately trained persons at 7 to 8 mph, and elite runners at 10 to 11 mph. The other protocols have a warm-up built into the protocol and begin as illustrated in Figure 6–1.

Figure 6–2 illustrates different rates of increase in $\dot{V}O_2$ (METs) with the various protocols, but similar maximal values.[46] Few differences among tests are noted with other maximal values, e.g., blood pressure, RPP, respiratory exchange ratio (RER), $\dot{V}_E$, and rating of perceived exertion (RPE). At a submaximal level, the rate of increase differs among tests when results are compared by time of the test (Fig. 6–2). When work loads are standardized among tests (equal MET values), testing protocols vary little at submaximal levels (see Fig. 6–3).[59] Some controversy exists concerning testing protocols, in that the Bruce protocol, which has a more abrupt increase in work load between stages of the test, may be more sensitive to picking up ischemic ECG responses than the protocols that have slower incremental increase

(Naughton).[60] These findings have not been replicated or validated on a large sample; thus, at this time it is suggested that a variety of protocols can be used and similar results should be expected.

How can a laboratory make a logical decision about what protocol to use for GXT? Special factors—e.g., population (patient, athlete, young, or old) and available time—should be considered. In general, a continuous, multistage test that starts at a low MET level (2 to 3 METs), has 1- to 3-minute stages, and increases the work load by no more than 1 to 3 METs per stage is recommended.[6,7] The test should allow time for a warm-up and general cardiovascular-respiratory adaptation period and enough time and stages to allow for an incremental HR, blood pressure, ECG, and RPE response curve. A test with a minimum time of 6 minutes and no longer than 15 to 20 minutes is recommended. A period longer than 15 minutes is generally not necessary to attain the needed physiological and clinical information and may add more discomfort to the patient (mouthpiece, etc.) and cause subjects to stop prematurely owing to boredom (motivation), plasma volume shifts, etc. Certainly, laboratories that evaluate a diverse population and use a common protocol should not be criticized. For research and other long-term comparative purposes, there are advantages in using the same protocol.

Experience with cardiac patients and, in particular, with patients who are relatively close to their event (1 to 12 weeks after myocardial infarction [MI] or surgery), an incremental work load of approximately 1 MET that starts at approximately 2 METs is advisable. Under this condition, the standard Bruce or Balke protocols start at too high a MET level. The Naughton protocol is particularly well suited for this situation. Bruce has designed a lower level 12-minute test for use with patients of low fitness.[61] The test includes four 3-minute stages: stage I, 1.2 mph, 0 per cent grade; stage II, 1.2 mph, 3 per cent grade; stage III, 1.2 mph, 6 per cent grade; and stage IV, 1.7 mph, 6 per cent grade. In addition, some have modified the Bruce test by adding two 3-minute stages to the existing test protocol: step I, 1.7 mph, 0 per cent grade, and step II, 1.7 mph, 5 per cent grade.[62] The Balke protocol has been modified by adding a preliminary 2 to 3-minute stage at 2 mph, 0 per cent grade.

From the criteria listed previously, it is obvious that the modified Åstrand protocol is not suitable for diagnostic testing. This protocol was designed to evaluate $\dot{V}O_2$ max in normal, healthy individuals and is particularly well suited for use with runners.

In summary, there are many excellent treadmill protocols, and the one used is often dictated by the population being evaluated and by personal preference. The Bruce and Ellestad tests have been shown to be the most flexible tests to be used with a diverse population (men-women, nonathlete-athlete, young–middle-aged).

Although these tests are very popular (particularly the Bruce test), they are not without criticism. For example, the Bruce test is often criticized because of its abrupt increase in work load between stages and because stage IV for men (4.2 mph, 16 per cent grade) and stage III for women (3.4 mph, 14 per cent grade) are awkward in speed, and thus it is difficult to decide whether to walk or run. One of the major advantages for using the Bruce test is its wide use and, thus, abundance of comparative data.

The main criticism of the Balke test is its duration. The same would be true of the Naughton test if it were used with healthy and fit individuals. Because of a shorter stride length, the modified Balke (3.0 mph) protocol may be preferable for use with women.[59] The Naughton test has been most

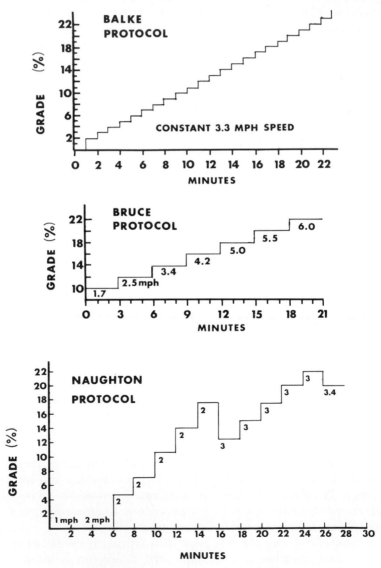

Figure 6–1. *See legend on opposite page.*

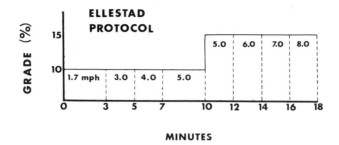

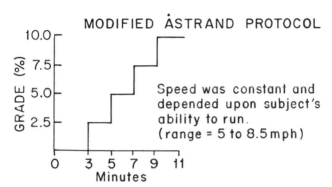

Figure 6–1. The Balke,[53] Bruce,[95] Naughton,[58] Ellestad,[30] and Åstrand[40] treadmill protocols are the most commonly used. Ellestad has modified his testing protocol. The treadmill speed of 5 mph is maintained from minutes 10 to 12 and is increased to 6 mph from minutes 12 to 14, and so on. (Reprinted with permission from Pollock, M.L., Wilmore, J.H., and Fox, S.M.: Health and Fitness Through Physical Activity. New York, copyright © John Wiley and Sons, 1978; Pollock, M. L., Schmidt, D.H., and Jackson, A.S.: Measurement of cardiorespiratory fitness and body composition in the clinical setting. From Comprehensive Therapy, Vol. 6, No. 9, pp. 12–27. Published with permission of The Laux Company, Inc., Harvard, MA.)

suitable for predischarge testing of cardiac patients and other patients and elderly persons who have low functional capacities (< 6 METs).

CYCLE, ARM ERGOMETER AND STEP TEST PROTOCOLS. Although the mode of testing is different with cycle and arm ergometers and with step test protocols, the general guidelines for GXT mentioned for treadmill testing are similar. Cycle ergometers are less expensive than treadmills. The advent of electronically controlled cycle ergometers has narrowed the price differential with treadmills. Whether the treadmill or cycle ergometer is used, frequent calibration for speed, grade, and resistance (kpm/min or watts) is necessary. The manufacturer's instruction manual and the recommendations established by the American Heart Association[63] provide information and guidelines on the calibration of ergometric equipment. The purchase of equipment that cannot be readily calibrated is not recommended.

The cycle ergometer test for determination of $\dot{V}O_2$ max is usually performed on a mechanically or electronically braked cycle ergometer that is calibrated at 100 to 150 kpm/min (17- to 25-watt) increments. Most multistage protocols would have 2- to 3-minute stages, with initial resistance for

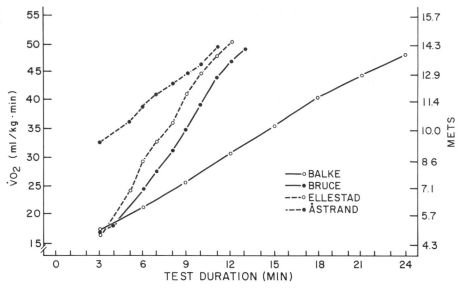

RATE OF INCREASE IN OXYGEN INTAKE IN FOUR STRESS TEST PROTOCOLS
ON 51 MEN, AGED 35–55 YEARS

Figure 6–2. Rate of increase in oxygen uptake in four GXT protocols on 51 men, aged 35 to 55 years. Data for women show similar results.[59] (Reprinted with permission from Pollock, M.L., et al.: A comparative analysis of four protocols for maximal treadmill stress testing. Am. Heart J. *92:*39–46, 1976.)

leg testing being set at 100 or 150 to 300 kpm/min. Power output would increase by 100- to 150-kpm/min increments per stage. Middle-aged, less fit, cardiac patients generally begin at 100 or 150 to 300 kpm/min and increase their power output by 100 to 150 kpm/min per stage. Younger, more fit persons usually begin at 300 to 600 kpm/min (50 to 100 watts) and increase their power output by 150- to 300-kpm/min (25 to 50 watts) increments.

Cycle ergometers that do not internally adjust the work load to compensate for change in pedaling rate have to be pedaled at a constant rate, i.e., revolution per minute (rpm). Some tests recommend a pedal rate of 50 rpm,[14, 64] but at the same power output efficiency varies little between 50 and 80 rpm.[64] Competitive cyclists generally pedal at a minimum of 90 rpm and often up to 120 rpm.[65] Most of the commercially built cycle ergometers are not designed to test elite cyclists. In cycle ergometers that do not internally adjust resistance to compensate for a change in pedal speed, the use of a metronome will assist the participant in keeping the proper pedal speed. Metronomes should be checked for calibration. In addition, calibration of all mechanical types of cycle ergometers is important. The friction type is the easiest to calibrate. With this kind of cycle ergometer, the friction belt expands as heat is generated by the fly wheel, and thus periodic tightening of the belt corrects for change in work load.

Another important point to remember when using a cycle ergometer is to make sure the height of the seat is properly adjusted. The seat should be

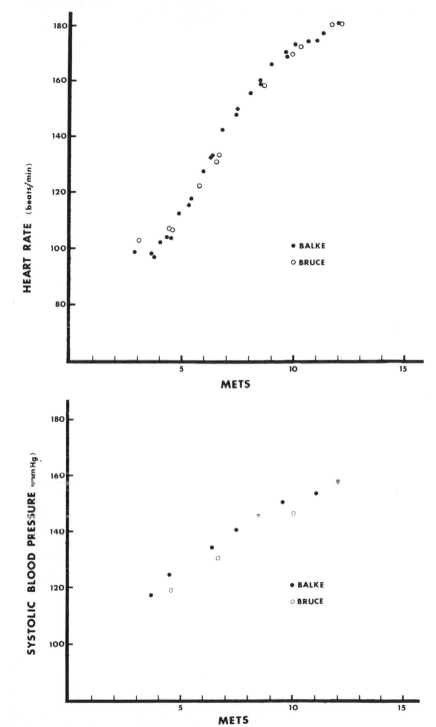

Figure 6–3. Rate of increase in heart rate (upper figure) and systolic blood pressure (lower figure) by MET increments on the Bruce and Balke GXT protocols. (Reprinted with permission from Pollock, M.L., et al.: Comparative analysis of physiologic responses to three different maximal graded exercise test protocols in healthy women. Am. Heart J. *103:*363–373, 1982.)

adjusted so that there is a slight bend in the knee joint when the ball of the foot is on the pedal with the pedal in its lowest position.[65]

In comparison to the treadmill, there are some advantages in using the cycle ergometer. It is generally more portable. In addition, they are quieter and may involve less upper body movement, and thus, blood pressure is easier to assess. This is particularly true at the higher work levels. When taking blood pressure of patients on a cycle ergometer, have them relax their grip and arm on the side being measured. Finally, in some cases, ECG recordings may show less skeletal muscle interference with cycle ergometry.

The major disadvantage of cycle ergometer testing is that most Americans are unaccustomed to cycle riding; hence their maximal values (HR and $\dot{V}O_2$ max) are often undermeasured. The lower values found on cycling can range from 5 to 25 per cent, depending upon the participant's conditioning and leg strength.[59,66-68] Since a lower measurement of functional capacity has obvious limitations in evaluation and exercise prescription, most testers prefer to use the treadmill. Persons trained on bicycles or cycle ergometers can often elicit equally high maximal physiological values on the cycle ergometer and the treadmill.[68]

Arm ergometry can be substituted when traditional leg testing is not possible owing to disability. Commercial arm ergometers are available, and cycle ergometers can be modified for use with the arms.[69-71] Either arm cranking or push-pull (Airdyne) types of devices are appropriate for GXT.[70,72]

Some disadvantages of arm ergometry when compared with leg testing (treadmill and cycle) are as follows: a smaller muscle mass is used—thus $\dot{V}O_2$ max is lower by 20 to 30 per cent;[69-72] HR max is lower; blood pressure is difficult to assess; ECG quality is often affected; and it is not recommended initially for patients with recent MI or heart surgery.[73] Arm training will increase the arm $\dot{V}O_2$ max relative to the leg $\dot{V}O_2$ max by 5 to 10 per cent.[71] Probably as a result of a greater use of muscle mass (arms and back muscles), the Airdyne apparatus (arms only) appears to elicit a higher $\dot{V}O_2$ max compared with arm cranking.[72] Although $\dot{V}O_2$ max and $\dot{V}_E$ max do not differ with wheelchair ergometry compared with arm cranking, power output and HR max are significantly reduced with wheelchair ergometry.[74] Although not many data are available on the value of arm ergometry in evaluating arrhythmias and ischemic responses to exercise, enough data exist to support its use.[75,76]

The same protocol recommended for leg ergometry can be used with arm ergometry, except that the initial power output and the incremental increases in power output between stages are lower for arm ergometry. For patients who are considered to be of low fitness, the initial power output may be set at zero, and for moderately fit individuals, it may be set at 75 to 150 kpm/min (12 to 25 watts). Incremental increases in power output between stages of 75 and 100 kpm/min are generally recommended.

Since $\dot{V}O_2$ max and HR max are significantly lower for arm work than for leg work, estimation of maximum values of leg work from arm work and its use for prescribing exercise for leg work are not recommended. With arm training, $\dot{V}O_2$ max and HR max significantly increase.[71] In prescribing exercise for arm training, the arm ergometer results should be used, and the same method of calculating training HRs should be used as recommended for leg exercise (see Chapter 7). When the percentage of HR max reserve is calculated from arm ergometry and compared with treadmill results, the same RPE score is often found, i.e., approximately 13 at 70 per cent of HR max reserve and 15 to 16 at 85 per cent.[72]

When neither a treadmill nor a cycle ergometer is available, a *graded step test* can be used as an alternative. The graded step test designed by Nagle, Balke, and Naughton[53] is recommended by the American Heart Association.[7] An adjustable platform permits the height to be varied from 2 to 50 cm while the patient continues to exercise. The platform height is initially set at 3 cm. At the end of the second minute, the platform is raised 2 cm; it is raised 4 cm each minute thereafter. The rhythm of stepping is regulated by a metronome at 30 steps/min. For elderly patients or persons with low exercise tolerance, slower stepping rates can be used (Table 6–5). The stepping procedure is completed in four counts: At counts one and two, the patient steps up to an erect standing position with both feet on the platform; at counts three and four, he or she returns to the starting position standing in front of the platform. To help avoid local muscle fatigue, the lead leg may be changed periodically. The test is terminated when the patient is unable to maintain the required rhythm.

SUBMAXIMAL TESTING PROTOCOLS AND FIELD TESTS TO DETERMINE FUNCTIONAL CAPACITY

The submaximal exercise testing protocols recommended here are found under plan C (Table 6–2). The tests do not monitor ECG and blood pressure and are not used for diagnostic purposes. The tests under plan C are generally used for physical fitness testing of apparently healthy, low-risk youth and adults. They are primarily used by agencies that do mass testing, e.g., schools or military, or that do not have extensive equipment or personnel with advanced training in test administration and interpretation, e.g., YMCA, Jewish Community Center, and health clubs. They also can be used as a follow-up test for persons who have had a diagnostic test and are considered at low risk and free from heart disease.

SUBMAXIMAL CYCLE TESTS. The most commonly used submaximal cycle ergometer tests used include a multistage physical work capacity test developed by Sjöstrand[77] and a single-stage test by Åstrand and Ryhming.[64] Both tests are based on the fact that HR and $\dot{V}O_2$ are linearly related over a broad range.[51] The premise is that a younger or more fit individual will have a lower submaximal steady-state HR at any given level of power output (kpm/min, watts).

These tests were designed to plot submaximal HRs versus power output on a cycle ergometer at HRs between 110 and 150 beats/min. This HR range seems to have the best linear relationship with $\dot{V}O_2$ over a wide variety of ages and fitness levels. Once the steady-state submaximal HR–power output relationship has been determined, $\dot{V}O_2$ max can be estimated. Although both tests have moderate-to-good predictability, multistage tests have been shown to be more valid than single-stage tests.[45]

The YMCAs of America have modified the Sjöstrand test by using two or three 3-minute continuous stages.[14] To administer the test properly, two HR–power output data points are needed within the 110 to 150 beat/min range. The test can start once a participant has had a chance to become familiar with the ergometer and the proper seat height has been adjusted. The metronome should be set so that one can pedal at 50 rpm, and the test subject should be allowed to warm up by pedaling for 1 minute at zero work load. Figures 6–4 and 6–5 can be used as a guide to set the initial and subsequent work loads for both men and women. As shown in the directions (Figs. 6–4 and 6–5), if the initial work load elicits a HR of 110 beats/min

GUIDE TO SETTING WORKLOADS

FOR MALES ON THE BICYCLE ERGOMETER

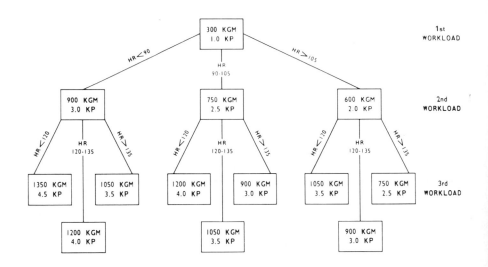

DIRECTIONS

1. Set the 1st workload at 300 kgm/min (1.0 KP)

2. If HR in 3rd min is: Less than (<) 90, set 2nd load at 900 kgm (3 KP)
   Between 90 and 105, set 2nd load at 750 kgm (2.5 KP)
   Greater than (>) 105, set 2nd load at 600 kgm (2.0 KP)

3. Follow the same pattern for setting 3rd and final load.

4. NOTE: If the 1st workload elicits a HR of 110 or more, it is used on the graph, and only ONE more workload will be necessary.

Figure 6–4. Guide for setting work loads for men on submaximal cycle ergometer test. (Reprinted with permission from Golding, L.A., Myers, C.R., and Sinning, W.E., editors: The Y's Way to Physical Fitness, revised. Chicago, The YMCA of the USA, 1982.)

or more, only one more work load will be needed to complete the two plots. In most cases, the HR will be lower than 110 beats/min on the initial work load, and then the values for the second and third work loads will be used. Each work load is timed for 3 minutes, with the HR being counted during the last half of the second and third minutes. At the end of each HR count, the scores are recorded on a form such as the one shown in Figure 6–6. The HR in the second and third minutes should not differ by more than 5 beats/min. If they do, extend the test period for an additional minute. When plotting the results, use the HR value for the third or final minute of each stage.

The HR is determined by measuring the length of time it takes to count 30 heartbeats. This is usually done with a stopwatch and a stethoscope. Once the test is completed, a 1- to 2-minute recovery period of low-to-zero resistance pedaling is recommended.

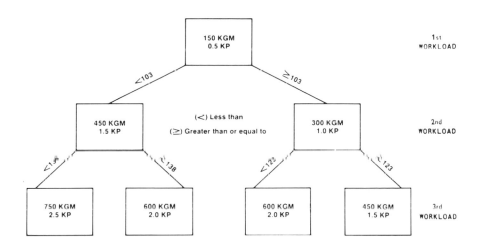

GUIDE TO SETTING WORKLOADS

FOR FEMALES ON THE BICYCLE ERGOMETER

DIRECTIONS

1. Set the first workload to 150 kgm/min (.5 KP).

2. If steady-state heart rate is < 103, set 2nd load at 450 kgm/min (1.5 KP).
   If steady-state heart rate is ≥ 103, set 2nd load at 300 kgm/min (1.0 KP).

3. Follow this same pattern for setting the third and final load.

4. NOTE: If the 1st workload elicits a HR of 110 or more, it is used on the graph, and only ONE more workload will be necessary.

Figure 6–5. Guide to setting work loads for women on submaximal cycle ergometer test. (Reprinted with permission from Golding, L.A., Myers, C.R., and Sinning, W.E., editors: The Y's Way to Physical Fitness, revised. Chicago, The YMCA of the USA, 1982.)

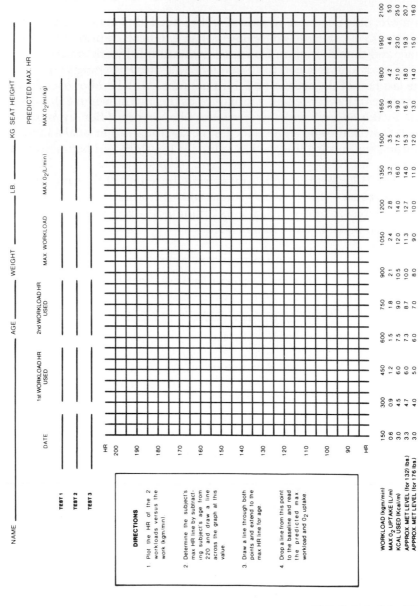

MAXIMUM PHYSICAL WORKING CAPACITY PREDICTION

Figure 6–6. Work sheet used to plot and calculate VO₂ from submaximal cycle ergometer test. (Reprinted with permission from Golding, L.A., Myers, C.R., and Sinning, W.E., editors: The Y's Way to Physical Fitness, revised. Chicago, The YMCA of the USA, 1982.)

The directions for calculating maximum working capacity and $\dot{V}O_2$ max are shown in Figure 6–6.[14] Plot only the last two HR–power output values determined. The lower horizontal axis shows the estimated $\dot{V}O_2$ max (L/min), Kcal/min, and METs for a given work load. Finally, to express $\dot{V}O_2$ max by $ml/kg \cdot min^{-1}$, divide the L/min value by body weight in kilograms.

SUBMAXIMAL BENCH STEPPING TEST.   The prediction of $\dot{V}O_2$ max also can be determined by a submaximal bench stepping test.[27,78,79] The basic assumption of this test is similar to that of the submaximal cycle test. Given an equal amount of work to accomplish (stepping up and down on a bench at the same rate and total time), the participant with a lower HR will be in better physical condition and therefore will have a higher $\dot{V}O_2$ max.

Katch and McArdle[79] describe a submaximal bench stepping test for predicting $\dot{V}O_2$ max in college-age men and women. The test is accomplished by stepping up and down on a bench 16.25 inches high (generally the height of a bleacher seat) for a total of 3 minutes. Men step at a rate of 24 steps/min and women at 22 steps/min. Again, it is best to use a metronome. On the completion of the 3-minute test, the participant remains standing while the pulse is counted for a 15-second interval, beginning 5 seconds after termination of the test. To convert the recovery HR to beats/min, the 15-second HR is multiplied by four. The equations for estimating $\dot{V}O_2$ max, expressed in $ml/kg \cdot min^{-1}$, are as follows.

Men: $\dot{V}O_2$ max = 111.33 – (0.42 X step test pulse rate, beats/min)
Women: $\dot{V}O_2$ max = 65.81 – (0.1847 X step test pulse rate, beats/min)

For ease in estimating the proper value, see Table A–11, Appendix A. The standards shown in the same table are from data collected on college-age men and women; hence, information collected on middle-aged participants could give slightly lower oxygen uptake values.

A submaximal bench stepping test for healthy, middle-aged adults was developed by Kasch.[14, 18] It is a 3-minute test conducted at 24 steps/min on a bench 12 inches high. After completion of the test, the participant sits down, and the pulse is counted for 1 minute, beginning 5 seconds into the recovery. Norms for adult men and women[14] and police officers[81] are available.

RUNNING FIELD TESTS.   The field type of test was designed to estimate $\dot{V}O_2$ max on large groups of healthy young men and women. A high correlation between the laboratory-determined $\dot{V}O_2$ max and distance run was first reported by Balke[21] (15-minute run) and later popularized by Cooper[82,83] (12-minute run and 1.5-mile run). For many years, the national test for cardiorespiratory endurance used with school children was the 600-yard run test developed by the American Alliance for Health, Physical Education, Recreation, and Dance (AAHPERD).[84] It was subsequently shown that run tests below 1 mile (approximately 9 minutes) had low correlations with laboratory-determined $\dot{V}O_2$ max and moderate-to-high correlations above this distance.[27,85] Thus, the latest tests used on school children recom-

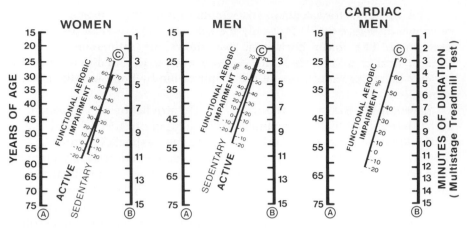

Figure 6–7. Nomograms for evaluating functional aerobic impairment (FAI) of men (Panel A), women (Panel B), and cardiac men (Panel C) according to age, by duration of exercise on Bruce protocol for sedentary and active groups. To find FAI, apply a straight-edge to age and duration and read intercepts on diagonal. (Reprinted with permission from Bruce, R.L., Kusumi, F., and Hosmer, D.: Maximal oxygen intake and nomographic assessment of functional aerobic impairment in cardiovascular disease. Am. Heart J. *85:*545–562, 1973.)

mended by AAHPERD is a 1-mile or 9-minute run for children 12 years old and under and a 1.5-mile or 12-minute run for children in junior and senior high school grades (13 years old and above).[48]

The most widely used field tests (schools, universities, and armed forces) are the 12-minute and 1.5-mile runs. The two tests have a very high intercorrelation, and because the 1.5-mile run test is easier to administer, it is the most preferred.

Like other unmonitored tests, the field test should not be used as a diagnostic tool and should be administered only to healthy, young persons. An exception to this would be its use with trained middle-aged participants who have already been thoroughly evaluated for heart disease and potential risk. Best results are found when participants have had a few weeks of preliminary training. This allows time for some adaptation to training and practice in pacing oneself. The test is normally administered on a smooth, level surface (track) and is performed in tennis or running shoes. Table 6–3 shows the estimation of $\dot{V}O_2$ max based on the time to run 1.5 miles.

INTERPRETATION OF GRADED EXERCISE TEST RESULTS

The interpretation of GXT results are to be discussed in relation to the prediction of $\dot{V}O_2$ max (functional capacity), knowledge of level of cardiorespiratory fitness, and the determination of medical status of participants entering health enhancement or preventive/rehabilitation programs.

AEROBIC CAPACITY. To determine the level of aerobic fitness, two sets of norms are available in Appendix A (Table A–1 to A–10 and A–12 to

A–13). The norms shown in Tables A–1 to A–10 were developed from a large sample of generally healthy men and women who were tested (first visit data only) at the Cooper Clinic in Dallas, Texas.[8, 86] The advantage of these standards compared with others is that they are age-specific by decades and include a large cell size for each age classification. Although the data from the two sets of norms were collected from different tests, maximal treadmill testing at the Cooper Clinic and a submaximal cycle ergometer test with subsequent prediction of $\dot{V}O_2$ max for the YMCA norms,[14] they show similar results.

Figure 6–7 illustrates another popular method of classifying men and women of various ages.[23] The functional aerobic impairment (FAI) scale was developed from treadmill performance time on the Bruce test and distinguishes between sedentary, active, and cardiac populations. In contrast to the Cooper Clinic and YMCA norms, much of the data reported by Bruce comes from a hospital setting wherein many more persons are evaluated because of potential CAD. In addition, the FAI is applicable only to the Bruce test.

The clinical classification scale as it relates to various GXT protocols was developed by the American Heart Association (see Table 6–6).[62] Although widely used by clinicians, its generally broad categories make it less precise in determining fitness status. Because norms are population-specific, the scale that most represents the participants tested should be used.

The fitness classifications shown in Table 6–3 are not to be confused with normative data. The categories developed in this table put potential participants who are interested in becoming involved in an aerobic exercise program into homogeneous subgroupings. This should help facilitate the physician or program director in determining the exercise prescription. The fitness classifications shown in Table 6–3 match up with the variety of recommended 6-week starter and 20-week training regimens described in Chapter 7.

The meaning of $\dot{V}O_2$ max standards for various groups (sedentary, active, and athletic), variability of the measure (sex, heredity, age, and so forth) and expected training responses are reviewed in Chapter 3. These factors should be taken into account when interpreting test results.

PREDICTION OF $\dot{V}O_2$ MAX. As mentioned earlier, $\dot{V}O_2$ max can be predicted with relative accuracy from performance time and standard submaximal work load tests. Maximal performance tests usually yield higher predictive scores ($r = 0.70$ to 0.95, SEE $\pm$ 2.5 to 4ml/kg·min^{-1}) than submaximal tests ($r = \sim 0.75$, SEE $\pm$ 4 to 5 ml/kg·min^{-1}).[27] Laboratory-controlled maximal tests using performance time on a treadmill show the highest correlation with laboratory-determined $\dot{V}O_2$ max ($r = \sim 0.9$, SEE $= 2.5 - 4$ ml/kg·min^{-1}).[23,46,59] Factors that significantly affect the results of laboratory performance tests are population specificity of equations, familiarity with treadmill and test procedures (habituation), hanging onto the handrails, and inappropriate endpoints for test termination.

Bruce et al.[23] and others[11,46,89] have shown that the prediction of $\dot{V}O_2$ max from standardized tests is population-specific. This is based on the statistical premise that a prediction equation best predicts (highest correlation and lowest standard error) at the mean value of the population

TABLE 6–6. CLINICAL CLASSIFICATION AS IT RELATES TO VARIOUS EXERCISE STAGES OF COMMONLY USED PROTOCOLS

FUNCTIONAL CLASS	CLINICAL STATUS	O₂ REQUIREMENTS ml O₂/kg/min	STEP TEST NAGLE, BALKE, NAUGHTON* (2 min stages 30 steps/min)	TREADMILL TESTS BRUCE† (3-min stages)		KATTUS‡ (3-min stages)		BALKE** (% grade at 3.4 mph)	BALKE** (% grade at 3 mph)	BICYCLE ERGOMETER**
		56.0	(Step height increased 4 cm q 2 min)					26		For 70 kg body weight
		52.5				mph %gr		24		kgm/min
		49.0		mph %gr		4	22	22		1500
NORMAL AND I	PHYSICALLY ACTIVE SUBJECTS	45.5	Height (cm)	4.2	16			20		
		42.0	40			4	18	18	22.5	1350
		38.5	36					16	20.0	1200
		35.0	32			4	14	14	17.5	1050
	SEDENTARY HEALTHY	31.5	28	3.4	14			12	15.0	900
		28.0	24			4	10	10	12.5	
		24.5	20	2.5	12	3	10	8	10.0	750
	DISEASED, RECOVERED	21.0	16					6	7.5	600
II	SYMPTOMATIC PATIENTS	17.5	12	1.7	10	2	10	4	5.0	450
		14.0	8					2	2.5	300
III		10.5	4						0.0	150
		7.0								
IV		3.5								

Oxygen requirements increase with work loads from bottom of chart to top in various exercise tests of the step, treadmill, and bicycle ergometer types.

* Nagle, F.S., Balke, B, and Naughton, J.P.[53]

† Bruce, R.A.[62]

‡ Kattus, A.A., Jorgensen, C.R., Worden, R.E., and Alvaro, A.B.[87]

§ Fox, S.M., Naughton, J.P., and Haskell, W.L.[88]

(From Exercise Testing and Training of Apparently Healthy Individuals: A Handbook for Physicians. Dallas, American Heart Association. By permission of the American Heart Association, copyright ©, 1972.)

used.[27,90] If data are curvilinear, then gross prediction errors are made on participants who deviate significantly from the mean of the population from which the equation was derived (see Fig. 6–8). For example, equations developed on average sedentary men or women underestimate $\dot{V}O_2$ max of highly active and elite endurance athletes and overpredict cardiac patients and persons of low fitness. This regression effect toward the mean is common among tests and will be discussed again under body composition evaluation.[27,90]

Population-specific equations for predicting $\dot{V}O_2$ max from treadmill performance time are available for middle-aged active and sedentary men and women for the Bruce test[23,46,59] and cardiac patients for the Bruce test.[23]

More recently, Foster et al.[89] (see Fig. 6–8 for Bruce protocol) developed a generalized equation for the Bruce and modified Naughton protocols that can be used for active and sedentary men and male cardiac patients. The prediction equation for the Naughton protocol is as follows: $\dot{V}O_2$ max $= 1.61$ (treadmill time : min) $+ 3.60$ ($r = 0.97$, SE $= \pm 2.60$).[91] The modification of the Naughton protocol included 2-minute stages. Using one generalized equation has the advantage of eliminating the judgmental factor of which equation to use for an individual and of having a slightly lower standard error of measurement. Other equations are available for predicting $\dot{V}O_2$ max for the Balke,[46,59,62] Ellestad,[7,46] and Naughton[58,62] protocols.

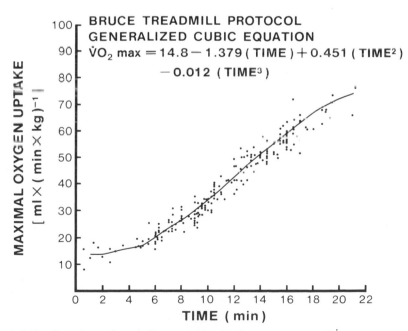

Figure 6–8. Data shows the curvilinear relationship between measured $\dot{V}O_2$ max to treadmill performance of persons of varied abilities ($n = 200$). The generalized cubic equation derived from the Bruce protocol[23] shows an $r = 0.98 \pm 3.35$ ml/kg · min⁻¹.[89] Treadmill time is expressed in minutes. (From Foster, C., et al.: Generalized equations for predicting functional capacity from treadmill performance. Am. Heart J. [in press].)

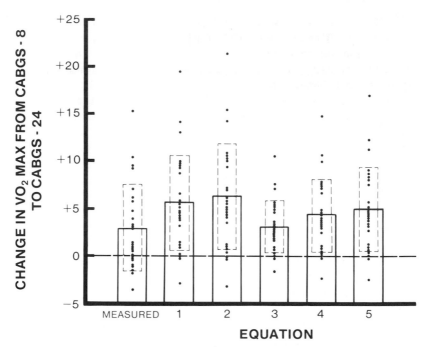

Figure 6–9. The actual measured change in $\dot{V}O_2$ max (*left bar*) is shown for coronary artery bypass graft surgery (CABGS) patients after 16 weeks of aerobic training.[92] The data shown for equations 1 and 2 are from Pollock et al.[46] on healthy sedentary and active individuals, and equations 3 to 5 are from Bruce et al.[23] on cardiac patients (3) and sedentary (4) and active (5) healthy men. Notice all equations that were derived from noncardiac populations overestimate the actual change in $\dot{V}O_2$ max. (Reprinted with permission from Foster, C., et al.: Prediction of oxygen uptake during exercise testing in cardiac patients and healthy adults. J. Cardiac Rehab. [in press].)

The treadmill times and estimation of $\dot{V}O_2$ max shown for the various protocols in Table 6–3 are based on the results of various prediction equations. They have been cross-validated with a varied population of patients and elite, active, and sedentary young and middle-aged populations (unpublished data, M.L. Pollock). Although fewer data are available for the elderly populations, Table 6–3 also has been validated for use with active Master's runners.

Another important factor related to using population-specific prediction equations for estimating $\dot{V}O_2$ max is their ability to predict training changes accurately. Figure 6–9 shows data from a 16-week training study conducted on cardiac patients.[92] The amount of change in $\dot{V}O_2$ max was similar for actual measured $\dot{V}O_2$ compared with prediction equation 3, Figure 6–9 which was derived from cardiac patients. The other equations (1, 2, 4, and 5, in Fig. 6–9), which were derived from healthy, sedentary, and active populations, consistently overpredicted the actual amount of $\dot{V}O_2$ max change.[92]

Some clinicians have used steady-state $\dot{V}O_2$ values at various standard work loads to estimate $\dot{V}O_2$ max [20] Using this technique can also lead to gross

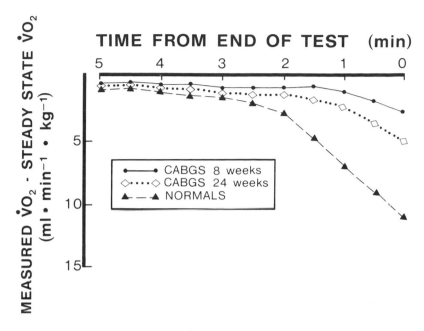

Figure 6–10. Foster et al.[92] show serial $\dot{V}O_2$ responses during the last 5 minutes of exercise on Bruce protocol for patients recovering from coronary artery bypass graft surgery (CABGS) and in healthy volunteers. See text for a detailed explanation of figure. (Reprinted with permission from Foster, C., et al.: Prediction of oxygen uptake during exercise testing in cardiac patients and healthy adults. J. Cardiac Rehab. [in press].)

errors of estimation.[92] For the normal population, it has been shown that $\dot{V}O_2$ often plateaus (depending upon the protocol used, 50 to 80 per cent of the time[46]) from 1 to 3 minutes before the end of the test.[93,94] Foster et al.[92] showed that during the clearly submaximal portions of the Bruce protocol, both cardiac and normal subjects accurately follow the estimated steady-state $\dot{V}O_2$ curve for each work load. In contrast, within 3 minutes from test termination (volitional maximum), the pattern deviated; i.e., predicted $\dot{V}O_2$ max was significantly greater than the actually measured $\dot{V}O_2$ max. This overprediction of $\dot{V}O_2$ max was particularly evident when equations developed for normal subjects were used for cardiac patients. The measured $\dot{V}O_2$ versus steady-state $\dot{V}O_2$ values as tabulated for uphill walking by the American College of Sports Medicine[6] are shown in Figure 6–10 for healthy volunteers and cardiac patients.[92] The pattern of response shows a progressive difference in measured $\dot{V}O_2$ versus steady-state $\dot{V}O_2$. Therefore, if steady-state $\dot{V}O_2$ values are used to predict $\dot{V}O_2$ max, backing off 2 to 4 minutes from the endpoint may be necessary. Protocols that have abrupt increases in $\dot{V}O_2$ from stage to stage (Bruce or Ellestad) have greater potential error when steady-state values are used for predicting $\dot{V}O_2$ max than protocols that have smaller incremental increases (Balke, Naughton). The data from Tables 6–4 and 6–5 are based on steady-state $\dot{V}O_2$ values and thus should not be used for predicting $\dot{V}O_2$ max.

Habituation and hanging onto the handrails are two important factors that significantly affect prediction of $\dot{V}O_2$ max from performance time.[11,27–30,43,44,95] Froelicher et al.[25] found treadmill performance to improve significantly when subjects were tested three times, a week apart on three different treadmill protocols. Although laboratory measurement of $\dot{V}O_2$ max did not change from week to week, treadmill time did. In this study, the use of treadmill time to predict $\dot{V}O_2$ max would have produced a 5 to 6 ml/kg·min^{-1} increase in $\dot{V}O_2$ max. Although not supported by the Froelicher et al.[25] study, other investigations suggest that one practice period should be sufficient to eliminate this prediction error.[8,96]

Although holding onto the handrails may have little significant effect on the diagnostic aspects of the GXT, its use invalidates any prediction of aerobic capacity from treadmill performance time.[43,44,93] Zeimetz et al.[43] demonstrated an overprediction error of up to 3.2 METs with holding onto the handrails. There was also a significant reduction in HR and $\dot{V}O_2$ at standard submaximal work loads. Therefore, if actual $\dot{V}O_2$ max is not measured and aerobic capacity is being estimated, holding onto the handrails should be avoided.

Whether actually measured or predicted from maximal performance time, $\dot{V}O_2$ max is most accurately assessed when participants go to volitional maximum. In addition to significant clinical signs and symptoms, maximal endpoints include the following: plateauing of $\dot{V}O_2$ with an increase in work load, RER above 1.0, blood lactate levels above 90 mg/100 ml (10 mM), HR aproaching or above age-predicted maximum, signs of exercise intolerance (fatigue, staggering, inability to keep up with work load, facial pallor, and so on), and RPE above 18 or 19.[11,30,51,52,94,95,97] Although more difficult to measure at peak excercise, systolic blood pressure will often decrease at maximum exercise.[30] Thus, unless a standard submaximal or maximal endpoint is used, measuring or predicting $\dot{V}O_2$ max becomes less accurate, and interpretation of serial results may become impossible. Although HR associated with a standard work load is often acceptable for comparing serial results, in itself HR is usually a poor criterion to use as an endpoint for maximum GXT.

As mentioned earlier, the prediction of $\dot{V}O_2$ max by the time taken to run a certain distance (1 to 2 miles) or by the distance covered in 9 to 12 minutes has a correlation with laboratory-determined $\dot{V}O_2$ max of $\pm$ 0.5 to 0.91 (average $r = 0.75$ to 0.85). A summary of these studies is tabulated by Baumgartner and Jackson.[27] In discussing the variance of results from the reported studies, they list the following factors that seem to alter the correlation between distance running performance and laboratory-measured $\dot{V}O_2$ max.

1. Several studies tested only a few subjects, this despite the fact that large samples are more reliable in correlation studies. In these studies, the number was limited by the difficulty of measuring the maximal oxygen uptake of a large group of subjects.

2. As stated in Chapter 3, a test can be valid for one group but not

for another. The high correlation (0.90) reported by Cooper (1968) may be due to the extreme variability of the group tested, which ranged in age from 17 to 52 and in body weight from 114 to 270 pounds. In general, the more variable the group, the higher the correlations. With a more homogenous group, we could expect lower correlations.

3. To achieve maximal performance on a distance run, students must learn to pace themselves. In a laboratory, pace is standardized by the motor-driven treadmill or bicycle ergometer.

4. Psychological factors have a pronounced effect on distance run tests. Students must be motivated to exert themselves fully on distance runs.

5. Cureton and his associates (1977) have shown that body composition is a major factor in distance running. The concurrent validity correlations . . . have not been adjusted for body composition differences, which probably would alter them.[27]

Cooper[86] recommends that middle-aged beginners need approximately 6 weeks of preliminary training before taking the 12-minute or 1.5-mile tests. High school and college students and military recruits probably need less preparation for these tests.

RATING OF PERCEIVED EXERTION (RPE) SCALE. The RPE scale, as shown in Figure 6–11, was first conceived and introduced by Borg.[98, 99] The scale is a 15-point category scale ranging from 6 to 20, with a descriptive verbal anchor at every odd number. RPE and HR are linearly related to each other and to work intensity across a variety of exercise modalities and conditions.[99–105] RPE also relates well to various physiological factors: A multiple correlation of 0.85 was found with $\dot{V}_E$, HR, lactate, and $\dot{V}_{O_2}$.[106] (Note that only individual correlations are found in this reference. Multiple correlations are available from authors.)

The original concept was developed from young adults; addition of a zero to each of the points in the scale would reflect the HR value under various levels of work intensity. For example, 6 would become 60 and represent HR at rest, and 19 and 20 would represent HR max (190 to 200 beats/min).[98,99] When the scale was applied to persons of various ages, it was found that the same linear relationship with work intensity existed at all ages, but the HR was consistently lower at each older age increment used.[99] When subjects were placed on atropine or practolol, the HR was significantly increased or decreased in relation to the control test, but the HR values under these conditions remained linear and parallel with increased intensity of exercise.[103] Another study using propranolol showed the same results as practolol.[96] In all cases (age differences, drug effects on HR, obese versus lean subjects)[96,99,100–104,107] when RPE was expressed in terms of relative work (per cent of $\dot{V}_{O_2}$ max or per cent of HR max reserve), the RPE values were similar. Thus, when the RPE scale is used under a variety of conditions as described previously, the use of the RPE scale under its original conception (RPE of 15 = HR of 150 beats/min, and so on) is

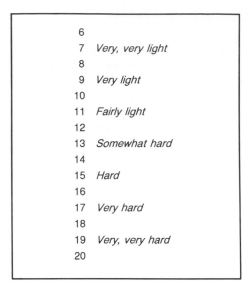

6	
7	*Very, very light*
8	
9	*Very light*
10	
11	*Fairly light*
12	
13	*Somewhat hard*
14	
15	*Hard*
16	
17	*Very hard*
18	
19	*Very, very hard*
20	

Figure 6–11. The rating of perceived exertion scale (RPE) developed by Borg. (Reprinted with permission from Borg, G.: Subjective effort in relation to physical performance and working capacity. *In* Pick, H.L., editor: Psychology: From Research to Practice. New York, Plenum Publishing Corp., 1978, pp. 333–361.)

not valid. The scale is valid, though, in relation to its various anchor points (see Fig. 6–11) and when HR is expressed relative to a percentage of maximum.[72,97,100–104,107]

The importance of the RPE scale is its high relationship to factors indicating relative fatigue. In this regard, the scale has been used for approximately 25 years in exercise testing laboratories. It has become more popularly used in the clinical setting during the past 5 years.[108] Its use in exercise prescription is detailed in Chapters 7 and 8.

As described previously, the RPE scale has been shown to be a valid indicator of the level of physical exertion (relative fatigue). It has also been shown to be reliable[99, 100] and thus can be used effectively in repeat testing. For example, if a patient rates the endpoint of a GXT 18 on one occasion, the 18 on subsequent tests should be interpreted the same way relative to the patient's feelings of fatigue. This has important implications for GXT when lactate, $\dot{V}O_2$, and $\dot{V}_E$ are not measured. RPE gives the tester an objective indicator through which to compare the relative degree of fatigue attained from test to test.[104] Thus, if aerobic capacity and treadmill performance significantly increased or decreased, and the endpoint RPE remained the same between test results, the tests could be then interpreted as representing a true change in cardiorespiratory fitness or medical status and not a reflection of whether the patient pushed as hard. Knowing the

RPE is also helpful to the clinician in judging when the patient may want to terminate the test.

Few persons rate maximum at 20, with 17 to 19 being selected most often.[97] Pollock et al.[97] found that young, healthy subjects rated maximum at 19, middle-aged healthy subjects at 18, and cardiac patients at 17.

Although the previous information shows the value of the RPE scale, it must be interpreted in the proper context. First, there are under- and overraters and it has been estimated that about 10 per cent of the population cannot use the scale with any accuracy.[109] Use of proper instructions is important. Morgan[109] has pointed out that different psychological states can also affect RPE ratings. When the Borg scale is first introduced, the use of the following written instructions can be helpful.

> You are now going to take part in a graded exercise test. You will be walking or running on the treadmill while we are measuring various physiological functions. We also want you to try to estimate how hard you *feel* the work is; that is, we want you to rate the degree of perceived exertion you feel. By perceived exertion we mean the total amount of exertion and physical fatigue. Don't concern yourself with any one factor such as leg pain, shortness of breath, or work grade, but try to concentrate on your *total, inner* feeling of exertion. Try to estimate as honestly and objectively as possible. Don't underestimate the degree of exertion you feel, but don't overestimate it either. Just try to estimate as accurately as possible.*

The written instructions can then be reinforced verbally. It is advisable to remind participants not to focus on any one problem but rather on a general fatigue. For patients with angina, claudication, orthopedic problems, and so on, rating their specific problem separately is helpful. It is also helpful to remind the participant of the various anchor points listed on the scale: 6 or 7 is resting, 13 to 15 is moderately difficult, and most persons rate maximum between 17 and 20.

Participants tend to rate treadmill and cycle ergometer exercise approximately the same.[101] If relative work is taken into account, arm ergometer activity is rated similarly to leg work, i.e., per cent of $\dot{V}O_2$ max or HR on each respective test mode.[72,102]

The Borg 15-point scale is not linear in relation to equal increments of increased intensity.[98,99,104] The scale is rather flat through a rating of 10 and then becomes curvilinear.[99,104] Above 15 on the scale, it takes very little added intensity to increase the RPE rating. Many participants do not discriminate well at the lower end of the scale. Smutok et al.[110] suggested that RPE was accurate to use in exercise prescription at running speeds or HR above 150 beats/min (80 per cent HR max) but was inaccurate and unreliable at slower speeds, such as used in walking programs. Contrary results have been reported by Gutmann et al.[111] and Pollock et al.,[72] i.e., patients

---

*William Morgan, Ed.D., University of Wisconsin, Madison, WI. Published with permission.

were able to discriminate accurately at 11 to 13 on the RPE scale. The difference in results was probably related to the subjects in the latter studies having had multiple practice periods in using the scale before data collection.

Borg[104] has recently published a new 10-step category scale for differential use that has positive attributes of a general-ratio scale. This scale is linear in relation to categories and increased intensity and may someday take the place of his original scale. A review of recent advances in the study and clinical use of perceived exertion is available.[104, 105, 108, 112, 113]

In light of all the discussion concerning the RPE scale, it should not be used or interpreted within a vacuum. It is not a perfect scale and should be used in conjunction with common sense and other pertinent clinical, psychological, and physiological information. Borg's summarization of this point follows.[104]

> **In defense of the use of perceived exertion it may be said that there is little evidence that a certain heart rate is a better indicator of "dangerous strain" than a certain perceived exertion. On any given day one may run and achieve a heart rate of 150 and feel "fine" with an RPE of 13, while on another day the same exertion may cause the runner to feel "bad" with an RPE of 17 as a result of physical and emotional negative factors.**
>
> **The elevated RPE value may be used equally with heart rate in determining a "risk factor." Neither a single RPE value nor a heart rate measure may be used alone as an accurate indicator of "dangerous strain." They complement each other.**
>
> **A "perfect" or "excellent" indicator of "dangerous strain" must involve an integration of all important risk factors, such as arrhythmias, blood pressure elevations, ST depressions, body temperature changes, blood lactate levels, and hormonal excretions. A single heart rate must be used in relation to the other strain variables and understood to be just one factor in a complicated pattern of interacting factors. A patient's perceived exertion is considered in exercise prescription because it is related closely to the heart rate but it also integrates some other important strain variables.**

PREPARATION FOR EXERCISE TESTING FOR DIAGNOSTIC PURPOSES

The diagnostic GXT is usually performed with a multiple-lead electrocardiographic (ECG) system.[11,30] As shown from Table 6–7 approximately 70 to 89 per cent of the abnormal ST-segment responses to exercise can be picked up by lead V_5 alone.[114] It appears that the addition of at least one precordial (horizontal) lead, V_1–V_3, and an inferior (vertical) lead II, III, or V_F adds significantly to the diagnosis.

Figure 6–12 shows the Mason-Likar 12-lead ECG system, and Figure 6–13 illustrates a 3-lead system popularized by Ellestad.[30] Each of these systems has been popularly used and is well accepted. In comparison to the

TABLE 6-7. SIX SERIES OF PATIENTS STUDIED WITH
MULTILEAD EXERCISE TESTS EVALUATING RELATIVE
YIELD OF ABNORMAL RESPONSES IN LEADS OTHER THAN V_5

STUDY	V_5 ALONE	OTHER LEADS ALONE
Blackburn and Katigbak[115]	89%	4% (aV_F), 2% (II), 1% (V_3) 2% (V_4), 2% (V_6)
Mason et al.[116]	70%	7% (II, III), 3.6% (V_3) 7% (V_4), 12.5% (V_6)
Phibbs and Buckels[117]		
Series A	85.5%	8.5% (II, aV_F, III), 4% (V_6)
Series B	79%	15% (II, aV_F, III), 3% (V_6), 2% (V_4) One each in I, V_1, and V_{2-3-4}
Robertson et al.[118]	75% →	10% (II, aV_F, III), 5% (V_4), 5% (V_6), 5% (mixed)
Tucker et al.[119]	70% ›	17% (aV_F), 13% (other)

(From American College of Sports Medicine: Guidelines for Graded Exercise
Testing and Exercise Prescription, 2nd ed. Philadelphia, Lea and Febiger, 1980.)

standard 12-lead system, which uses the conventional ankle and wrist attachments, placing the limb leads at the shoulders and base of the torso can eliminate most of the movement artifact found during GXT. Although the modified electrode placement systems offer an ECG pattern similar to the conventional lead system, they display a more rightward axis of the ECG. Caution should be taken if the limb leads, as shown in Figure 6-12, are moved more onto the abdomen and chest. It may eliminate additional movement artifact, but it will further distort the ECG.[11]

For the most part, standard commercial ECG recorders offer acceptable frequency responses to obtain ECGs of diagnostic quality (0 to 100 Hz). Alternation of the 25 to 45 Hz frequency response is the most common cause of the distortion of the ST segment.[11] See the American Heart Association standards for ECG recording equipment and Froelicher[11, 63] for more details concerning proper frequency responses, ECG distortion, and calibration checking of ECG equipment.

Recent advances in the manufacturing of electrodes and cable connectors for GXT have helped reduce movement artifact. Both nondisposable and disposable electrodes can be used. Silverplate or silver-silver chloride crystal pellets are used as electrode materials. Nondisposable electrodes are recessed and have to be filled with electrode paste while disposable electrodes are pregelled. The disposable electrodes are more convenient but are significantly more expensive. To obtain a good skin-to-electrode contact, the outer epidermal layer of skin must be removed. This can be accomplished by the use of an emery cloth, light abrasions with a stick or drill (dental burr). In men, the area for electrode placement must first be shaved. Usually the patient is placed in the supine position, the anatomical landmarks for electrode placement are noted (marked), the skin is cleansed with

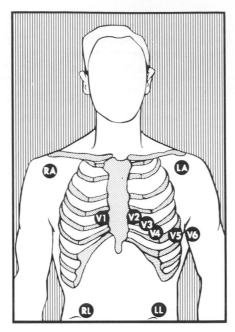

Figure 6–12. The Mason-Likar 12-lead exercise ECG lead system. (Reproduced with permission from Froelicher, V.F.: Exercise Testing and Training. Copyright © August 1983 by Year Book Medical Publishers, Inc., Chicago.)

an alcohol-saturated gauze pad, the epidermal layer of skin is removed, and the electrodes are firmly placed. Do not underestimate the importance of proper skin preparation. The use of an alternating current (AC) impedance meter (ohmeter) will aid in evaluating skin resistance. A force of less than 5,000 ohms is recommended, and each electrode is tested against a common electrode.

Once the electrodes are in place, the blood pressure cuff is attached. Baseline ECG tracings are determined in the supine, sitting, and standing positions. Another tracing is recorded after 30 to 60 seconds of hyperventilation. Because of an occasional problem with hypotension (faintness), hyperventilation should be done in the sitting position. Changes in ECG or blood pressure caused by orthostasis and hyperventilation should be noted before beginning the test.[11,30]

DIAGNOSTIC ASPECTS OF GRADED EXERCISE TESTING

This section will cover some of the basic aspects of GXT and its diagnostic value. A more detailed description of the medical aspects of the electrocardiogram (ECG)[3, 11, 16, 17, 30, 114–125] and radionuclide angiography[126–130] is found elsewhere. See Figure A–5, Appendix A, for an example of a GXT data collection form.

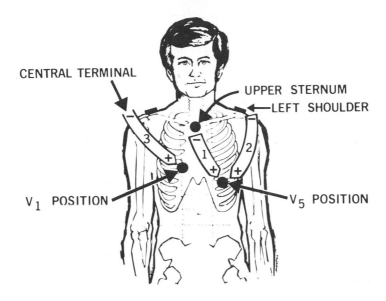

CENTRAL TERMINAL

UPPER STERNUM

LEFT SHOULDER

V_1 POSITION

V_5 POSITION

1. BIPOLAR — STERNUM TO V_5 (CM$_5$)
2. BIPOLAR — LEFT SHOULDER TO V_5 (VERTICAL)
3. CENTRAL TERMINAL TO V_1 (HORIZONTAL)

Figure 6–13. A three-lead ECG monitoring system described and used by Ellestad.[30] It shows the location of the two bipolar electrode systems and the V_1 attachment. This system provides not only the most sensitive single monitoring lead (CM$_5$), but a vertical and horizontal lead system as well. (Reprinted with permission from Ellestad, M.S.: Stress Testing Principles and Practice, 2nd ed. Philadelphia, F.A. Davis Co., 1980.)

Many aspects of the GXT have been shown to be important for diagnostic and prognostic purposes. Significant ST-segment depression or elevation, abnormal HR and/or blood pressure response to exercise, angina pectoris, dysrhythmia, and poor effort tolerance ($\dot{V}o_2$ max) have been shown to be of significant value in predicting future cardiac events.[11,30] Significant ST-segment depression has a high correlation with cardiac ischemia; usually, a minimum of 1.5 to 2 mm of upsloping and 1 mm of flat or downsloping ST-segment depression, 0.08 seconds from the J point, is considered significant.[11,30,122] It should be noted that for the normal recording speed of 25 mm/sec and 1 cm deflection with 1 mv of electrical impulse, each small 1-mm square of the ECG paper represents 0.04 seconds horizontally and 0.10 mV vertically. Figure 6–14 shows a normal (left panel) and an abnormal ECG (right panel). Figure 6–15, upper panel, shows an example of significant upsloping ST-segment depression and Figure 6–16, lower panel, non-significant upsloping ST-segment depression. Figure 6–15, lower panel, shows an example of significant downsloping ST-segment depression and Figure 6–16, mid panel, shows significant horizontal ST-segment depression.

There are different classification systems and degrees of significance

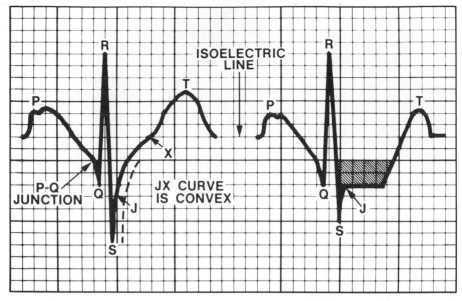

Figure 6–14. *Left,* the normal exercise electrocardiographic complex. It can be noted that the PQ segment is deflected below the isoelectric line. This point is considered to be a baseline for determining ST-segment abnormalities. *Right,* a horizontal ST-segment depression of 2.0 mm as measured from the PQ segment. (Reprinted with permission from Ellestad, M.S.: Stress Testing Principles and Practice, 2nd ed. Philadelphia, F.A. Davis Co., 1980.)

used for rating dysrhythmias.[131-133] Significant or complex dysrhythmias usually include the following: frequent unifocal (more than 10 beats/min) or multifocal (more than 4 beats/min) premature ventricular contractions (PVCs), ventricular couplets (two in sequence), R-on-T ventricular extrasystoles (early premature contraction on T wave), ventricular tachycardia (three or more consecutive PVCs), atrial tachycardia or fibrillation, and second- or third-degree heart block.

Figure 6–15 shows an example of a single PVC (lower panel). Figure 6–16 illustrates a multifocal PVC (mid panel), ventricular couplet (upper panel), and ventricular tachycardia (lower panel). When referring to the significance of dysrhythmia in regard to sudden death, Lown and Wolf[132] have developed the grading system shown in Table 6–8. Grades are designated according to severity of risk, with grades 4 and 5 considered most significant. Controversy exists over the use of this system.[134] In addition, electrophysiologists find it difficult to agree on any one system. See the chapter by Akhtar, Wolf, and Denker[135] for further details on dysrhythmias and sudden death. Whatever the system used, it is agreed that patients with significant (complex) dysrhythmias and left ventricular dysfunction (an ejection fraction of less than 0.50) are at higher risk for sudden death than patients with less complex dysrhythmias or left ventricular dysfunction alone.

Heart rate and systolic blood pressure rise linearly with increased levels

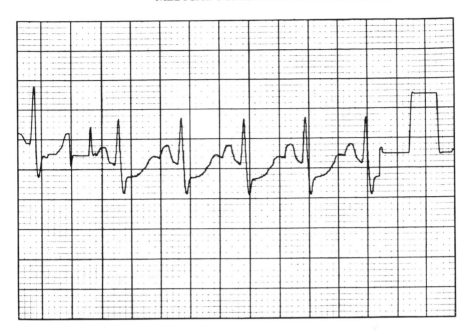

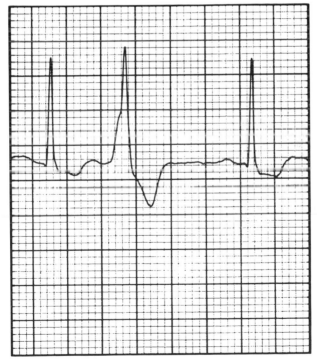

Figure 6–15. The upper panel shows an example of 2-mm upsloping ST-segment depression, and the lower panel shows 1.6-mm downsloping ST-segment depression. The lower panel also shows an example of a single premature ventricular contraction.

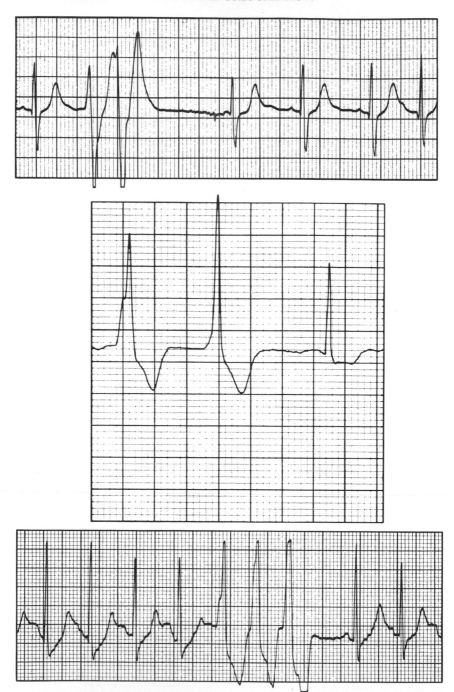

Figure 6–16. The upper panel shows an example of a ventricular couplet, the mid panel a multifocal premature ventricular contraction, and the lower panel a ventricular tachycardia. The mid panel also shows an example of 2-mm horizontal ST-segment depression.

TABLE 6-8. THE LOWN AND WOLF
GRADING SYSTEM

LOWN GRADE	DEFINITION
0	No PVCs
1	Fewer than 30 PVCs/hr
2	30 or more PVCs/hr
3	Multiform PVCs
4A	Paired PVCs
4B	Ventricular tachycardia
5	R-on-T PVCs

Data taken from Lown, B.: Sudden cardiac death: the major challenge confronting contemporary Cardiology. Am. J. Cardiol. 43:313-328, 1979; Lown, B., and Wolf, M.: Approaches to sudden death from coronary heart disease. Circulation 44:130-142, 1971.

of exercise, and diastolic blood pressure should decrease slightly or may remain rather constant.[51] Froelicher[11] and Ellestad[30] show a wide variation in HR and systolic blood pressure responses to exercise. The standard deviation for HR max is approximately ±12 beats/min.[11,136] It has been suggested that the average HR and systolic blood pressure response to exercise is approximately 8 to 10 beats/min and 7 to 10 mm Hg, respectively, for each 1-MET increase in work load.[20] These standards were developed from the data collected on average men and are not relevant to elite endurance athletes. Subsequent data gathered on women show a 11 to 13 beat/min rise in HR and 5 to 6 mm Hg increase in systolic blood pressure per 1-MET increase in work load.[59] Although the HR response per MET is less for trained than sedentary persons, not much difference is found between groups for rises in systolic blood pressure.[46,59] Cardiac patients and patients on beta-blocking drugs have a blunted HR and systolic blood pressure response to increased exercise. Heart rate increased between 5 and 7 beats/min per MET (see Figure 8-7 for HR data on patients soon after coronary artery bypass graft surgery).[137] For patients not on beta-blocking medication, the blunted HR response to exercise for cardiac patients persists for approximately 3 to 6 months.[138] If a patient is apprehensive or unfamiliar with the GXT procedure, an artificially high HR and systolic blood pressure may be present initially. Under these conditions, a slight fall in these values may occur early in the test.[28,30]

A chronotropic (very low HR) response to GXT in untrained individuals reflects an abnormal response to exercise and has significant prognostic value.[11,30] Usually, depending on age, the HR max should reach a minimum of 130 to 150 beats/min. Do not look at HR alone for diagnosis. Pollock tested a highly fit Master's runner (52 years of age) who had a HR max of 138 beats/min. He had a good HR reserve, a resting HR of 35 beats/min, and a $\dot{V}O_2$ max of 53 ml/kg·min^{-1} (personal communication). When approaching maximum effort, the HR and systolic blood pressure responses will level off. At maximum effort, systolic blood pressure may begin to fall

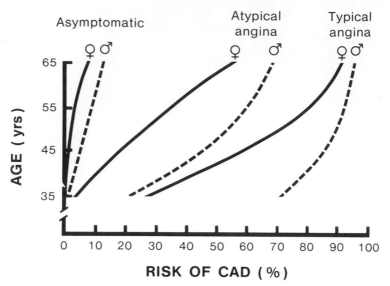

Figure 6–17. Influence of age, sex, and symptoms on risk of coronary artery disease (CAD) (derived from data of Diamond and Forrester).[16] (Reprinted with permission from Epstein, S.E.: Implications of probability analysis on the strategy used for noninvasive detection of coronary artery disease. Am. J. Cardiol. *46:*491–499, 1980.)

but should rebound within 30 to 60 seconds of recovery.[30] Systolic blood pressure for highly trained individuals may return to near pre-exercise levels within 1 to 2 minutes of recovery.

A drop in systolic blood pressure during the submaximal portion of the GXT (both at steady state and with increased work load) is clearly an abnormal response. A systolic blood pressure response above 240 mm Hg has been suggested as an endpoint for GXT[20], but values of 250 to 280 mm Hg have been recorded without incidence.[11] Bruce et al.[3] have shown that a maximum systolic blood pressure response of less than 130 mm Hg, along with cardiomegaly or a functional capacity of less than 4 METs, significantly increased the annual morbidity and mortality rate in the Seattle Heart Watch project.

Development of angina pectoris during exercise is the most significant finding associated with ischemia (CAD).[11,30] Approximately 90 per cent of patients with angina have been shown to have significant CAD by angiography.[11,17] See Figure 6–17.

PREDICTIVE VALUE OF THE GRADED EXERCISE TEST

The prognostic and diagnostic value of the GXT is dependent not only on the various abnormal findings of the GXT as described in the previous sections but also on the pretest likelihood or prevalence of CAD of the population tested. Bayes' theorem states "that the odds of a patient having

TABLE 6–9. RELATION OF PREVALENCE OF A DISEASE
AND PREDICTIVE VALUE OF A TEST*

ACTUAL DISEASE PREVALENCE (%)	PREDICTIVE VALUE OF A POSITIVE TEST (%)	PREDICTIVE VALUE OF A NEGATIVE TEST (%)
1	16.1	99.9
2	27.9	99.9
5	50.0	99.7
10	67.9	99.4
20	82.6	98.7
50	95.0	95.0
75	98.3	83.7
100	100.0	—

*Sensitivity and specificity rates each equal 95 per cent.
(From Vecchio, T.H.: Predictive value of a single diagnostic test in unselected populations. N. Engl J. Med. 274:1171–1177, 1966. Reprinted by permission of the New England Journal of Medicine.)

TABLE 6–10. DEFINITIONS AND CALCULATION OF TERMS USED
TO DEMONSTRATE THE DIAGNOSTIC VALUE OF A TEST

$$\text{Sensitivity} = \frac{TP}{TP + FN} \times 100$$

$$\text{Relative risk} = \frac{\dfrac{TP}{TP + FP}}{\dfrac{FN}{TN + FN}}$$

$$\text{Specificity} = \frac{TN}{FP + TN} \times 100 \qquad \text{Predictive value of abnormal test} = \frac{TP}{TP + FP} \times 100$$

TP = true positives or those with abnormal test and disease; FN = false negatives or those with normal test and with disease; TN = true negatives or those with normal test and no disease; FP = false positives in those with abnormal test and no disease.

Predictive value of an abnormal response is the percentage of individuals with an abnormal test who have disease.

Relative risk, or risk ratio, is the relative rate of occurrence of a disease in the group with an abnormal test compared to those with a normal test.

(Reproduced with permission from Froelicher, V.F.: Exercise Testing and Training. Copyright © August 1983 by Year Book Medical Publisher, Inc., Chicago.)

the disease after a test will be the product of the odds before the test and the odds that the test provided true results."[11] For example, Table 6–9 shows the relation of disease prevalence in regard to the prediction value of a positive (abnormal) or negative (normal) test.

To understand Bayes' theorem more clearly, the definitions that are used to demonstrate the diagnostic value of a test have been described. [11,16,17,30,139] In Table 6–10, Froelicher[11] gives the definitions for sensitivity, specificity, relative risk, and the predictive value of a test. The terms sensitivity and specificity are commonly used to determine how reliable a test is in differentiating between patients with or without CAD. Sensitivity of a test refers to the percentage of patients with disease who have an abnormal test result. Specificity of a test refers to the percentage of participants without disease who have a normal test result. The problem with diagnostic testing is that no test is ever perfect and must be interpreted in both the context of the test results (post-test likelihood of disease) and the population from which the patient is being tested (pretest likelihood of disease).

Epstein,[17] using the data of Diamond and Forrester,[16] showed how age, symptomatology, and risk factors are used to determine the pretest likelihood of having CAD. Figure 6–17 shows the risk of CAD in relation to age, sex, and angina pectoris. Note that for both atypical and typical angina, women are significantly more difficult to diagnose and determine risk. The same is true for women when using the results of the GXT (ST-segment change) and testing with radionuclides (static and dynamic imaging).

Epstein[17] illustrates well that once the pretest likelihood of disease and the results from various tests are available (post-test likelihood of disease), then a family of curves can be drawn to estimate the likelihood of disease. The use of intercepting lines based on the appropriate sensitivity and specifity permits a revised (post-test) likelihood of disease. Figure 6–18 illustrates the likelihood of CAD with increased ST-segment depression, and Figure 6–19 is based on the ECG results of a GXT (ECG EX) plus thallium perfusion scanning (TL SCAN) and radionuclide cineangiography (RN CINE). Thus, it is easy to surmise from these figures that increased ST-segment depression, and the addition of TL SCAN and RN CINE increases the likelihood of correctly categorizing patients in regard to the probability of having disease.

For those not familiar with nuclear cardiology, two of the noninvasive procedures used to evaluate cardiac function will be briefly described.[11,140] As mentioned previously, they include TL SCAN and RN CINE. The TL SCAN is usually performed in conjunction with a GXT. In this case, an intravenous (IV) line is placed into the right arm before the test, and the GXT proceeds as previously described. During the last minute of exercise, approximately 15 m CI of [201]thallium is injected intravenously. After an abbreviated recovery (usually less than 5 minutes), the patient is immediately placed under a gamma camera, and images are acquired in the anterior, 45-degree left anterior oblique, and left lateral positions or 70-degree left anterior oblique position. The measurements are repeated approximately 4 hours later. The technique is based on the premise that the potassium analog [201]thallium goes where capillary perfusion (blood flow) is adequate to avoid ischemia. This generally depends on two factors, capillary perfusion and cell viability. Necrotic or scar tissue and ischemic areas will not perfuse, whereas viable tissue will (see Fig. 6–20). Thus, by evaluating the immediate postexercise TL SCAN and comparing it with the resting values (4 hours after exercise), normal, scarred, and ischemic areas may be differentiated.

The RN CINE evaluates the dynamic action of the heart.[11,140] Although different techniques may be used (gated or first pass), both derive an outer perimeter of the left ventricular chamber during systole (end-systolic vol-

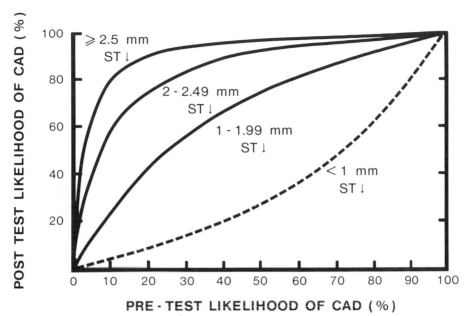

Figure 6–18. Family of ST-segment depression curves (based on data derived from Diamond and Forrester[16]) and likelihood of coronary artery disease (CAD). ST↓ = ST-segment depression. (Reprinted with permission from Epstein, S. E.: Implications of probability analysis on the strategy used for noninvasive detection of coronary artery disease. Am. J. Cardiol. 46:491–499, 1980.)

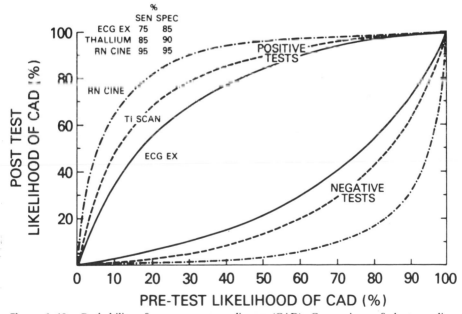

Figure 6–19. Probability of coronary artery disease (CAD). Comparison of electrocardiographic exercise testing (ECG EX), thallium perfusion scanning (TI SCAN), and radionuclide cineangiography (RN CINE). (Sensitivity [SEN] and specificity [SPEC] values are approximations derived from published series.) (Reprinted with permission from Epstein, S.E.: Implications of probability analysis on the strategy used for noninvasive detection of coronary artery disease. Am. J. Cardiol. 46:491–499, 1980.)

ume) and diastole (end-diastolic volume) (see Fig. 6–21). The test is performed with a patient seated or supine, with exercise being performed on a modified cycle ergometer. Patients exercise with a gamma camera placed against the chest, and a radionuclide (^{99m}technetium, for example) is introduced into the venous system (usually via the antecubital or jugular vein). The scintillation camera picks up the counts as the radioactive materials pass through the heart. The RN CINE method is particularly good for determination of ejection fraction and regional wall motion. See Schmidt et al.[140] and

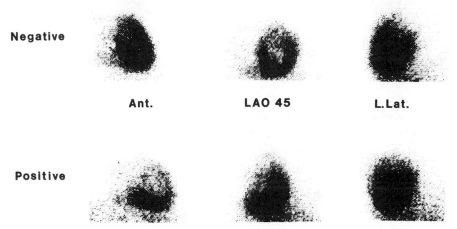

Negative

Ant.   LAO 45   L.Lat.

Positive

Figure 6–20. A normal (*upper panel*) and an abnormal (*lower panel*) thallium scintigram. The normal scan reveals a relatively homogeneous distribution of the indicator, whereas the abnormal study reveals an anteroseptal defect seen best in the anterior and LAO views. (Reprinted with permission from Schmidt, D.H., and Port, S.: The clinical and research application of nuclear cardiology. *In* Pollock, M.L., and Schmidt, D.H., editors: Heart Disease and Rehabilitation, 2nd ed. New York, copyright © John Wiley and Sons [in press].)

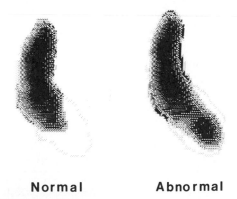

Normal   Abnormal

Figure 6–21. Radionuclide angiograms done in the right anterior oblique position. A normal study (*left*) and an abnormal study (*right*) are shown. Wall motion is represented by the distance between the end-diastolic perimeter and the end-systolic image. (Reprinted with permission from Schmidt, D.H., and Port, S.: The clinical and research application of nuclear cardiology. *In* Pollock, M.L., and Schmidt, D.H., editors: Heart Disease and Rehabilitation, 2nd ed. New York, copyright © John Wiley and Sons [in press].)

Froelicher[11] for more details concerning methodology and interpretation of radionuclide procedures.

BODY COMPOSITION

This section will deal with the various techniques used for measuring body composition. Both laboratory and field techniques will be described and illustrated. Determination of ideal weight and interpretation of results will be discussed.

MEASUREMENT OF BODY COMPOSITION

Many methods are currently available for estimating body density (percentage of body fat).[141] The most common are the underwater weighing, volume displacement, radiographic analysis, potassium-40, isotopic dilution, and ultrasound techniques. Behnke and Wilmore[141] describe the principles and methodologies for these techniques. Because of time, equipment, and space requirements, these methods are not generally used in clinical practice. Anthropometric measures (skinfold fat and body circumference and diameter measures) are more practical for use in a clinical or nonlaboratory setting.

UNDERWATER WEIGHING: PRINCIPLE, EQUATIONS, AND MEASUREMENT ERRORS

Of the various laboratory techniques used for determining body density, only the underwater weighing method will be described. This technique is the most widely used laboratory procedure for measuring body density. The underwater weighing technique is based on Archimedes' principle. The principle states that "a solid heavier than a fluid, if placed in it, descends to the bottom of the fluid, and the solid will, when weighed in the fluid, be lighter than its true weight by the weight of the fluid displaced."[8] In other words, an object placed in water must be buoyed up by a counterforce that equals the weight of the water it displaces. The density of bone and muscle tissue (1.2 to 3.0) is higher than that of water, whereas fat (0.90) is less dense than water.[141,142] Therefore, a person with proportionally more bone and muscle mass for the same total body weight will weigh heavier in water and thus have a higher body density (lower percentage of body fat). This was illustrated in Figure 2–1.

To determine body density from underwater weighing, the following equation has been derived:[141,143]

$$Db = \frac{Wa}{\dfrac{(Wa-Ww) - (RV + 100 \text{ ml})}{Dw}}$$

whereby Db = body density; Wa = body weight out of the water; Ww = weight in the water; Dw = density of water; and RV = residual volume. The 100 ml is the estimated air volume of the gastrointestinal tract. Although this volume can fluctuate, Buskirk[144] has suggested the use of a constant correction factor.

The other body gas volume that is needed to calculate body density is residual volume (RV). The RV is the amount of air left in the lungs after a maximal expiration. Residual volume is normally measured by an open circuit nitrogen washout technique or by a closed circuit oxygen or helium dilution method.[141] Residual volume can also be estimated by average population values based upon age, sex, and height[145] or by an estimated percentage of the vital capacity (approximately 25 to 30 per cent).[146] If the RV of a large population were measured by the three methods (actual per cent measurement; value based on age, sex, and height; or value based on a percentage of vital capacity), RV would vary little among them.[147] Wilmore[147] showed that the difference in mean body density calculated among groups using actual and estimated values for RV was less than 0.001 g/ml. Thus, for screening purposes or when measuring large groups, the estimation of RV would be an acceptable technique. However, RV is quite variable at any given age, height, or vital capacity and may result in errors of up to 5 per cent body fat (see example in Table 6–11). Therefore, for individual analysis and counseling, the actual measured RV is recommended.[141,147,148]

When determining body density, if an estimation of RV is used, the following equations developed by Goldman and Becklake[145] are recommended:

Male, RV = 0.017 (age, yr) + 0.06858 (height, inches) − 3.477
Female, RV = 0.009 (age, yr) + 0.08128 (height, inches) − 3.9

The density of water also has to be accounted for in the equation to determine body density. Water density varies with temperature and requires a standard conversion factor.[144] Table 6–12 lists water density at various common water temperatures from 23°C to 37°C.[149] For subject comfort, measuring underwater weight at temperatures between 32°C and 35°C is recommended. Although water density is important to determine, its slight variation within the temperature range used for underwater weighing makes its effect negligible on the error of measurement within the calculation of body density.

Figure 6–22 is an example of a body composition and pulmonary function form used to record data for determining body density by underwater weighing. The form shows actual values of a 20-year-old male subject. Residual volume was measured twice outside the water with the subject in a sitting position. Two values are determined for verification purposes. If repeat values differ by more than 100 to 200 ml, then a third measure should be taken. The amount of accuracy that is acceptable when determining RV will depend upon the equipment and technique used and purpose of the test

TABLE 6-11. THE EFFECT OF ERRORS IN RESIDUAL
VOLUME (RV), SCALE WEIGHT IN THE WATER (Ww), AND
BODY WEIGHT OUT OF THE WATER (Wa) ON
DETERMINATION OF BODY DENSITY (Db)
FROM UNDERWATER WEIGHING

MEASURE	ACTUAL*	ERRORS[†]		
		1	2	3
RV, L	1.200	1.400	1.700	2.200
Db, gm/cc	1.0606	1.0631	1.0669	1.0734
Fat, %	16.72	15.62	13.95	11.16
Ww, kg	13.08	13.58	14.08	15.08
Db, gm/cc	1.0606	1.0612	1.0618	1.0631
Fat, %	16.72	16.46	16.18	15.61
Wa, kg	88.70	88.80	89.20	89.70
Db, gm/cc	1.0606	1.0605	1.0602	1.0598
Fat, %	16.72	16.77	16.91	17.08

* Actual values are from Figure 6-22.
† Each error for Db and per cent fat is calculated with the other two
variables from the actual values.

TABLE 6-12. CONVERSION CHART FOR
DETERMINING WATER DENSITY (Dw) AT VARIOUS
WATER TEMPERATURES (W TEMP)

W TEMP (°C)	Dw	W TEMP (°C)	Dw
23	0.997569	31	0.995372
24	0.997327	32	0.995057
25	0.997075	33	0.994734
26	0.996814	34	0.994403
27	0.996544	35	0.994063
28	0.996264	36	0.993716
29	0.995976	37	0.993360
30	0.995678		

(screening or research). For calculation purposes, the RV values listed in
Figure 6-22 were averaged.

To determine underwater weight, multiple trials of 6 to 10 are recommended.[150] As shown with the data in Figure 6-22, there is a learning curve.
When the data level off and remain so, even with continued encouragement
from the tester, the test can be terminated. What criteria should be used in
picking the actual underwater weight? Behnke and Wilmore[141] have used
the following method: (1) select the highest observed weight if it is obtained
more than once; (2) if criterion 1 is not met, select the second highest weight
if it is observed more than once; and (3) if criteria 1 and 2 are not met, select
the third highest measure. With the data in Figure 6-22, trials 6 and 7 were
used in the calculation of body density. Although it is apparent from the

BODY COMPOSITION AND PULMONARY FUNCTION

Name: _____ Date: _____10/5/82_____

Age: 20   Body Wt: 88.70 X kg   Ht: 177.8 X cm   Bar. Pr. _____746.1_____

_____lb   _____ in

Group: _____ Sex: M

	Trial 1	Trial 2		Trial 1	Trial 2
PF	_____	_____	Temp	22.0	22.0
$FEV_{1.0}$	_____	_____	E_{N2}	0.073	0.069
VC	_____	_____	I_{N2}	0.003	0.002
$(FEV_{1.0}/VC) \cdot 100$	_____	_____	A_{iN2}	0.771	0.769
$FEV_{2.0}$	_____	_____	A_{fN2}	.079	.072
$FEV_{3.0}$	_____	_____	DS	.09	.09
MVV	_____	_____	PREDICTED RV	.	.
Temp. (°C)	_____	_____	CALCULATED RV	1.225	1.174
			AVERAGE RV =	1.200	

UNDERWATER WEIGHT

Trial	Wt (kg)	Temp. (°C)	Trial	Wt (kg)	Temp. (°C)
①	12.96	34.0		_____	_____
2	13.00	34.0		_____	_____
3	13.02	34.0		_____	_____
4	13.08	34.0		_____	_____
5	13.06	34.0		_____	_____
⑥	13.08	34.0		_____	_____
⑦	13.08	34.0		_____	_____
⑧	13.06	34.0		_____	_____
⑨	_____	_____		_____	_____
10	_____	_____		_____	_____

Chair and belt wt.	8.84*	_____	Chair and belt wt.	_____	_____
Db	1.0606	_____	Db	_____	_____
Calculated % fat (Siri)	16.72	_____	Calculated % fat (Siri)	_____	_____

*To be subtracted from the underwater weight to derive the net underwater weight of the subject.

Figure 6–22. Body composition and pulmonary function form used in determining body density by underwater weighing. (Courtesy of The Human Performance Laboratory, Mount Sinai Medical Center, Milwaukee, WI.)

subject's data in Figure 6–22 that he leveled off after trial 4, additional trials were determined to verify his best effort.

What is meant by the chair and belt weight shown in Figure 6–22? This is simply the weight of the chain, chair, weight belt, and so on that is subtracted from the total observed weight (see Fig. 6–23). This measure is usually obtained after the underwater weight is determined, with the chair lowered to the level at which the underwater weight was observed. For the calculation of underwater weight from the data in Figure 6–22, 8.84 kg (chair and weight belt) is subtracted from 13.08 kg (total weight observed).

As an example of calculating body density by underwater weighing, the subject's data shown in Figure 6–22 are substituted into the equation used to derive body density.

$$Db = \frac{88.70}{(88.7 - 4.24) - (1.20 + .100)}{0.994}$$

$$Db = 1.0606$$

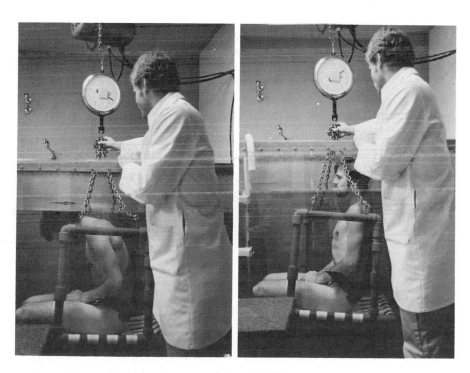

Figure 6–23. The right panel shows subject seated in underwater weighing tank. The left panel shows the subject placing his head under water and being measured for underwater weight. The above tank is 4 X 5 X 5 feet. It is constructed of ¼-inch stainless steel bottom and sides with one side of ¾-inch Plexiglas. The tank has its own filtering and heating system. The chair is constructed from 2-inch PVC pipe. (Courtesy of Mount Sinai Medical Center, Milwaukee, WI.)

Percentage of fat is usually predicted from one of the two following equations:

Brozek et al.[142]: % body fat $= \left[\left(\dfrac{4.570}{Db}\right) - 4.142\right] 100$

and

Siri[151]: % body fat $= \left[\left(\dfrac{4.950}{Db}\right) - 4.500\right] 100$

Both equations are based on the general assumption that various body components—e.g., muscle, bone, and fat—are of a constant density and that total body water is of a constant nature. Both percentage of body fat equations correlate highly ($r = 0.995 - 0.999$) and give similar mean values.[141] With the body density value determined from the subject in Figure 6–22 (1.0606), percentage of body fat values calculated by the Siri and Brozek equations are 16.72 per cent and 16.69 per cent, respectively. Thus, either equation is recommended for use, but consistency with the use of a particular equation should be maintained. When comparing percentage of body fat results (norms, research studies, and so on), knowledge of the equation used to derive the comparative data should be known. The percentage of body fat norms shown in Appendix A, Tables A–1 to A–10, were derived from the Siri equation.

Although the Brozek and Siri equations are universally accepted, they are not without problems. Both equations were based on the results of direct compositional analysis through dissection of fresh human cadavers.[141] Only a few cadavers were used, and they did not represent a distribution of the normal population. All assumptions of compositional analysis used to derive the percentage of fat equations have not been validated on children and youth and the elderly. Lohman[152] and others[48, 141, 153, 154] have discussed the problems of using percentage of body fat equations with youth and children. Bone density is less during this period of life, and total body water is higher.[155] After 40 to 50 years of age for women and 50 years of age for men, bone density decreases.[156] Loss of muscle mass is also evident in the elderly. Because of this problem, percentage of body fat equations are not valid for use in children and youth up to 16 or 17 years of age and are questionable for use in the elderly. Because of this invalidity, the new Health Related Physical Fitness Test Manual[48] developed by the American Alliance for Health, Physical Education, Recreation and Dance for use with school children and youth aged 6 to 18 years uses the sum of two skinfold fat measures for body fat analysis and comparison and does not make a conversion to percentage of body fat.

Recently, Martin et al.[157] have completed extensive dissections of 12 male and 13 female adult cadavers. Although only preliminary data have been presented, the work shows a significant variance among cadavers for the various body components. These data could well lead to more refined equations for predicting percentage of body fat in adults.

In regard to potential errors in determining body density from the underwater weighing technique, RV, scale weight (Ww), and body weight (Wa) are critical factors. Table 6–11 shows body density and percentage of body fat calculated from the actual RV, scale weight, and body weight shown in Figure 6–22. To determine the potential error of each of the three factors on the calculation of body density, the following additions were made to the actual values: RV, 200, 500, and 1,000 ml; Ww, 50, 100, and 200 g; and Wa, 100, 500, and 1,000 g, respectively. The ramifications for each error factor will be discussed separately.

The errors related to actually measuring or estimating RV from age and height or from vital capacity were discussed earlier. As shown from Table 6–11, errors in RV can make a dramatic difference in the results. A 2 to 5.5 per cent error in body fat was found with 500- to 1,000-ml differences in estimating RV. Another potential error in measuring RV is whether the measure is actually determined in the water at the time of the underwater weighing or separately, out of the water. Although 200- to 300-ml differences in RV have been reported between the two methods, if care is taken to have the subject exhale fully and replicate the body position for the measurements (sitting and so on), the error is probably smaller.[141,158] Nevertheless, even if a 200-ml difference is found, only an approximate 1 per cent error in body fat is found (Table 6–11). This error is certainly acceptable for clinical and research purposes, and if replicated consistently, it is adequate for serial analysis, i.e., RV should be a constant error in one direction.

Normally, a 50-gram error in underwater scale weight would be unusually large: thus, the error should be less than 0.5 per cent fat (Table 6–11). Scales not being calibrated, subjects being unable to coordinate the underwater weighing procedure, and oscillations created by water movement are the most common problems associated with reading the scale weight. Periodic calibration of the scale with known weights can easily correct the first problem, and multiple practice trials can correct the second. A stable, comfortable chair will aid in increasing the subject's ability to minimize underwater motion. Water oscillations are more problematic in large bodies of water (swimming pools) than in smaller tanks. Having the subject move slowly in the water and be relaxed in the chair seat, as well as the use of a weighted belt, enhances the accuracy in reading the scale. Usually some oscillation is present, but interpolation should be within 20 to 60 g and rarely more than 100 g. If a small water tank is used and techniques are adequate, the scale stylus should have imperceptible movement in approximately 50 per cent of adult subjects.

Body weight can be quite variable and changes with time of day, dietary pattern, state of hydration, and illness. Best results are obtained in the morning before breakfast and exercise. A scale graduated to 100-g increments is quite satisfactory for use in this procedure and would account for a very small error of measurement (see Table 6–11). Excessive hydration or dehydration (exercise, sauna, diarrhea, or menstruation) can have a significant effect on body density.[34] For example, a 2- to 3-kg weight gain or loss would cause a 0.75 to 1.0 per cent change in percentage of body fat.

The scale used in Figure 6–23 is a 15-kg scale, calibrated in 20-g increments. This type of scale or a 9-kg (10-gram increments) scale is adequate for use with the underwater weighing procedure. In the figure, the scale is attached to a quarter-ton hoist. The hoist is helpful in adjusting the seat height to the proper level. In the same figure, the technician is helping to hold (stabilize) the scale when the subject is hyperventilating (before going under the water), placing his head underwater, and bringing his head out of the water. This helps to keep the subject from accidentally swallowing water and reduces water oscillations during the procedure. The hand is removed from the scale (chain) once the subject is in position and stable under water.

Using a strain gauge or load cell that is directly connected to a recorder is a more sophisticated (and expensive) technique in measuring the underwater weight. In this case, the chair can still be suspended from the ceiling or set directly on the load cells. Although the use of a load cell system makes the measurement more objective and has the advantage of supplying a permanent record of the procedure, it has not been shown to be more accurate with experienced technicians.[159] Fahey and Schroeder,[159] using trained subjects and trained technicians, showed a mean of 2.30 ± 0.48 kg versus 2.29 ± 0.45 kg (nonsignificant) when comparing the load cell and autopsy scale methods, respectively. Fluctuations in the reading were less with the load cell system and thus may be a better system for use with less experienced technicians.

UNDERWATER WEIGHING: PROCEDURE

The underwater weighing procedure can be accomplished in almost any body of fresh water that is at least 3 to 4 feet deep. Water tanks may be as diverse as an Olympic size swimming pool, a small, framed crib that is placed in a swimming pool (decreases water turbulence),[150] a wine vat, a 120-gallon gas drum, a canvas bag, a specially built small swimming pool, or a stainless steel or fiberglass–enforced tank. With this in mind, the cost can vary from nothing to $10,000 to $15,000. A tank no smaller than 4 feet X 4 feet X 4 feet is recommended. A 5-foot depth has been helpful in testing subjects over 6 feet 8 inches in height. A water heater and filtering system are recommended. In addition, an easily accessible emergency water drainage system should be built in. If possible, the tank should be recessed into the floor, or, if not possible, a platform should be built on at least one side so that the top of the tank is about waist to chest high and the weight scale is approximately at eye level (see Fig. 6–23).

The underwater weighing procedure can also be performed with the subject in the standing or prone position. Different specifications for tank size are needed for other body positions.

For best results, instructions to and preparation of the subject before underwater weighing is important. A normal diet, drinking, and exercise pattern is recommended. Subjects should avoid foods that can cause excessive amounts of gas to develop in the gastrointestinal tract. Situations that cause unusual hydration or dehydration should be avoided. There should be no eating or smoking for at least 2 to 3 hours before testing. If eating is necessary before testing, just a moderate portion is recommended.

Men should be measured in the nude or in a supporter or swimming brief. Women should wear a two-piece tank suit or bikini type of bathing suit. A regular two-piece bathing suit can be acceptable for use, but more caution is needed to avoid air trapping. Air trapping from a bathing suit (top or bottom) can lead to a significant error in underwater weight.

Before beginning the procedure, subjects should be asked to void and defecate. Once this has been accomplished, body weight should be measured. If anthropometric measures are to be taken, they should be done next, followed by the underwater weighing. Doing the underwater weighing procedure first and then having the subject dry off changes the texture of the skin and thus may influence the skinfold fat measurement.

The underwater weighing procedure to be described is with the tank and accessory apparatus shown in Figure 6–23. After subjects are standing in the tank and before they sit on the chair (water about chest depth), have them slowly rub their hands over the surface of all body parts, stirring the water as little as possible, to help eliminate air bubbles attached to the skin. Starting with one foot and leg and then the other, and culminating with dipping the head under the water and rubbing the shoulders and head. Wiggling the top and bottom of the swim suit will help release any trapped air. Once this has been completed, take the weight belt and secure it around the waist. A scuba type of weight belt with approximately 3 to 5 kg of weight attached is satisfactory. The subject will then sit on the chair and assume a comfortable position. The seat height is then adjusted to bring the chin-mouth to water level.

Explain the total procedure, and use the first trial as a talk-through rehearsal. Have the subject do the following:

1. Hyperventilate five to six times and expel most of the air while in the upright position.

2. Continue to expel air from the lungs and slowly lower the head under the water until the top of the head clears the surface. If the head is not completely submerged, the technician should tap the top of the subject's head until it does clear the surface.

3. Place hands on top of thighs and relax once all of the air has been forcefully expelled. Often an imbalance is experienced (unsteadiness in water) if the subject pulls self down by holding on to the knees or chair.

4. Lift the head back out of the water when measurement has been determined. Knocking on the side of the tank can generally be used as a signal to come up.

5. Repeat the procedure 6 to 10 times. A critique and review of problem points between trials will improve accuracy. Brief rest periods may be necessary if subject gets tired.

TABLE 6-13. MEANS AND STANDARD DEVIATIONS OF HYDROSTATICALLY DETERMINED BODY DENSITY AND CONCURRENT VALIDITY OF REGRESSION EQUATIONS FOR MALES AND FEMALES

SOURCE	SAMPLE		BODY DENSITY		REGRESSION ANALYSIS	
	Age*	n	$\bar{x}$	s	R	SE
Males						
Brozek and Keys (1951)[161]	20.3	133	1.077	.014	.88	.007
	45–55	122	1.055	.012	.74	.009
Cureton et al. (1975)[162]	8–11	49	1.053	.013	.77	.008
Durnin and Rahaman (1967)[163]	18–33	60	1.068	.013	.84	.007
	12–15	48	1.063	.012	.76	.008
Durnin and Wormsley (1974)[164]	17–19	24	1.066	.016	†	.007
	20–29	92	1.064	.016	†	.008
	30–39	34	1.046	.012	†	.009
	40–49	35	1.043	.015	†	.008
	50–68	24	1.036	.018	†	.009
Forsyth and Sinning (1973)[165]	19–29	50	1.072	.010	.84	.006
Haisman (1970)[166]	22–26	55	1.070	.010	.78	.006
Harsha et al. (1978)[167]	6–16	79‡	1.046	.018	.84	.010
	6–16	49§	1.055	.020	.90	.009
Jackson and Pollock (1978)[168]	18–61	308	1.059	.018	.92	.007
Katch and McArdle (1973)[169]	19.3	53	1.065	.014	.89	.007
Katch and Michael (1969)[170]	17.0	40	1.076	.013	.89	.006
Parizkova (1961)[171]	9–12	57	†	†	.92	.011
Pascale et al. (1956)[172]	22.1	88	1.068	.012	.86	.006
Pollock et al. (1976)[173]	18–22	95	1.068	.014	.87	.007
	40–55	84	1.043	.013	.84	.007
Sloan (1967)[174]	18–26	50	1.075	.015	.85	.008
Wilmore and Behnke (1969)[175]	16–36	133	1.066	.013	.87	.006
Wright and Wilmore (1974)[176]	27.8	297	1.061	.014	.86	.007
Females						
Durnin and Rahaman (1967)[163]	18–29	45	1.044	.014	.78	.010
	13–16	38	1.045	.011	.78	.008
Durnin and Wormsley (1974)[164]	16–19	29	1.040	.017	†	.009
	20–29	100	1.034	.021	†	.011
	30–39	58	1.025	.020	†	.013
	40–49	48	1.020	.016	†	.011
	50–68	37	1.013	.016	†	.008
Harsha et al. (1978)[167]	6–16	52‡	1.033	.016	.85	.008
	6–16	39§	1.041	.019	.90	.008
Jackson et al. (1980)[177]	18–55	249	1.044	.016	.87	.008
Katch and McArdle (1973)[169]	20.3	69	1.039	.015	.84	.009
Katch and Michael (1968)[178]	19–23	64	1.049	.011	.70	.008
Parizkova (1961)[171]	9–12	56	†	†	.81	.012
	13–16	62	†	†	.82	.010
Pollock et al. (1975)[179]	18–22	83	1.043	.014	.84	.008
	33–50	60	1.032	.015	.89	.007
Sinning (1978)[180]	17–23	44	1.064	.010	.81	.006
Sloan et al. (1962)[181]	20.2	50	1.047	.012	.74	.008
Wilmore and Behnke (1970)[182]	21.4	128	1.041	.010	.76	.007
Young (1964)[183]	53.0	62	1.020	.014	.84	.008
Young et al. (1962)[184]	17–27	94	1.034	.009	.69	.007

* Age is expressed as the mean or range.
† Data not provided.
‡ White.
§ Black.

(From Baumgartner, J.A., and Jackson, A.S.: Measurement and Evaluation in Physical Education, 2nd ed. Copyright © 1975, 1982 Wm. C. Brown Publishers, Dubuque, Iowa. All Rights Reserved. Reprinted by permission.)

A few subjects may have to use a nose clip during the underwater weighing procedure. It should be noted that a few individuals may not be able to complete the procedure satisfactorily (approximately 2 to 3 per cent). Patience and making the subject feel comfortable in the water are key factors. For beginners, the RV procedure may take 10 to 15 minutes, and he underwater weighing, 30 to 40 minutes.

ANTHROPOMETRIC MEASURES

Anthropometry is the science that deals with the measurement of size, weight, and proportions of the human body. In the areas of body composition, measurement, exercise science, and sports medicine, skinfold fat, circumferences, and body diameter measures have been utilized.[141,155] As mentioned earlier in the book and in this section, anthropometric measures are used to predict body density and percentage of body fat. In some cases, and in particular with school children, the sum of skinfold measures should be used. In addition, various individual skinfold fat and circumference measures when taken serially over weeks or months can demonstrate a shift in body composition. For example, the gluteal and waist circumference measures are excellent in showing reductions in body fat with aerobic training, and biceps circumference increases with strength training.

Although the aforementioned laboratory methods of assessing body density are considered most accurate, they are often not practical for the clinical setting or for mass testing. Anthropometric measurement correlates well with the underwater weighing method and has several advantages: The necessary equipment is inexpensive and needs little or no space, and the measures can be obtained easily and quickly.[141] The results from many studies using skinfold fat or combinations of skinfold fat, circumferences, and diameters are shown in Table 6–13. These data represent studies conducted on both men and women and on persons of various ages and body fatness (density).

In general, the results show that the correlations for predicting body density from height and weight are below 0.6, the best combination of height and weight indices, e.g., the body mass index,[160] 0.65 to 0.7, and multiple regression equations using a combination of skinfolds, or skinfold, circumference, and diameter measures at or above 0.8.[27] In addition, see Table 6–14 for comparisons of correlations of various anthropometric measures with body density.[24]

The first body composition regression equations using anthropometric techniques were published in 1951 by Brozek and Keys,[161] who used skinfolds to estimate body density for young and middle-aged men. In the early 1960s, Sloan et al.[181] and Young et al.[183, 184] published similar equations for women of selected age groups. These equations were developed by using various combinations of skinfold fat measurements. From the middle 1960s to the 1970s, numerous researchers published additional equations

TABLE 6-14. CORRELATION BETWEEN HYDROSTATICALLY
DETERMINED BODY DENSITY (Db) AND ANTHROPOMETRIC VARIABLES

ANTHROPOMETRIC VARIABLE	FEMALE SAMPLE (N = 249)			MALE SAMPLE (N = 308)		
	r	SE (Db)	SE (% F)	r	SE (Db)	SE (% F)
Age	−.35	0.015	6.7	−.38	0.017	7.4
Height	−.08	0.016	7.2	.01	0.018	8.0
Weight	−.63	0.012	5.6	−.62	0.014	6.3
Body mass index[a]	−.70	0.011	5.1	−.69	0.013	5.8
Sum of seven skinfolds	−.85	0.008	3.8	−.88	0.009	3.8
Sum of Three I[b]	−.84	0.009	3.9	−.89	0.008	3.6
Sum of Three II[c]	−.83	0.009	4.0	−.86	0.009	4.1

[a] Body mass Index = Wt/Ht^2, where weight is in kilograms and height is in meters.

[b] Sum of three skinfold fat measures: Females: triceps, suprailium, and thigh. Males: chest, abdomen, and thigh.

[c] Sum of three skinfold fat measures: Females: triceps, abdomen, and suprailium. Males: chest, triceps, and subscapula.

(From Pollock, M.L., Schmidt, D.H., and Jackson, A.S.: Measurement of cardiorespiratory fitness and body composition in the clinical setting. Comprehensive Therapy, Vol. 6, No. 9, pp. 12–27, 1980. Published with permission of The Laux Company, Inc., Harvard, MA.)

for women and men (see Table 6–13). The objective of this research was to produce more accurate prediction equations. In addition to skinfold measurements, several body circumferences and, in some instances, bone diameters were used as independent variables. During this era, electronic computers and stepwise multiple regression computer programs became readily available to researchers. This increased computing capacity made it easy to analyze a large number of variables and select the combination of anthropometric variables that produced the highest multiple correlation. The equations consisting of skinfolds, circumferences, and diameters were more accurate than the earlier equations using only skinfolds; this was especially true for women and middle-aged men.[173,179]

The research leading to the development of population-specific equations has shown that age and gender are important sources of body density variation. Body density differences between men and women can largely be traced to essential fat variance.[141] In addition, population-specific equations for gender have been important because of the differences in subcutaneous fat distribution for men and women.[185] Bone density changes are related to aging; bone density increases up to age 20 and decreases after age 50.[152,156] Lohman[152] showed how the relationship between body density and subcutaneous fat is affected by gender and age. Using published data involving men and women who varied in age,[173,179] Lohman examined skinfold thickness with body density adjusted to 1.050 g/ml (21.4 per cent fat, Siri). With this common body density, the skinfold thicknesses of women were lower than men, and older subjects had less subcutaneous fat than their younger counterparts. Since skinfold thickness is the primary variable used in body density equations, the analysis by Lohman showed that equations developed on one group will be biased when applied to subjects who differ in gender, age, and fatness. Equations developed on younger subjects will underestimate the body density of older subjects. Using gender-specific equations and applying them to the opposite sex will produce a constant prediction error of about 0.025 g/ml (11 per cent fat).[152] The findings from the research on population-specific equations show that gender, age, and degree of fatness need to be considered when estimating body density from anthropometric variables.[152,164,185–187]

Not only are the population-specific equations sensitive to differences in age, gender, and degree of fatness, but also they are subject to error regarding a basic assumption that hydrostatically determined body density is linearly related to skinfold fat. Figure 6–24 clearly shows that the latter relationship is curvilinear rather than linear.[168] This means that population-specific equations predict most accurately at the mean of the population in which the data were collected and the equation developed. As subjects differ from the mean, the standard error of measurement increases significantly.[187] This concept is diagrammatically shown in Figure 6–25.

DEVELOPMENT OF GENERALIZED EQUATIONS FOR PREDICTING BODY DENSITY FROM ANTHROPOMETRIC MEASURES

The more recent trend has been to develop generalized rather than population-specific equations. These specific equations provide valid estimates with subjects representative of defined populations. Durnin and Wormersley[164] were the first to consider the generalized approach. They published equations with a common slope but adjusted the intercept to account for aging. More recently, Jackson and Pollock published generalized equations for adult men[168] and women.[177] Their research was an extension of the Durnin and Wormersley work and was designed to further overcome some of the limitations of population-specific equations. The newer generalized equations by Jackson and Pollock added age in the prediction equation to account for potential changes in the ratio of internal to external fat and bone density.

Tables 6–14 and 6–15 illustrate the differences in the prediction accuracy of body density and percentage of body fat using the best body height-weight index or body mass index (BMI) and linear and curvilinear equations. The data were from 249 women, 18 to 55 years of age (average, 31.4 years), who ranged from 4 to 44 per cent fat (average, 24.1 per cent), and 308 men, 18 to 61 years of age (average, 32.6 years), who ranged from 1 to 33 per cent fat (average, 17.7 per cent).[24] The zero-order correlations and standard error of measurement between selected anthropometric variables and body density determined by underwater weighing are shown in Table 6–14. Height was the only variable not related to body density. The BMI had only a slightly better correlation than body weight alone. The sum of skinfold fat measures represented the highest correlations. In addition, the correlation between the various combinations of the sum of three skin-

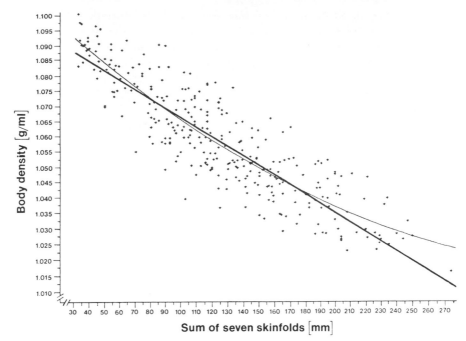

Figure 6–24. Scattergram of body density and sum of seven skinfolds with the linear and quadratic regression lines for adult men age 18 to 61 years. (From Jackson, A.S., and Pollock, M. L.: Generalized equations for predicting body density of men. Br. J. Nutr. *40:*497–504, 1978. Reprinted by permission of Cambridge University Press.)

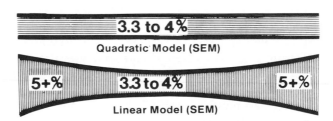

Figure 6–25. The figure diagrammatically illustrates the differences of the standard error of measurement (SEM) for predicting percentage of body fat (body density) using the linear and quadratic regression models. Note that the SEM are similar at the population means but vary significantly away from the mean for the linear model. The linear model tends to underestimate body density in lean subjects and overestimate it in fatter than average subjects. (Reprinted with permission from Jackson, A.S., and Pollock, M.L.: Steps toward the development of generalized equation for predicting body composition of adults. Can. J. Appl. Sport Sci. *7:* 189–196, 1982.)

fold measures exceeds 0.97.[24,168,186,187] Certain circumference measures, such as gluteal (buttocks) for women, show slightly higher correlations in combination with skinfolds.[177] Inclusion of circumference measures in the prediction equations shown in Table 6–15 was of minimal additional value. The sum of skinfolds provides a more representative sample of subcutaneous body fat and is more highly correlated with body density than are individual sites.

TABLE 6–15. GENERALIZED REGRESSION EQUATIONS FOR PREDICTING BODY DENSITY (Db)* FOR ADULT FEMALES AND MALES

VARI-ABLES			REGRESSION EQUATION	r	SE (Db)	SE (% F)
			Adult Females[a]			
Σ	7, Age	Db =	$1.0970 - 0.00046971\ (X_1)$ $+ 0.00000056\ (X_1)^2 - 0.00012828\ (X_6)$	0.85	0.008	3.8
Σ	3, Age	Db =	$1.0994921 - 0.0009929\ (X_2)$ $+ 0.0000023\ (X_2)^2 - 0.0001392\ (X_6)$	0.84	0.009	3.9
Σ	3, Age	Db =	$1.0902369 - 0.0009379\ (X_5)$ $+ 0.0000026\ (X_5)^2 - 0.0001087\ (X_6)$	0.84	0.009	3.9
			Adult Males[a]			
Σ	7, Age	Db =	$1.11200000 - 0.00043499\ (X_1)$ $+ 0.00000055\ (X_1)^2 - 0.00028826\ (X_6)$	0.90	0.008	3.5
Σ	3, Age	Db =	$1.1093800 - 0.0008267\ (X_3)$ $+ 0.0000016\ (X_3)^2 - 0.0002574\ (X_6)$	0.91	0.008	3.4
Σ	3, Age	Db =	$1.1125025 - 0.0013125\ (X_4)$ $+ 0.0000055\ (X_4)^2 - 0.0002440\ (X_6)$	0.89	0.008	3.6

*Db = body density.

[a] X_1 = Sum of seven skinfolds (mm); X_2 = sum of triceps, suprailium, and thigh skinfolds (mm); X_3 = sum of chest, abdomen, and thigh skinfolds (mm); X_4 = sum of chest, triceps, and subscapular skinfolds (mm); X_5 = sum of triceps, suprailium, and abdomen skinfolds (mm); X_6 = age in years.

(From Pollock, M.L., Schmidt, D.H., and Jackson, A.S.: Measurement of cardiorespiratory fitness and body composition in the clinical setting. Comprehensive Therapy, Vol 6, No. 9, pp. 12–7, 1980. Published with permission of The Laux Company, Inc., Harvard, MA.)

It should be noted that the use of the quadratic component and age in the generalized equation shown in Table 6–15 did not increase the correlation substantially over the linear equation shown in Table 6–14. The value of the generalized equations over the linear equation is that they minimize large prediction errors that occur at the extremes of the body density distribution. This is shown in Figures 6–24 and 6–25.

It is important to recognize that every measurement method has defined sources of error. Bakker and Struikenkamp[188] have raised this issue with hydrostatically determined measures of lean body weight and have demonstrated that the method had defined degrees of inaccuracy. More recently, Lohman[152] has estimated the standard error for hydrostatically determined percentage of body fat of specific populations to be 2.7 per cent. Since error variances are uncorrelated, it means that the generalized equations add only about 1 per cent to the measurement error of percentage of body fat.

To determine body density from anthropometric measures, select an equation from Table 6–15. Once body density is found, then convert to percentage of body fat in the same manner as was described for underwater weighing, i.e., use either the Siri or the Brozek equation. For ease of determination, actual calculated percentages of body fat using age and the sum of triceps, suprailium, and thigh skinfolds for women and the sum of chest, abdomen, and thigh skinfolds for men are shown in Tables 6–16 and 6–17,

TABLE 6–16. PERCENTAGE OF BODY FAT ESTIMATION FOR WOMEN FROM AGE AND TRICEPS, SUPRAILIUM, AND THIGH SKINFOLDS*

SUM OF SKINFOLDS (mm)	AGE TO THE LAST YEAR								
	Under 22	23 to 27	28 to 32	33 to 37	38 to 42	43 to 47	48 to 52	53 to 57	Over 58
23–25	9.7	9.9	10.2	10.4	10.7	10.9	11.2	11.4	11.7
26–28	11.0	11.2	11.5	11.7	12.0	12.3	12.5	12.7	13.0
29–31	12.3	12.5	12.8	13.0	13.3	13.5	13.8	14.0	14.3
32–34	13.6	13.8	14.0	14.3	14.5	14.8	15.0	15.3	15.5
35–37	14.8	15.0	15.3	15.5	15.8	16.0	16.3	16.5	16.8
38–40	16.0	16.3	16.5	16.7	17.0	17.2	17.5	17.7	18.0
41–43	17.2	17.4	17.7	17.9	18.2	18.4	18.7	18.9	19.2
44–46	18.3	18.6	18.8	19.1	19.3	19.6	19.8	20.1	20.3
47–49	19.5	19.7	20.0	20.2	20.5	20.7	21.0	21.2	21.5
50–52	20.6	20.8	21.1	21.3	21.6	21.8	22.1	22.3	22.6
53–55	21.7	21.9	22.1	22.4	22.6	22.9	23.1	23.4	23.6
56–58	22.7	23.0	23.2	23.4	23.7	23.9	24.2	24.4	24.7
59–61	23.7	24.0	24.2	24.5	24.7	25.0	25.2	25.5	25.7
62–64	24.7	25.0	25.2	25.5	25.7	26.0	26.7	26.4	26.7
65–67	25.7	25.9	26.2	26.4	26.7	26.9	27.2	27.4	27.7
68–70	26.6	26.9	27.1	27.4	27.6	27.9	28.1	28.4	28.6
71–73	27.5	27.8	28.0	28.3	28.5	28.8	28.0	29.3	29.5
74–76	28.4	28.7	28.9	29.2	29.4	29.7	29.9	30.2	30.4
77–79	29.3	29.5	29.8	30.0	30.3	30.5	30.8	31.0	31.3
80–82	30.1	30.4	30.6	30.9	31.1	31.4	31.6	31.9	32.1
83–85	30.9	31.2	31.4	31.7	31.9	32.2	32.4	32.7	32.9
86–88	31.7	32.0	32.2	32.5	32.7	32.9	33.2	33.4	33.7
89–91	32.5	32.7	33.0	33.2	33.5	33.7	33.9	34.2	34.4
92–94	33.2	33.4	33.7	33.9	34.2	34.4	34.7	34.9	35.2
95–97	33.9	34.1	34.4	34.6	34.9	35.1	35.4	35.6	35.9
98–100	34.6	34.8	35.1	35.3	35.5	35.8	36.0	36.3	36.5
101–103	35.3	35.4	35.7	35.9	36.2	36.4	36.7	36.9	37.2
104–106	35.8	36.1	36.3	36.6	36.8	37.1	37.3	37.5	37.8
107–109	36.4	36.7	36.9	37.1	37.4	37.6	37.9	38.1	38.4
110–112	37.0	37.2	37.5	37.7	38.0	38.2	38.5	38.7	38.9
113–115	37.5	37.8	38.0	38.2	38.5	38.7	39.0	39.2	39.5
116–118	38.0	38.3	38.5	38.8	39.0	39.3	39.5	39.7	40.0
119–121	38.5	38.7	39.0	39.2	39.5	39.7	40.0	40.2	40.5
122–124	39.0	39.2	39.4	39.7	39.9	40.2	40.4	40.7	40.9
125–127	39.4	39.6	39.9	40.1	40.4	40.6	40.9	41.1	41.4
128–130	39.8	40.0	40.3	40.5	40.8	41.0	41.3	41.5	41.8

*Percentage of fat calculated by the formula of Siri. Percentage of fat = $[(4.95/Db) - 4.5] \times 100$, where Db = body density.

(From Pollock, M.L., Schmidt, D.H., and Jackson, A.S.: Measurement of cardiorespiratory fitness and body composition in the clinical setting. Comprehensive Therapy, Vol. 6, No. 9, pp. 12–27, 1980. Published with permission of The Laux Company, Inc., Harvard, MA.)

respectively.[24] For example, if the sum of three skinfolds for a 35-year-old woman was 63 mm, her percentage of body fat would be 25.5 per cent and if a 50-year-old man had 60 mm, he would be 20.2 per cent fat. Using age and the same sum of three skinfolds for men and women, as shown in Tables 6–16 and 6.17, Baun et al.[189] developed a nomogram for estimating percentage of body fat. Because thigh skinfolds are difficult for some technicians

TABLE 6-17. PERCENTAGE OF BODY FAT ESTIMATION FOR MEN FROM AGE AND THE SUM OF CHEST, ABDOMINAL, AND THIGH SKINFOLDS*

SUM OF SKINFOLDS (mm)	AGE TO THE LAST YEAR								
	Under 22	23 to 27	28 to 32	33 to 37	38 to 42	43 to 47	48 to 52	53 to 57	Over 58
8-10	1.3	1.8	2.3	2.9	3.4	3.9	4.5	5.0	5.5
11-13	2.2	2.8	3.3	3.9	4.4	4.9	5.5	6.0	6.5
14-16	3.2	3.8	4.3	4.8	5.4	5.9	6.4	7.0	7.5
17-19	4.2	4.7	5.3	5.8	6.3	6.9	7.4	8.0	8.5
20-22	5.1	5.7	6.2	6.8	7.3	7.9	8.4	8.9	9.5
23-25	6.1	6.6	7.2	7.7	8.3	8.8	9.4	9.9	10.5
26-28	7.0	7.6	8.1	8.7	9.2	9.8	10.3	10.9	11.4
29-31	8.0	8.5	9.1	9.6	10.2	10.7	11.3	11.8	12.4
32-34	8.9	9.4	10.0	10.5	11.1	11.6	12.2	12.8	13.3
35-37	9.8	10.4	10.9	11.5	12.0	12.6	13.1	13.7	14.3
38-40	10.7	11.3	11.8	12.4	12.9	13.5	14.1	14.6	15.2
41-43	11.6	12.2	12.7	13.3	13.8	14.4	15.0	15.5	16.1
44-46	12.5	13.1	13.6	14.2	14.7	15.3	15.9	16.4	17.0
47-49	13.4	13.9	14.5	15.1	15.6	16.2	16.8	17.3	17.9
50-52	14.3	14.8	15.4	15.9	16.5	17.1	17.6	18.2	18.8
53-55	15.1	15.7	16.2	16.8	17.4	17.9	18.5	19.1	19.7
56-58	16.0	16.5	17.1	17.7	18.2	18.8	19.4	20.0	20.5
59-61	16.9	17.4	17.9	18.5	19.1	19.7	20.2	20.8	21.4
62-64	17.6	18.2	18.8	19.4	19.9	20.5	21.1	21.7	22.2
65-67	18.5	19.0	19.6	20.2	20.8	21.3	21.9	22.5	23.1
68-70	19.3	19.9	20.4	21.0	21.6	22.2	22.7	23.3	23.9
71-73	20.1	20.7	21.2	21.8	22.4	23.0	23.6	24.1	24.7
74-76	20.9	21.5	22.0	22.6	23.2	23.8	24.4	25.0	25.5
77-79	21.7	22.2	22.8	23.4	24.0	24.6	25.2	25.8	26.3
80-82	22.4	23.0	23.6	24.2	24.8	25.4	25.9	26.5	27.1
83-85	23.2	23.8	24.4	25.0	25.5	26.1	26.7	27.3	27.9
86-88	24.0	24.5	25.1	25.7	26.3	26.9	27.5	28.1	28.7
89-91	24.7	25.3	25.9	25.5	27.1	27.6	28.2	28.8	29.4
92-94	25.4	26.0	26.6	27.2	27.8	28.4	29.0	29.6	30.2
95-97	26.1	26.7	27.3	27.9	28.5	29.1	29.7	30.3	30.9
98-100	26.9	27.4	28.0	28.6	29.2	29.8	30.4	31.0	31.6
101-103	27.5	28.1	28.7	29.3	29.9	30.5	31.1	31.7	32.3
104-106	28.2	28.8	29.4	30.0	30.6	31.2	31.8	32.4	33.0
107-109	28.9	29.5	30.1	30.7	31.3	31.9	32.5	33.1	33.7
110-112	29.6	30.2	30.8	31.4	32.0	32.6	33.2	33.8	34.4
113-115	30.2	30.8	31.4	32.0	32.6	33.2	33.8	34.5	35.1
116-118	30.9	31.5	32.1	32.7	33.3	33.9	34.5	35.1	35.7
119-121	31.5	32.1	32.7	33.3	33.9	34.5	35.1	35.7	36.4
122-124	32.1	32.7	33.3	33.9	34.5	35.1	35.8	36.4	37.0
125-127	32.7	33.3	33.9	34.5	35.1	35.8	36.4	37.0	37.6

*Percentage of fat calculated by the formula of Siri. Percentage fat = $[(4.95/Db) - 4.5] \times 100$, where Db = body density.

(From Pollock, M.L., Schmidt, D.H., and Jackson, A.S.: Measurement of cardiorespiratory fitness and body composition in the clinical setting. Comprehensive Therapy, Vol. 6, No. 9, pp. 12-27, 1980. Published with permission of The Laux Company, Inc., Harvard, MA.)

to measure, other equations not using thigh skinfolds are available.[14, 24] For women, triceps, abdomen, and suprailium are used, and for men, chest, axilla, abdomen, and suprailium are used.[14] If fat calipers are not available, a relatively accurate estimation of percentage of body fat for men was developed by Wilmore et al.[8, 175] from body weight and waist circuference measures (see Fig. A–7, Appendix A).

MEASUREMENT OF ANTHROPOMETRIC MEASURES

A description of anatomical landmarks and measurement of skinfold fat, circumference, and diameter measures follows.

Skinfold Fat

Chest: a diagonal fold taken one half of the distance between the anterior axillary line and the nipple for men and one third of the distance from the anterior axillary line and the equivalent position for women (Fig. 6–26).
Axilla: a vertical fold on the midaxillary line at the level of the xiphoid process of the sternum (Fig. 6–27).
Triceps: a vertical fold on the posterior midline of the upper arm (over triceps

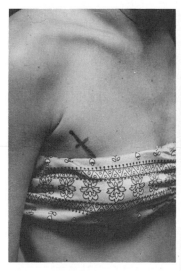
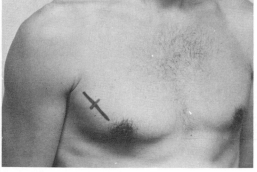
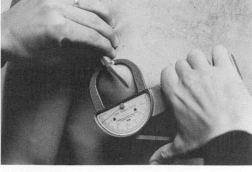

Figure 6–26. Chest skinfold fat site for males and females. (From Pollock, M.L., Schmidt, D.H., and Jackson, A.S.: Measurement of cardiorespiratory fitness and body composition in the clinical setting. Comprehensive Therapy. Vol. 6, No. 9, pp. 12–27, 1980. Published with permission of The Laux Company, Inc., Harvard, MA.)

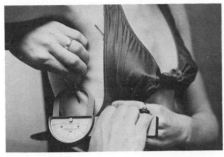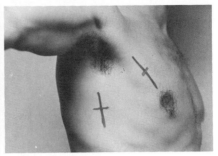

Figure 6–27. Axilla skinfold fat site. (From Pollock, M.L., Schmidt, D.H., and Jackson, A.S.: Measurement of cardiorespiratory fitness and body composition in the clinical setting. Comprehensive Therapy, Vol. 6, No. 9, pp. 12–27, 1980. Published with permission of The Laux Company, Inc., Harvard, MA.)

muscle), halfway between the acromion and olecranon processes; the elbow should be extended and relaxed (Fig. 6–28).

Subscapular: a fold taken on a diagonal line coming from the vertebral border to 1 to 2 cm from the inferior angle of the scapula (Fig. 6–28).

Abdominal: a vertical fold taken at a lateral distance of approximately 2 cm from the umbilicus (Fig. 6–29).

Suprailium: a diagonal fold above the crest of the ilium at the spot where an imaginary line would come down from the anterior axillary line (Fig. 6–29). It should be noted that many recommend that the measure be taken more laterally at the midaxillary line.[141] Data for generalized equations of Jackson and Pollock[168,177] were determined at the anterior axillary line.

Thigh: a vertical fold on the anterior aspect of the thigh, midway between hip and knee joints (Fig. 6–29).

Circumference Measures

Shoulder: taken in the horizontal plane at the maximum circumference of the shoulders at the level of the greatest lateral protrusion of the deltoid muscles.

Chest—High: taken in the horizontal plane at the largest circumference above the breasts (women).

Chest—Middle: taken in the horizontal plane at the nipple line at mid–tidal volume.

Chest—Low: taken in the horizontal plane just below the breasts (women).

Abdominal: taken in a horizontal plane at the smallest circumference in the abdominal region, generally 2 to 4 inches above the umbilicus.

Waist: taken in the horizontal plane at the level of the umbilicus.

Gluteal: taken in the horizontal plane at the largest circumference around the buttocks. Subjects stand with feet together and gluteals tense (Fig. 6–30).

Thigh: taken in the horizontal plane just below the gluteal fold or maximum thigh girth. Thigh flexed.

Calf: taken in the horizontal plane at the maximum girth of the calf with muscle tensed.

Ankle: taken in the horizontal plane at the smallest point above the malleoli.

Arm: taken at maximum girth of the midarm when flexed to the greatest angle with the underlying muscles fully contracted.

Forearm: taken at the largest circumference with the forearm parallel to the floor, the elbow joint at a 90-degree angle, the hand in the supinated position, and the muscles flexed.

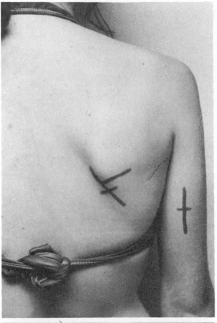

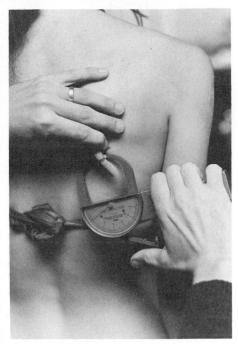

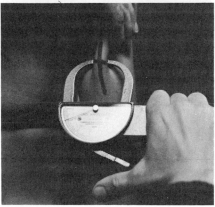

Figure 6–28. Triceps and subscapular skinfold fat sites. (From Pollock, M.L., Schmidt, D.H., and Jackson, A.S.: Measurement of cardiorespiratory fitness and body composition in the clinical setting. Comprehensive Therapy, Vol. 6, No. 9, pp. 12–27, 1980. Published with permission of The Laux Company, Inc., Harvard, MA.)

Wrist: taken over the styloid process of the radius and ulna with the arm extended in front of the body and fist loosely clenched, relaxed, and pronated.

Diameter Measures

Shoulder: distance between the outermost protrusions of the shoulder (deltoid muscles).

Biacromial: distance between the most lateral projections of the acromial processes.

Chest: arms abducted slightly for placement of the anthropometer at the level of the xiphoid process.

Bi-iliac: distance between the most lateral projections of the iliac crests.

Bitrochanteric: distance between the most lateral projections of the greater trochanters.

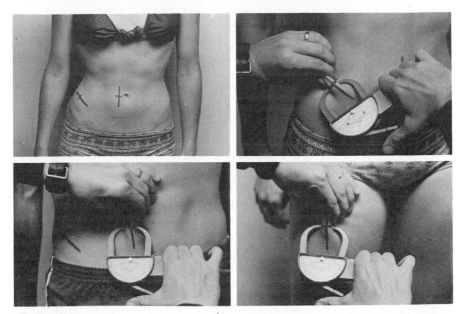

Figure 6–29. Abdominal, suprailium, and front thigh skinfold fat sites. (From Pollock, M.L., Schmidt, D.H. and Jackson, A.S.: Measurement of cardiorespiratory fitness and body composition in the clinical setting. Comprehensive Therapy, Vol. 6, No. 9, pp. 12–27, 1980. Published with permission of The Laux Company, Inc., Harvard, MA.)

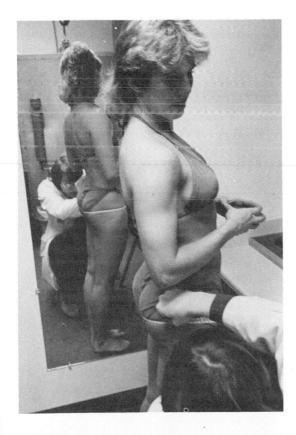

Figure 6–30. Measuring gluteal circumference with a 2-meter steel tape. Mirror in background assists the technician in adjusting tape at the proper level.

Knee: 45-degree angle measurement at the smallest width of the knee, which is taken with the right foot placed on a small stool so that the knee is flexed at a 90-degree angle.

Wrist: distance between the radial and ulna styloid processes.

An example of a data collection form used for recording anthropometric measures is shown in Figure A–6, Appendix A.

A caliper that is accurately calibrated and has a constant pressure of 10 g/mm^2 throughout the full range of the caliper opening is recommended for taking skinfold fat measures. Caliper specifications and recommended standards for measurement are well documented.[190-192]

Recent data have suggested that the use of cheaper calipers often gives results similar to those achieved with the recommended constant pressure type of calipers.[193-195] Although this may be true, more information is needed regarding long-term use (durability), quality control, and so on. Some evidence suggests that even the highly recommended calipers may give different results. Lohman et al.[195] found that the Lange caliper yielded higher values than the Harpenden caliper. Although experienced technicians collected the data, none had equal experience in using both calipers; thus, a bias may have been present. In general, it appears that a variety of calipers may be satisfactorily used, but because of possible differences among calipers, use of the caliper with which the data for the specific body density equation were developed is recommended. The Lange caliper was used for the equations developed by Jackson and Pollock.[168,177]

The accuracy of predicting body density from skinfold fat measures is subject to large intertester error.[196] A difference of as much as 12 mm on one skinfold fat site and up to 3 per cent in body fat can be noted even by experienced testers.[197] When testers practice together and take care to standardize their testing procedures, however, intertester error usually results in less than a 1 per cent fat calculated error.[198] A recent review suggests that the largest error found among investigators results from the nonstandardization of sites and differences in selecting a skinfold site.[196]

A flexible steel tape is generally used for taking circumference measures. The tape should be approximately 2 meters in length and should be easily retractable. A sliding broad-breadth caliper (anthropometer) is used for assessing diameters. Usually circumference and diameter measures are recorded to the nearest 0.1 cm. Further discussion of procedures and description of sites of anthropometric measures are provided by Hertzberg et al. and by Behnke and Wilmore.[141,190]

In measuring skinfold fat, the skinfold is grasped firmly by the thumb and index finger; the caliper is perpendicular to the fold at approximately 1 cm (¼ to ½ inch) from the thumb and finger.[141,191] Then, while maintaining a grasp of the skinfold, allow the caliper grip to be released so that the full tension is exerted on the skinfold. In grasping the skinfold, the pads at the tip of the thumb and finger are used. Testers should trim their nails. The dial is read to the nearest 0.5 mm (Lange) and 0.1 mm (Harpenden) approximately 1 to 2 seconds after the grip has been released. A minimum of two measurements should be taken at each site. If the repeated measurement varies by more than 1 mm, a third should be taken. If consecutive fat measurements become increasingly smaller, the fat is being compressed; this occurs mainly with fleshy people. If this occurs, the tester should proceed to the next site and return to the trouble spot after finishing the other measurements; the final value will be the average of the two that seem to represent the skinfold fat site best. It is better to take measurements when the skin is dry because when the skin is moist or wet the tester may grasp extra skin (fat) and get larger values. Practice is necessary to grasp the same size of skinfold consistently at exactly the same location every time. Most skinfold fat equations or sums of skinfold norms are based on taking measurements on the right side of the body.

CALCULATION OF DESIRED/TARGET WEIGHT

Desired or target weight was described in Chapter 2. If 23 per cent fat for women and 16 per cent fat for men are used as the desired body fat standards, then the following equations can be used.

$$\text{Women, desired weight} = \frac{[\text{weight} - (\text{weight} \times \% \text{ fat})/100]}{0.77}$$

$$\text{Men, desired weight} = \frac{[\text{weight} - (\text{weight} \times \% \text{ fat})/100]}{0.84}$$

For example, a 35 year old male patient who is 23 per cent fat and weighs 210 pounds would have to reduce to 192.5 pounds to attain his goal of 16 per cent fat. A 45-year-old woman who is 28 per cent fat and weighs 145 pounds would have to reduce to 135.6 pounds to attain her desired goal of 23 per cent fat. For ease in computation of desired weight based on 23 per cent fat for women and 16 per cent fat for men, see Tables A–14 and A–15, Appendix A.

The numerator of the formulas subtracts the fat weight from the total body weight, leaving the fat-free weight. The denominator adds back the desired amount of fat weight to the fat-free weight. If another desired weight (per cent of fat goal) is wanted, it is simply necessary to change the fraction value in the denominator. This technique for estimating desirable weight is not without error, and it is suggested that 2 pounds be added and subtracted from the desired weight to provide a desired weight range. For the preceding examples, this would mean 190.5 to 194.5 pounds for the man and 133.6 to 137.6 for the woman.

Although these desired weight formulas are useful in working with patients and giving them objective goals for fat and weight loss, they have certain limitations. Weight loss depends on caloric intake and expenditure, but diet and exercise affect body composition differently.[199] When weight loss comes from diet alone, both fat and lean tissue are reduced, whereas exercise alone will increase or maintain lean body weight and reduce body fat. Therefore, the accuracy of the desired weight formulas depends on how weight and fat are lost. Periodic checks of body composition during the weight reduction program will help refine estimations.

Normative data on skinfolds and other anthropometric measures are available for school children and youth 6 to 17 years of age and adults up to 79 years of age through the National Center for Health Statistics.[200] Normative data for skinfold fat of school children and youth are also available elsewhere.[48,201] Percentile rankings for percentage of fat and for chest, abdomen, suprailium, axilla, triceps, subscapula, and front thigh skinfolds are available for both males and females less than 35 years of age, 36 to 45 years of age, and 46 years and older in *The Y's Way to Physical Fitness.*[14]

MUSCULAR STRENGTH AND ENDURANCE, AND FLEXIBILITY

STRENGTH

As mentioned in Chapter 5, strength relates to both dynamic and static contractions. Strength testing has usually been conducted by the use of weights (free standing or various apparatus), dynamometers, cable tensiometers (static), isokinetic devices, and elaborately designed force transducers and recorders.[202-204] A thorough description of these methods and discussion concerning reliability and validity can be found in several texts.[27,202-204] Elaborate strength and endurance type of equipment can be expensive and may not always provide a substantial improvement in measurement accuracy. For the purpose of this section, only the field type tests listed in Table 6–2 will be described in detail. More sophisticated testing of muscular strength and endurance and the testing of athletes are described by Berger,[204] Wilmore,[202] Riley,[205] and Darden.[206]

Strength can be easily assessed by the one-repetition maximum test (1-RM).[27,204] The basic muscle or muscle group to be tested is selected, and then the individual is given a series of trials to determine the greatest weight able to be lifted only once for that particular lift. This test is conducted largely through trial and error when subjects are inexperienced in lifting weights. The subject starts with a weight that can be lifted comfortably, and then weight is added progressively until the weight can be lifted correctly just one time. If this weight can be lifted more than once, more weight needs to be added until a true 1-RM is reached.

If one test only is to be selected, use the 1-RM bench press. Berger[204,207] showed moderately high intercorrelations between back hyperextension, bench press, standing military press, sit-up, squat, upright rowing, and curl exercises. Using 174 college-age men, he found that the best single lifts for predicting total dynamic strength (sum of 1-RM of seven exercises listed previously) were bench press ($r = 0.84$) and standing military press

TABLE 6-18. STRENGTH STANDARD VALUES RECOMMENDED FOR
FOUR WEIGHT-LIFTING EXERCISES FOR VARIOUS BODY WEIGHTS
(DATA BASED ON THE 1-RM TEST)[a,b]

BODY WEIGHT (LB)	BENCH PRESS		STANDING PRESS		CURL		LEG PRESS	
	Male	Female	Male	Female	Male	Female	Male	Female
80	80	56	53	37	40	28	160	112
100	100	70	67	47	50	35	200	140
120	120	84	80	56	60	42	240	168
140	140	98	93	65	70	49	280	196
160	160	112	107	75	80	56	320	224
180	180	126	120	84	90	63	360	252
200	200	140	133	93	100	70	400	280
220	220	154	147	103	110	77	440	308
240	240	168	160	112	120	84	480	336

[a]Note: Data collected on Universal Gym apparatus. Information collected on other apparatus could modify results.

[b]Data expressed in pounds.

(Reprinted with permission from Pollock, M.L., Wilmore, J.H., and Fox, S.M.: Health and Fitness Through Physical Activity. New York, copyright © John Wiley and Sons, 1978.)

($r = 0.87$). For safety and administrative purposes, the 1-RM bench press was selected for use.

Although the bench press can be used for assessing strength, test batteries usually select three or four exercises that represent the body's major muscle groups. Table 6-18 gives a series of values for selected strength exercises for both males and females on the basis of body weight.[8] Although strength requirements will differ for each sport or activity, or even for position or event within each sport, these values are optimal for the average person who is training mainly for general fitness purposes. Specific standards for each sport have yet to be developed.

MUSCULAR ENDURANCE

Muscular endurance has been measured in a number of different ways, including the greatest number of sit-ups that can be performed in a fixed period of time (usually 30 seconds or 1 minute) or the maximum number of push-ups, pull-ups, or bar dips that can be performed continuously in an indefinite time period.[14,27,202,204] Many of these tests penalize the participant who has long legs, short arms, or a heavy body weight. To eliminate this, a concept has evolved that uses a fixed percentage of the individual's body weight as the resistance; the individual lifts this as many times as possible until he or she reaches the point of fatigue or exhaustion.[204] Firm guidelines have yet to be established with regard to what the actual fixed percentages of the individual's body weight should be for each of the muscle groups tested. In fact, it is debatable whether the weight used in the test

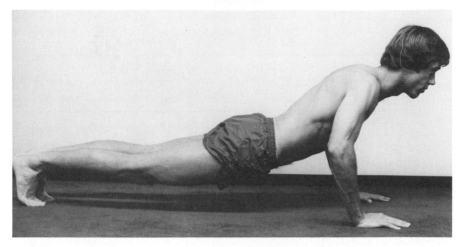

Figure 6–31. Standard or full push-up. (Reprinted with permission from Pollock, M.L., Wilmore, J.H., and Fox, S.M.: Health and Fitness Through Physical Activity. New York, copyright © John Wiley and Sons, 1978.)

should be a fixed percentage of the individual's body weight or a fixed percentage of the individual's 1-RM or absolute strength. As an example, if the endurance test for the bench press movement was conducted using 50 per cent of the individual's body weight as the resistance, the 180-pound man would be asked to lift 90 pounds as many times as he could. A strong man of this body weight would be able to lift this 90-pound weight 20 or more times, whereas the relatively weak man who weighs 180 pounds may not be able to lift the 90-pound weight even one single repetition, i.e., the designated weight exceeds his 1-RM. In this case, the test for muscular endurance would be highly dependent on strength. To isolate muscular endurance as a pure component, where the test is not so dependent on the individual's strength, it is advocated that the test battery be established on the basis of the individual's strength, not body weight.

In accordance with the previous recommendation, it is suggested that a fixed percentage of 70 per cent of the maximum strength be used to test muscle endurance. This percentage would be the same for all movements tested.[8] Since this is a relatively new concept, norms or standards have yet to be established but could be easily developed for each specific population to be tested. On the basis of limited test data, the recreational athlete or health-seeking exerciser should be able to perform 12 to 15 repetitions, and the competitive athlete should be able to do 20 to 25 repetitions at 70 per cent of his or her maximum strength for each of the movements tested.[8]

Two tests that have been traditionally used to measure muscular endurance are the push-up and sit-up tests, to assess upper body (triceps, anterior deltoids, and pectoralis major) and abdominal muscular endurance, respectively.[14, 27, 48, 84] The push-up test is administered with the individual in the standard "up" position for a full push-up (Fig. 6–31). Testers place their fist on the floor beneath the individual's chest, and the individual lowers himself

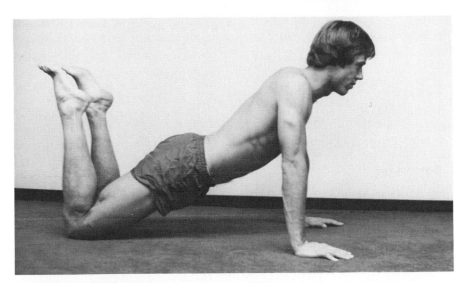

Figure 6–32. Modified knee push-up. (Reprinted with permission from Pollock, M.L., Wilmore, J.H., and Fox, S.M.: Health and Fitness Through Physical Activity. New York, copyright © John Wiley and Sons, 1978.)

or herself down until the chest touches the tester's fist, keeping the back straight, and then raising back to the up position. The maximum number of correctly completed push-ups is counted and then compared with Table 6–19, which lists standards relative to age and sex. Women can perform this test from the bent-knee position (Fig. 6–32).[27,84]

In the sit-up test, individuals start by lying on their back, knees bent, feet flat on the floor, with heels between 12 and 18 inches from the buttocks. Hands should be interlocked behind the neck. The tester holds the person's feet down. The individual performs as many correct sit-ups (Fig. 6–33) as possible in a 60-second period. Elbows should be touched to the knees in the up position, and this must be followed by a complete return to the full lying position before starting the next sit-up. The total number of sit-ups performed in 60 seconds is recorded and compared with Table 6–20, which lists standards relative to age and sex. Other norms for the 1-minute sit-up test have been developed for both men and women by three age categories (see Tables A–16 and A–17, Appendix A).[14] Data and standards for school children 5 to 17 years of age are also available.[27,48,84,201]

FLEXIBILITY

Probably the most accurate tests of flexibility currently available are those that assess the actual range of motion of the various joints. Although this is easily accomplished by instruments such as the Leighton Flexometer[208] and the electrogoniometer,[209] these pieces of equipment are not readily available.[27]

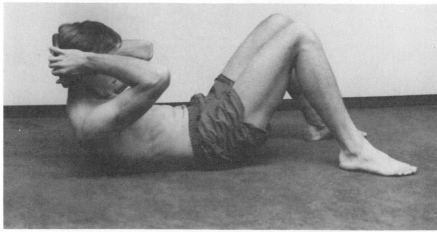

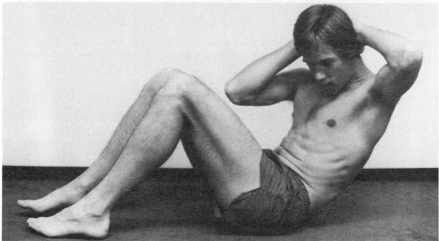

Figure 6–33. Sixty-second sit-up. (Reprinted with permission from Pollock, M.L., Wilmore, J.H., and Fox, S.M.: Health and Fitness Through Physical Activity. New York, copyright © John Wiley and Sons, 1978.)

TABLE 6–19. PUSH-UP MUSCULAR ENDURANCE TEST STANDARDS[a]

	MALES					FEMALES[b]				
AGE	Excellent	Good	Average	Fair	Poor	Excellent	Good	Average	Fair	Poor
20–29	55–above	45–54	35–44	20–34	0–19	49–above	34–48	17–33	6–16	0–5
30–39	45–above	35–44	25–34	15–24	0–14	40–above	25–39	12–24	4–11	0–3
40–49	40–above	30–39	20–29	12–19	0–11	35–above	20–34	8–19	3–7	0–2
50–59	35–above	25–34	15–24	8–14	0–7	30–above	15–29	6–14	2–5	0–1
60–69	30–above	20–29	10–19	5–9	0–4	20–above	5–19	3–4	1–2	0

[a]These values represent approximations, since actual norms are not available.
[b]Modified push-up.

(Reprinted with permission from Pollock, M.L., Wilmore, J.H., and Fox, S.M.: Health and Fitness Through Physical Activity. New York, copyright © John Wiley & Sons, 1978.)

TABLE 6-20. SIT-UP MUSCULAR ENDURANCE TEST STANDARDS[a, b]

	MALES					FEMALES				
AGE	*Excellent*	*Good*	*Average*	*Fair*	*Poor*	*Excellent*	*Good*	*Average*	*Fair*	*Poor*
20-29	48-above	43-47	37-42	33-36	0-32	44-above	39-43	33-38	29-32	0-28
30-39	40-above	35-39	29-34	25-28	0-24	36-above	31-35	25-30	21-24	0-20
40-49	35-above	30-34	24-29	20-23	0-19	31-above	26-30	19-25	16-18	0-15
50-59	30-above	25-29	19-24	15-18	0-14	26-above	21-25	15-20	11-14	0-10
60-69	25-above	20-24	14-19	10-13	0-9	21-above	16-20	10-15	6-9	0-5

[a]These values represent approximations, since actual norms arc not available.
[b]Test is timed for 60 seconds.
(Reprinted with permission from Pollock, M.L., Wilmore, J.H., and Fox, S.M.: Health and Fitness Through Physical Activity. New York, copyright © John Wiley and Sons, 1978.)

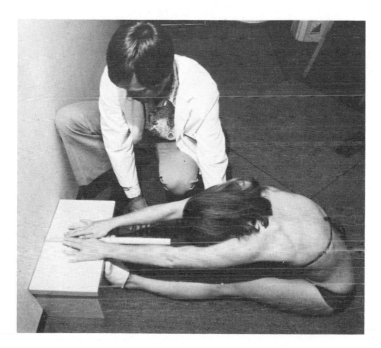

Figure 6-34. The Sit and Reach Test to determine flexibility of the low back and posterior thigh muscles. (Reprinted with permission from Pollock, M.L., Wilmore, J.H., and Fox, S.M.: Health and Fitness through Physical Activity. New York, copyright © John Wiley and Sons, 1978.)

Since flexibility is specific to each joint, no generalized flexibility test is available.[27] Because the emphasis of this book is on adult physical fitness and related health aspects, lower back flexibility will be mentioned here. As stated earlier, low back pain and disability are prevalent among men and women in the adult population.[210] Much of this problem is related to the lack of flexibility in the back of the legs (hamstrings), hips, and lower back.[210,211] To measure this capability, a simple field test called the Sit and Reach Test can be used (Fig. 6-34).

TABLE 6-21. STANDARDS FOR THE SIT
AND REACH FLEXIBILITY TEST

	SIT AND REACH
Excellent	22 in or greater
Good	19–21 in
Average	14–18 in
Fair	12–13 in
Poor	11 in. or less

(Reprinted with permission from Health Improvement Program, National Athletic Health Institute, Inglewood, CA, 1975.)

In the Sit and Reach Test, the individual sits with the legs extended directly in front of him or her and the knees pressed against the floor. The feet are placed against a stool to which is attached a yardstick, with the 14-inch mark being placed at the point where the foot contacts the stool. The individual puts the index fingers of both hands together and reaches forward slowly as far as possible. The distance reached is noted on the yardstick and recorded. The knees must be kept in contact with the floor, and bouncing is to be discouraged. A short warm-up of four to six stretches is recommended before starting the test. Standards for the normal population are presented in Table 6–21. Other norms based on males and females of various ages are shown in Tables A–16 and A–17, Appendix A.[14] It must be noted that the norms shown in Appendix A are based on placing the yardstick at the 15-inch mark. Norms for school children and youth 5 to 17 years of age are also available.[48] Obviously, the Sit and Reach Test is influenced by the length of the arms and legs of the individual, in addition to flexibility.

SUMMARY

This chapter has presented an explanation and discussion of many of the factors involved in a comprehensive medical screening and physical fitness examination. In the first portion of the chapter, risk factors related to coronary heart disease and a coronary risk factor profile chart were shown. Within this profile chart, risk is estimated to be high or low. The established risk factor charts should be used as education tools, but their limitations with regard to validity should be understood.

Next, tests to evaluate cardiorespiratory fitness, body composition (leanness-fatness), strength, muscular endurance, and flexibility were described. The recommended tests were graded with regard to their sophistication and feasibility.

An important aspect of this chapter is its ability to explain to the participants how to assess their health and physical fitness status properly and safely. This information should give participants a secure basis for initiating an exercise program at the proper level or for monitoring the progress of the exercise program. To aid in evaluation of physical fitness, norm tables that are specific to age and sex were presented.

REFERENCES

1. Hurst, W. J.: The Heart, 5th ed. New York, McGraw-Hill, 1982.
2. Braunwald, E.: Heart Disease: A Textbook of Cardiovascular Medicine. Philadelphia, W.B. Saunders Co., 1980.
3. Bruce, R.A., DeRouen, T.A., and Hossack, K.F.: Value of maximal exercise tests in the risk assessment of primary coronary heart disease events in healthy men. Five years' experience of the Seattle heart watch study. Am. J. Cardiol. 46:371–378, 1980.
4. Chisholm, D.M., Collis, M.L., Kulak, L.L., Davenport, W., and Gruber, N.: Physical activity readiness. Br. Col. Med. J. 17:375–378, 1975.
5. Policy Statement Regarding the Use of Human Subjects and Informed Consent. Med. Sci. Sports Exer. 14:xii, 1982.
6. American College of Sports Medicine: Guidelines for Graded Exercise Testing and Exercise Prescription, 2nd ed. Philadelphia, Lea and Febiger, 1980.
7. Ellestad, M.H., Blomqvist, C.G., and Naughton, J.P.: Standards for adult exercise testing laboratories. Circulation 59:421A–430A, 1979.
8. Pollock, M.L., Wilmore, J.H., and Fox, S.M.: Health and Fitness Through Physical Activity. New York, John Wiley and Sons, 1978.
9. Fry, G., and Berra, K.: YMCArdiac Therapy. Chicago, National Council of the YMCA, 1981.
10. Wilson, P.K., Fardy, P.S., and Froelicher, V.F.: Cardiac Rehabilitation, Adult Fitness, and Exercise Testing. Philadelphia, Lea and Febiger, 1981.
11. Froelicher, V.F.: Exercise Testing and Training. New York, LeJacq Publishing Co., 1983.
12. Shephard, R.J.: The current status of the Canadian home fitness test. Br. J. Sports Med. 14:114–125, 1980.
13. Shephard, R.J., Bailey, D.A., and Mirwald, R.L.: Development of the Canadian home fitness test. Can. Med. Assoc. J. 114:675–679, 1976.
14. Golding, L.A., Myers, C.R., and Sinning, W.E., editors: The Y's Way to Physical Fitness, revised. Chicago, The YMCA of the USA, 1982.
15. The National Heart, Lung, and Blood Institute: Exercise and Your Heart. Washington, D.C., U.S. Government Printing Office 726 248, 1981.
16. Diamond, G.A., and Forrester, J.S.: Analysis of probability as an aid in the clinical diagnosis of coronary-artery disease. N. Engl. J. Med. 300: 1350–1358, 1979.
17. Epstein, S.E.: Implications of probability analysis on the strategy used for noninvasive detection of coronary artery disease. Am. J. Cardiol. 46:491–499, 1980.
18. Kannel, W.B., McGee, D., and Gordon, T.: A general cardiovascular risk profile: The Framingham study. Am. J. Cardiol. 38:46–51, 1976.
19. American Heart Association: Coronary Risk Handbook. Dallas, American Heart Association, 1973.
20. American Heart Association: Exercise Testing and Training of Individuals with Heart Disease or at High Risk for its Development: A Handbook for Physicians. Dallas, American Heart Association, 1975.
21. Balke, B.: A simple field test for the assessment of physical fitness. CARI Report 63-6. Civil Aeromedical Research Institute, Federal Aviation Agency, Oklahoma City, 1963.
22. Cooper, K.H.: Correlation between field and treadmill testing as a means of assessing maximal oxygen intake. J.A.M.A. 203:201–204, 1968.
23. Bruce, R.A., Kusumi, F., and Hosmer, D.: Maximal oxygen intake and nomographic assessment of functional aerobic impairment in cardiovascular disease. Am. Heart J. 85: 545–562, 1973.
24. Pollock, M.L., Schmidt, D.H., and Jackson, A.S.: Measurement of cardiorespiratory fitness and body composition in the clinical setting. Compr. Ther. 6:12–27, 1980.
25. Froelicher, V.F., Brammel, H., Davis, G., Noguera, I., Stewart, A., and Lancaster, M.C.: A comparison of reproducibility and physiologic response to three maximal treadmill exercise protocols. Chest 65:512–517, 1974.

26. Wilson, P.K., Bell, C.W., and Norton, A.C.: Rehabilitation of the Heart and Lungs. Fullerton, CA, Beckman Instruments, 1980.
27. Baumgartner, J.A., and Jackson, A.S.: Measurement and Evaluation in Physical Education, 2nd ed. Dubuque, IA, William C. Brown Co., 1982.
28. Taylor, H.L., Wang, Y., Rowell, L., and Blomqvist, G.: The standardization and interpretation of submaximal and maximal tests of working capacity. Pediatrics 32: (II):703–722, 1963.
29. Taylor, H.L., Haskell, W., Fox, S.M., and Blackburn, H.: Exercise tests: a summary of procedures and concepts of stress testing for cardiovascular diagnosis and function evaluation. In Blackburn, H., editor: Measurement in Exercise Electrocardiography. Springfield, IL, Charles C Thomas, 1969, 259–305.
30. Ellestad, M.S.: Stress Testing Principles and Practice, 2nd ed. Philadelphia, F.A. Davis Co., 1980.
31. Lipid Research Clinics Manual of Laboratory Operation, Vol. 1. Lipid and Lipoprotein Analysis. HEW Publication No. NIH 75–628. Washington, D.C., U.S. Government Printing Office, 1974.
32. Dufaux, B., Assmann, G., Order, U., Hoederath, A., and Hollman, W.: Plasma lipoproteins, hormones, and energy substrates during the first days after prolonged exercise. Int. J. Sports Med. 2:256–260, 1981.
33. Buskirk, E.R., Iampietro, P.F., and Bass, D.E.: Work performance after dehydration: effects of physical conditioning and heat acclimation. J. Appl. Physiol. 12:189–194, 1958.
34. Girandola, R.N., Wiswell, R.A., and Romero, G.: Body composition changes resulting from fluid ingestion and dehydration. Res. Q. 48:299–303, 1977.
35. Aronow, W.S., Cassidy, J., Vangrow, J.S., March, H., Kern, J.C., Goldsmith, J.R., Khemka, M., Pagano, J., and Vawter, M.: Effect of cigarette smoking and breathing carbon monoxide on cardiovascular hemodynamics in anginal patients. Circulation 50: 340–347, 1974.
36. American Heart Association: Recommendations for Human Blood Pressure Determination by Sphygmomanometers. Dallas, American Heart Association, 1980.
37. American Heart Association of Wisconsin: Blood Pressure Measurement Education Program. Milwaukee, AHA/Wisconsin Affiliate, 1981.
38. Lind, A.R., and McNicol, G.W.: Muscular factors which determine the cardiovascular responses to sustained and rhythmic exercise. Can. Med. Assoc. J. 96:706–713, 1967.
39. Bezucha, G.R., Lenser, M.C., Hanson, P.G., and Nagle, F.J.: Comparison of hemodynamic responses to static and dynamic exercise. J. Appl. Physiol. 53:1589–1593, 1982.
40. Consolazio, F.C., Johnson, R.E., and Pecora, L.J.: Physiological Measurements of Metabolic Functions in Man. New York, McGraw-Hill, 1963.
41. Wilmore, J.H., Davis, J.A., and Norton, A.C.: An automated system for assessing metabolic and respiratory function during exercise. J. Appl. Physiol. 40:619–624, 1976.
42. Wilmore, J.H., and Costill, D.L.: Semiautomated systems approach to the assessment of oxygen uptake during exercise. J. Appl. Physiol. 36:618–620, 1974.
43. Zeimetz, G.A., Moss, R.F., Butts, N., Wilson, P.K., and Obma, R.: Support versus nonsupport treadmill walking. Med. Sci. Sports 11:112 (abstract), 1979.
44. Ragg, K.E., Murray, T.F., Karbonit, L.M., and Jump, D.A.: Errors in predicting functional capacity from a treadmill exercise stress test. Am. Heart J. 100:581–583, 1980.
45. Wyndham, C.H.: Submaximal tests for estimating maximum oxygen intake. Can. Med. Assoc. J. 96:736–745, 1967.
46. Pollock, M.L., Bohannon, R.L., Cooper, K.H., Ayres, J.J., Ward, A., White, S.R., and Linnerud, A.C.: A comparative analysis of four protocols for maximal treadmill stress testing. Am. Heart J. 92:39–46, 1976.
47. Price, C.S., Pollock, M.L., Gettman, L.R., and Kent, D.A.: Physical Fitness Programs for Law Enforcement Officers: A Manual for Police Administrators. Washington, D.C., U.S. Government Printing Office, 1977.
48. American Alliance for Health, Physical Education, Recreation, and Dance: Health Related Physical Fitness Test Manual. Reston, VA, AAHPERD, 1981.
49. Drews, F.R., Bedynek, J.L., Rushatz, A.S., and Emerson, J.B.: Individual Fitness Handbook. Carlisle Barracks, PA, U.S. Army War College, 1983.
50. Haskell, W.L., and DeBusk, R.: Cardiovascular responses to repeated treadmill exercise testing soon after myocardial infarction. Circulation 60:1247–1251, 1979.
51. Åstrand, P.O., and Rodahl, K.: Textbook of Work Physiology, 2nd ed. New York, McGraw-Hill, 1977.

52. Mitchell, J.H., Sproule, B.J., and Chapman, C.B.: The physiological meaning of the maximal oxygen intake test. J. Clin. Invest. 37:538–547, 1958.
53. Nagle, F.S., Balke, B., and Naughton, J.P.: Gradational step tests for assessing work capacity. J. Appl. Physiol. 20:745–748, 1965.
54. Balke, B., and Ware, R.: An experimental study of physical fitness of Air Force personnel. U.S. Armed Forces Med. J. 10:675–688, 1959.
55. Blomqvist, C.G.: Exercise testing in rheumatic heart disease. Cardiovasc. Clin. 5:267–287, 1973.
56. James, F.W., Blomqvist, C.G., Freed, M.D., Miller, W.W., Moller, J.H., Nugent, E.W., Riopel, D.A., Strong, W.B., and Wessel, H.U.: Standards for exercise testing in the pediatric age group. Circulation 66:1377A–1397A, 1982.
57. Stuart, R. J., and Ellestad, M.H.: National survey of exercise stress testing facilities. Chest 77:94–97, 1980.
58. Naughton, J.P., and Haider, R.: Methods of exercise testing. In Naughton, J.P., Hellerstein, H.K., and Mohler, L.C., editors: Exercise Testing and Exercise Training in Coronary Heart Disease. New York, Academic Press, 1973, pp. 79–91.
59. Pollock, M.L., Foster, C., Schmidt, D.H., Hellman, C., Linnerud, A.C., and Ward, A.: Comparative analysis of physiologic responses to three different maximal graded exercise test protocols in healthy women. Am. Heart J. 103:363–373, 1982.
60. Starling, M.R., Crawford, M.H., and O'Rourke, R.A.: Superiority of selected treadmill exercise protocols predischarge and six weeks postinfarction for detecting ischemic abnormalities. Am. Heart J. 104:1054–1060, 1982.
61. Lerman, J., Bruce, R.A., Sivarajan, E., Pettet, G.E.M., and Trimble, S.: Low-level dynamic exercises for earlier cardiac rehabilitation: aerobic and hemodynamic responses. Arch. Phys. Med. Rehabil. 57:355–360, 1976.
62. American Heart Association: Exercise Testing and Training of Apparently Healthy Individuals: A Handbook for Physicians. Dallas, American Heart Association, 1972.
63. Hellerstein, H.K.: Specifications for exercise testing equipment. Circulation 59:849A–854A, 1979.
64. Åstrand, P.O., and Ryhming, I.A.: Nonogram for calculation of aerobic capacity from pulse rate during submaximal work. J. Appl. Physiol. 7:218–221, 1954.
65. Faria, I.E., and Cavanagh, P.R.: The Physiology and Biomechanics of Cycling. New York, John Wiley and Sons, 1978.
66. Hermansen, L., and Saltin, B.: Oxygen uptake during maximal treadmill and bicycle exercise. J. Appl. Physiol. 26:31–37, 1969.
67. Faulkner, J.A., Roberts, D.E., Elk, R.L., and Conway, J.: Cardiovascular response to submaximal and maximal effort cycling and running. J. Appl. Physiol. 30:457–461, 1971.
68. Pollock, M.L., Dimmick, J., Miller, H.S., Kendrick, Z., and Linnerud, A.C.: Effects of mode of training on cardiovascular function and body composition of adult men. Med. Sci. Sports. 7:139–145, 1975.
69. Åstrand, P.O., and Saltin, B.: Maximal oxygen uptake and heart rate in various types of muscular activity. J. Appl. Physiol. 16:977–981, 1961.
70. Sawka, M.N., Foley, M.E., Pimental, N.A., Tomer, M.M., and Pandolf, K.B.: Determination of maximal aerobic power during upper-body exercise. J. Appl. Physiol. 54:113–117, 1983.
71. Pollock, M.L., Miller, H.S., Linnerud, A.C., Laughridge, E., Coleman, E., and Alexander, E.: Arm pedaling as an endurance training regimen for the disabled. Arch. Phys. Med. Rehabil. 55:418–424, 1974.
72. Pollock, M.L., Foster, C., and Hare, J.: Metabolic and perceptual responses to arm and leg exercise. Med. Sci. Sports Exer. 15:140 (abstract), 1983.
73. Pollock, M.L., Foster, C., and Ward, A.: Exercise prescription for rehabilitation of the cardiac patient. In M.L., Pollock, and Schmidt, D.H. editors: Heart Disease and Rehabilitation. New York, John Wiley and Sons, 1979, pp. 413–445.
74. Glaser, R.M., Sawka, M.N., Brune, M.F., and Wilde, S.W.: Physiological responses to maximal effort wheelchair and arm crank ergometry. J. Appl. Physiol. 48:1060–1064, 1980.
75. Markiewicz, W., Houston, N., and DeBusk, R.: A comparison of static and dynamic exercise soon after myocardial infarction. Israel J. Med. Sci. 15:894–897, 1979.
76. DeBusk, R.F., Valdez, R., Houston, N., and Haskell, W.: Cardiovascular responses to dynamic and static effort soon after myocardial infarction. Application to occupational work assessment. Circulation 58:368–375, 1978.

77. Sjöstrand, T.: Changes in respiratory organs of workmen at an ore melting works. Acta. Med. Scand. Suppl. 196:687–695, 1947.
78. Kurucz, R.L., Fox, E.L., and Mathews, D.K.: Construction of a submaximal cardiovascular step test. Res. Q. 40:115–122, 1969.
79. Katch, F.I., and McArdle, W.D.: Nutrition, Weight Control, and Exercise, 2nd ed. Philadelphia, Lea and Febiger, 1983.
80. Kasch, F.W., and Boyer, J.L.: Adult Fitness Principles and Practices. San Diego, San Diego State College, 1968.
81. Price, C., Pollock, M.L., Gettman, L.R., and Kent, D.A.: Physical fitness programs for law enforcement officers: a manual for police administrators. Washington, D.C., U.S. Government Printing Office, No. 027–000–00671–0, 1978.
82. Cooper, K.H.: Aerobics. New York, M. Evans and Company, 1968.
83. Cooper, M., and Cooper, K.H.: Aerobics for Women. New York, M. Evans and Company, 1972.
84. American Alliance for Health, Physical Education, and Recreation: AAHPER Youth Fitness Test Manual. Washington, D.C., AAHPER, 1958.
85. Ribisl, P.M., and Kachadorian, W.A.: Maximal oxygen intake prediction in young and middle-aged males. J. Sports Med. Phys. Fitness 9:17–22, 1969.
86. Cooper, K.H.: The Aerobics Way. New York, M. Evans and Company, 1977.
87. Kattus, A.A., Jorgensen, C.R., Worden, R.E., and Alvaro, A.B.: S–T segment depression with near-maximal exercise in detection of preclinical coronary heart disease. Circulation 41: 585–595, 1971.
88. Fox, S.M., Naughton, J.P., and Haskell, W.L.: Physical activity and the prevention of coronary heart disease. Ann. Clin. Res. 3:404–416, 1971.
89. Foster, C., Jackson, A.S., Pollock, M.L., Taylor, M.M., Hare, J., Rod, J.L., Sarwar, M., and Schmidt, D.H.: Generalized equations for predicting functional capacity from treadmill performance. Am. Heart J. (in press).
90. Cohen, J., and Cohen, P.: Applied Multiple Regression/Correlation Analysis for the Behavioral Sciences. New York, John Wiley and Sons, 1975.
91. Foster, C., Pollock, M.L., Rod, J.L., Dymond, D.S., Wible, G., and Schmidt, D.H. Evaluation of functional capacity during exercise radionuclide angiography. Cardiology 70: 85–93, 1983.
92. Foster, C., Hare, J., Taylor, M., Goldstein, T., Anholm, J., and Pollock, M.L.: Prediction of oxygen uptake during exercise testing in cardiac patients and healthy adults. J. Cardiac Rehab. (in press).
93. Taylor, H.L., Buskirk, E., and Henschel, A.: Maximal oxygen intake as an objective measure of cardiorespiratory performance. J. Appl. Physiol. 8:77–83, 1955.
94. Mitchell, J.H., Sproule, B.J., and Chapman, C.B.: The physiological meaning of the maximal oxygen intake test. J. Clin. Invest. 37:538–547, 1958.
95. Haskell, W.L., Savin, N., Oldridge, N., and DeBusk, R.: Factors influencing estimated oxygen uptake during exercise testing soon after myocardial infarction. Am. J. Cardiol. 50:299–304, 1982.
96. Pollock, M.L., Foster, C., Rod, J., Stoiber, J., Hare, J., Schmidt, D.H.: Effects of propranolol dosage on the response to submaximal and maximal exercise. Am. J. Cardiol. 49:1000 (abstract), 1982.
97. Pollock, M.L., Foster, C., Rod, J.L., and Wible, G.: Comparison of methods for determining exercise training intensity for cardiac patients and healthy adults. In Kellerman, J.J., editor: Comprehensive Cardiac Rehabilitation. Basel, S. Karger, 1982, pp. 129–133.
98. Borg, G.: Physical Performance and Perceived Exertion. Lund, Sweden, Gleerup, pp. 1–63, 1962.
99. Borg, G.: Subjective effort in relation to physical performance and working capacity. In Pick, H.L., Jr., editor: Psychology: From Research to Practice. New York, Plenum Publishing Corp., 1978, pp. 333–361.
100. Skinner, J.S., Hutsler, R., Bergsteinova, V., and Buskirk, E.R.: The validity and reliability of a rating scale of perceived exertion. Med. Sci. Sports 5:94–96, 1973.
101. Skinner, J.S., Hutsler, R., Bergsteinova, V., and Buskirk, E.R.: Perception of effort during different types of exercise and under different environmental conditions. Med. Sci. Sports 5:110–115, 1973.
102. Sargeant, A.J., and Davies, C.T.M.: Perceived exertion during rhythmic exercise involving different muscle masses. J. Hum. Ergol. 2:3–11, 1973.

103. Davies, C.T.M., and Sargeant, A.J.: The effects of atropine and practolol on the perception of exertion during treadmill exercise. Ergonomics 22:1141–1146, 1979.
104. Borg, G.A.V.: Psychophysical bases of perceived exertion. Med. Sci. Sports Exer. 14: 377–381, 1982.
105. Pandolf, K.B.: Differentiated ratings of perceived exertion during physical exercise. Med. Sci. Sports. Exer. 14:397–405, 1982.
106. Morgan, W.P., and Pollock, M.L.: Psychologic characterization of the elite distance runner. Ann. N.Y. Acad. Sci. 301:382–403, 1977.
107. Pollock, M.L., and Foster, C.: Exercise prescription for participants on propranolol. J. Am. Coll. Cardiol. (abstract) 2:624, 1983.
108. Noble, B.J.: Clinical applications of perceived exertion. Med. Sci. Sports Exer. 14: 406–411, 1982.
109. Morgan, W.P.: Psychophysiology of self-awareness during vigorous physical activity. Res. Q. Exer. Sport 52:385–427, 1981.
110. Smutok, M.A., Skrinar, G.S., and Pandolf, K.B.: Exercise intensity: subjective regulation by perceived exertion. Arch. Phys. Med. Rehabil. 61:569–574, 1980.
111. Gutmann, M.C., Squires, R.W., Pollock, M.L., Foster, C., and Anholm, J.: Perceived exertion-heart rate relationship during exercise testing and training in cardiac patients. J. Cardiac Rehab. 1:52–59, 1981.
112. Cafarelli, E.: Peripheral contributions to the perception of effort. Med. Sci. Sports Exer. 14:382–389, 1982.
113. Robertson, R.J.: Central signals of perceived exertion during dynamic exercise. Med. Sci. Sports Exer. 14:390–396, 1982.
114. Koppes, G., McKiernan, T., Bassan, M., and Froelicher, V.F.: Treadmill exercise testing. Curr. Probl. Cardiol. 7:1–44, 1977.
115. Blackburn, H., and Katigbak, R.: What electrocardiographic leads to take after exercise? Am. Heart J. 67:184–191, 1963.
116. Mason, R.E., Likar, I., Biern, R.O., and Ross, R.S.: Multiple-lead exercise electrocardiography. Experience in 107 normal subjects and 67 patients with angina pectoris, and comparison with coronary cinearteriography in 84 patients. Circulation 36:517–525, 1967.
117. Phibbs, B., and Buckels, L.: Comparative yield of ECG leads in multistage stress testing. Am. Heart J. 90:275–281, 1975.
118. Robertson, D., Kostuk, W.J., and Ahuja, S.P.: The localization of coronary artery stenosis of 12 lead ECG response to graded exercise test: support for intercoronary steal. Am. Heart J. 91:437–444, 1976.
119. Tucker, S.C., Kemp, V.E., Holland, W.E., and Horgan, J.H.: Multiple lead ECG submaximal treadmill exercise tests in angiographically documented coronary heart disease. Angiology 27:149–155, 1976.
120. Bruce, R.A., De Rouen, T.A., and Hammermeister, K.E.: Noninvasive screening criteria for enhanced 4 year survival after aortocoronary bypass surgery. Circulation 60:638–646, 1979.
121. McNeer, J.F., Margolis, J.E., Lee, K.L., Kisslo, J.A., Peter, R.H., Kong, Y., Behar, V.S., Wallace, A.G., McCants, C.B., and Rosati, R.A.: The role of the exercise test in the evaluation of patients for ischemic heart disease. Circulation 57:64–70, 1978.
122. McHenry, P.L., and Morris, S.N.: Exercise electrocardiography—current state of the art. In Schlanti, R.C., and Hurst, J.W., editors: Advances in Electrocardiography, Vol. 2. New York, Grune and Stratton, 1976, pp. 265–304.
123. Chaitman, B.R., and Hanson, J.S.: Comparative sensitivity and specificity of exercise electrocardiographic lead systems. Am. J. Cardiol. 47:1335–1349, 1981.
124. Simoons, M.L., and Block, P.: Toward the optimal lead system and optimal criteria for exercise electrocardiography. Am. J. Cardiol. 47:1366–1374, 1981.
125. Weiner, D.A., McCabe, C.H., and Ryan, T.J.: Identification of patients with left main and three vessel coronary disease with clinical and exercise test variables. Am. J. Cardiol. 46:21–27, 1980.
126. Ritchie, J.L., Zaret, B.L., Strauss, H.W., Pitt, B., Berman, D.S., Shelbert, H.R., Ashburn, W.L., Berger, H.J., and Hamilton, G.W.: Myocardial imaging with thallium-201: a multicenter study in patients with angina pectoris or acute myocardial infarction. Am. J. Cardiol. 42:345–350, 1978.
127. Borer, J.S., Bacharach, S.L., Green, M.V., Kent, K.M., Epstein, S.E., and Johnston, G.S.: Real-time radionuclide cineangiography in the noninvasive evaluation of global and

regional left ventricular function at rest and during exercise in patients with coronary artery disease. N. Engl. J. Med. *296:*839–844, 1977.

128. Iskandrian, A.S., Hakki, A.H., DePace, N.L., Manno, B., and Segal, B.L.: Evaluation of left ventricular function by radionuclide angiography during exercise in normal subjects and in patients with chronic coronary heart disease. J. Am. Coll. Cardiol. *1:*1518–1529, 1983.

129. Port, S., Cobb, F.R., Coleman, R.E., and Jones, R.H.: Effect of age on the response of the left ventricular ejection fraction to exercise. N. Engl. J. Med. *303:*1133–1137, 1980.

130. Jones, R.H., McEwan, P., Newman, G.E., Port, S., Rerych, S.K., Scholz, P.M., Upton, M.T., Peter, C.A., Austin, E.H., Leong, K., Gibbons, R.J., Cobb, F.R., Coleman, R.E., and Sabiston, Jr., D.C.: Accuracy of diagnosis of coronary artery disease by radionuclide measurement of left ventricular function during rest and exercise. Circulation *64:*586–601, 1981.

131. Lown, B.: Sudden cardiac death: the major challenge confronting contemporary cardiology. Am. J. Cardiol. *43:*313–328, 1979.

132. Lown, B., and Wolf, M.: Approaches to sudden death from coronary heart disease. Circulation *44:*130–142, 1971.

133. DeMaria, A.N., Zakauddin, V., Amsterdam, E.A., Mason, D.T., and Massumi, R.A.: Disturbances of cardiac rhythm and conduction induced by exercise, diagnostic, prognostic and therapeutic implications. Am. J. Cardiol. *33:*732–736, 1974.

134. Bigger, J.T., and Weld, F.M.: Shortcomings of the Lown grading system for observational or experimental studies in ischemic heart disease. Am. Heart J. *100:*1081–1088, 1980.

135. Akhtar, M., Wolf, F., and Denker, S.: Sudden cardiac death. *In* Pollock, M.L., and Schmidt, D.H., editors: Heart Disease Rehabilitation, 2nd ed. New York, John Wiley and Sons (in press).

136. Cooper, K.H., Purdy, J.G., White, S.R., Pollock, M.L., and Linnerud, A.C.: Age-fitness adjusted maximal heart rates. *In* Brunner, D., and Jokl, E., editors: Medicine and Sport, Vol. 10, The Role of Exercise in Internal Medicine. Basel, S. Karger, 1977, pp. 78–88.

137. Rod, J.L., Squires, R.W., Pollock, M.L., Foster, C., and Schmidt, D.H.: Symptom-limited graded exercise testing soon after myocardial revascularization surgery. J. Cardiac Rehab. *2:*199–205, 1982.

138. Powles, A.C.P., Sutton, J.R., Wicks, J.R., Oldridge, N.B., and Jones, N.L.: Reduced heart rate response to exercise in ischemic heart disease: the fallacy of the target heart rate in exercise testing. Med. Sci. Sport *11:*227–233, 1979.

139. Vecchio, T.H.: Predictive value of a single diagnostic test in unselected populations. N. Engl. J. Med. *274:*1171–1177, 1966.

140. Schmidt, D.H., and Port, S.: The clinical and research application of nuclear cardiology. *In* Pollock, M. L., and Schmidt, D.H., editors: Heart Disease and Rehabilitation, 2nd ed. New York, John Wiley and Sons. (in press).

141. Behnke, A.R., and Wilmore, J.H.: Evaluation and Regulation of Body Build and Composition. Englewood Cliffs, NJ, Prentice-Hall, 1974.

142. Brozek, J., Grande, F., Anderson, T., and Keys, A.: Densitometric analysis of body composition; revision of some quantitative assumptions. Ann. N.Y. Acad. Sci. *110:*113–140, 1963.

143. Goldman, R.F., and Buskirk, E.R.: Body volume measurement by underwater weighing: description of a method. *In* Brozek, J. and Henschel, A., editors: Techniques for Measuring Body Composition. Washington, D.C., National Academy of Sciences, 1961, pp. 78–89.

144. Buskirk, E.R.: Underwater weighing and body density: a review of procedures. *In* Brozek, J., and Henschel, A., editors: Techniques for Measuring Body Composition. Washington, D.C., National Academy of Sciences, 1961, pp. 90–105.

145. Goldman, H.I., and Becklace, M.R.: Respiratory function tests: Normal values of medium altitudes and the prediction of normal results. Am. Rev. Tuber. Respir. Dis. *79:*457–467, 1959.

146. Clinical Spirometry. Braintree, MA, W.E. Collins, 1967.

147. Wilmore, J.H.: The use of actual, predicted and constant residual volumes in the assessment of body composition by underwater weighing. Med. Sci. Sports *1:*87–90, 1969.

148. Katch, F.I., and Katch, V.L.: Measurement and prediction errors in body composition assessment and the search for a perfect prediction equation. Res. Q. Exer. Sport *51:*249–260, 1980.

149. Weast, R.C., editor-in-chief: Handbook of Chemistry and Physics, 50th ed. Cleveland, The Chemical Rubber Co., 1969.

150. Katch, F.I.: Apparent body density and variability during underwater weighing. Res. Q. 39:993–999, 1968.

151. Siri, W.E.: Body composition from fluid spaces and density. In Brozek, J., and Henschel, A., editors: Techniques for Measuring Body Composition. Washington, D.C., National Academy of Science, 1961, pp. 223–244.

152. Lohman, T.G.: Skinfolds and body density and their relation to body fatness: A review. Hum. Biol. 53:181–225, 1981.

153. Wormersley, J., Durnin, J.V.G.A., Boddy, K., and Mahaffy, M.: Influence of muscular development obesity and age on the fat-free mass of adults. J. Appl. Physiol. 41:223–229, 1976.

154. Garn, S.M.: Some pitfalls in the quantification of body composition. Ann. N.Y. Acad. Sci. 110:171–174, 1963.

155. Lohman, T.G.: Body composition methodology in sports medicine. Phys. Sportsmed. 10:47–58, 1982.

156. Cureton, T.K.: Physical Fitness Appraisal and Guidance. St. Louis, C.V. Mosby Company, 1947.

157. Martin, A.D., Drinkwater, D.T., Clarys, J.P., and Ross, W.D.: Estimation of body fat: A new look at some old assumptions. Paper presented at the Pan American Congress of Sports Medicine. Miami, FL, May 1981.

158. Craig, A.B., and Ware, D.E.: Effect of immersion in water on vital capacity and residual volume of lungs. J. Appl. Physiol. 23:423–425, 1967.

159. Fahey, T.D., and Schroeder, R.: A load cell system for hydrostatic weighing. Res. Q. 49:85–87, 1978.

160. Keys, A., Fidanza, F., Karvonen, M.J., Kimura, N., and Taylor, H.L.: Indices of relative weight and obesity. J. Chronic Dis. 25:329–343, 1972.

161. Brozek, J., and Keys, A.: The evaluation of leanness-fatness in man: norms and intercorrelations. Br. J. Nutr. 5:194–206, 1951.

162. Cureton, K.J., Boileau, R.A., and Lohman, T.G.: A comparison of densiometric, potassium 40 and skinfold estimates of body composition in prepubescent boys. Hum. Biol. 47:321–336, 1975.

163. Durnin, J.V.G.A., and Rahaman, M.M.: The assessment of the amount of fat in the human body from measurements of skinfold thickness. Br. J. Nutr. 21:681–689, 1967.

164. Durnin, J.V.G.A., and Wormersley, J.: Body fat assessed from total body density and its estimation from skinfold thickness: measurements on 481 men and women aged from 16 to 72 years. Br. J. Nutr. 32:77–92, 1974.

165. Forsyth, M.L., and Sinning, W.E.: The anthropometric estimation of body density and lean body weight of male athletes. Med. Sci. Sports 5:174–180, 1973.

166. Haisman, M.F.: The assessment of body fat content in young men from measurements of body density and skinfold thickness. Hum. Biol. 42:679–688, 1970.

167. Harsha, D.W., Fredrichs, R.R., and Berenson, G.S.: Densitometry and anthropometry of black and white children. Hum. Biol. 50:261–280, 1978.

168. Jackson, A.S., and Pollock, M.L.: Generalized equations for predicting body density of men. Br. J. Nutr. 40:497–504, 1978.

169. Katch, F.I., and McArdle, W.D.: Prediction of body density from simple anthropometric measurements in college age women and men. Hum. Biol. 45:445–454, 1973.

170. Katch, F.I., and Michael, E.D.: Densitometric validation of six skinfold formulas to predict body density and percent fat of 17 year old boys. Res. Q. 40:712–716, 1969.

171. Parizkova, J.: Total body fat and skinfold thickness in children. Metabolism 10:794–807, 1961.

172. Pascale, L., Grossman, M., Sloane, H., and Frankel, T.: Correlations between thickness of skinfolds and body density in 88 soldiers. Hum. Biol. 28:165–176, 1956.

173. Pollock, M.L., Hickman, T., Kendrick, Z., Jackson, A., Linnerud, A.C., and Dawson, G.: Prediction of body density in young and middle-aged men. J. Appl. Physiol. 40:300–304, 1976.

174. Sloan, A.W.: Estimation of body fat in young men. J. Appl. Physiol. 23:311–315, 1967.

175. Wilmore, J.H., and Behnke, A.R.: An anthropometric estimation of body density and lean body weight in young men. J. Appl. Physiol. 27:25–31, 1969.

176. Wright, H.F., and Wilmore, J.H.: Estimation of relative body fat and lean body weight in a United States Marine Corps population. Aerospace Med. 45: 301–306, 1974.

177. Jackson, A.S., Pollock, M.L., and Ward, A.: Generalized equations for predicting body density of women. Med. Sci. Sports Exer. *12:*175–182, 1980.
178. Katch, F.I., and Michael, E.D.: Prediction of body density from skinfold and girth measurement of college females. J. Appl. Physiol. *25:*92–94, 1968.
179. Pollock, M.L., Laughridge, E., Coleman, B., Linnerud, A.C., and Jackson, A.: Prediction of body density in young and middle-aged women. J. Appl. Physiol. *38:*745–749, 1975.
180. Sinning, W.E.: Anthropometric estimation of body density, fat and lean body weight in women gymnasts. Med. Sci. Sports *10:*243–249, 1978.
181. Sloan, A.W., Burt, J.J., and Blyth, C.S.: Estimation of body fat in young women. J. Appl. Physiol. *17:*967–970, 1962.
182. Wilmore, J.H., and Behnke, A.R.: An anthropometric estimation of body density and lean body weight in young women. Am. J. Clin. Nutr. *23:*267–274, 1970.
183. Young, C.M.: Prediction of specific gravity and body fatness in older women. J. Am. Diet. Assoc. *45:*333–338, 1964.
184. Young, C.M., Martin, M., Tensuan, R., and Blondin, J.: Predicting specific gravity and body fatness in young women. J. Am. Diet. Assoc. *40:*102–107, 1962.
185. Parizkova, J.: Body Fat and Physical Fitness. The Hague, Martinus Nijhoff b.v., Publishers, 1977.
186. Jackson, A.S., and Pollock, M.L.: Steps toward the development of generalized equations for predicting body composition in adults. Can. J. Appl. Spt. Sci. *7:*189–196, 1982.
187. Jackson, A.S., and Pollock, M.L.: Factor analysis and multivariate scaling of anthropometric variables for the assessment of body composition. Med. Sci. Sports *8:*196–203, 1976.
188. Bakker, H.K., and Struikenkamp, R.S.: Biological variability and lean body mass estimates. Hum. Biol *49:*187–202, 1977.
189. Baun, W.B., Baun, M.R., and Raven, P.B.: A nomogram for the estimate of percent body fat from generalized equations. Res. Q. Exer. Sport *52:*380–384, 1981.
190. Hertzberg, H.T.E., Churchill, E., Dupertuis, C.W., White, R.M., and Damon, A.: Anthropometric Survey of Turkey, Greece, and Italy. New York, Macmillan, 1963.
191. Keys, A. (Chairman): Recommendations concerning body measurements for the characterization of nutritional status. Hum. Biol. *28:*111–123, 1956.
192. Edwards, D.A.W., Hammond, W.H., Healy, M.J.R., Tanner, J.M., and Whitehouse, R.H.: Design and accuracy of calipers for measuring subcutaneous tissue thickness. Br. J. Nutr. *9:*133–143, 1955.
193. Leger, L.A., Lambert, J., and Martin, P.: Validity of plastic skinfold caliper measurements. Hum. Biol. *54:*667–675, 1982.
194. Hawkins, J.D.: An analysis of selected skinfold measuring instruments. JOPERD *54:*25–27, 1983.
195. Lohman, T.G., Pollock, M.L., Slaughter, M.H., Brandon, L.J., and Boileau, R.A.: Methodological factors and the prediction of body fat in female athletes. Med. Sci. Sports Exer. (in press).
196. Pollock, M.L. Research progress in validation of clinical methods of assessing body composition. Med. Sci. Sports Exer. (in press).
197. Lohman, T.G., Wilmore, J.H., and Massey, B.H.: Interinvestigator reliability of skinfolds. AAHPERD Research Abstracts. Washington, D.C., AAHPERD, 1979, p. 102.
198. Jackson, A.S., Pollock, M.L., and Gettman, L.R.: Intertester reliability of selected skinfold and circumference measurements and percent fat estimates. Res. Q. *49:*546–551, 1978.
199. Zuti, W.B., and Golding, L.A.: Comparing diet and exercise as weight reduction tools. Phys. Sportsmed. *4:*49–53, 1976.
200. Johnston, F.E., Hamill, D.V., and Lemeshow, S.: Skinfold Thickness of Children 6-11 years—United States (series II No. 120, 1972), Skinfold Thickness of Youth 12–17 years (series II No. 132, 1974), and Skinfolds, Body Girths, Biacromial Diameter, and Selected Anthropometric Indices of Adults (series II No. 35, 1970), U.S. National Center for Health Statistics, HEW. Washington, D.C., U.S. Government Printing Office.
201. Monitoba Physical Fitness Performance Test Manual and Fitness Objectives. Winnipeg, Manitoba Department of Education, 1977.
202. Wilmore, J.H.: Training for Sport and Activity—The Physiological Basis of the Conditioning Process, 2nd ed. Boston, Allyn and Bacon, 1982.
203. Clarke, H.H.: Muscular Strength and Endurance in Man. Englewood Cliffs, NJ, Prentice-Hall, 1966.

204. Berger, R.A.: Applied Exercise Physiology. Philadelphia, Lea and Febiger, 1982.
205. Riley, D.P.: Strength Training for Football the Penn State Way, 2nd ed. West Point, NY, Leisure Press, 1982.
206. Darden, E.: Strength-Training Principles. Winter Park, FL, Anna Publishing, 1977.
207. Berger, R.A.: Classification of students on the basis of strength. Res. Q. *34:*514–515, 1963.
208. Leighton, J.: An instrument and technique for the measurement of joint motion. Arch. Phys. Med. Rehab. *36:*571–578, 1955.
209. Adrian, M.J.: An introduction to electrogoniometry. *In* Kinesiology Review. Washington, D.C., American Association of Health, Physical Education and Recreation, 1968
210. Kraus, H.: Clinical Treatment of Back and Neck Pain. New York, McGraw-Hill, 1970.
211. Melleby, A.: The Y's Way to a Healthy Back. Piscataway, NJ, New Century Publishers, 1982.

Chapter 7

PRESCRIBING EXERCISE FOR THE APPARENTLY HEALTHY

GUIDELINES AND PRELIMINARY CONSIDERATIONS

A clear understanding of the person involved is necessary in order to prescribe exercise safely and adequately. People vary greatly in status of health and fitness, structure, age, motivation, and needs; therefore, the individual approach to exercise prescription is recommended.

The needs and goals of elementary school children, college athletes, middle-aged men and women, and cardiac patients clearly differ. For example, an athlete often must get into condition quickly for a competition. In this case, many safeguards concerning intensity and progression of exercise are not closely followed. Although the abrupt approach is followed in certain instances, its general use is not recommended. The initial experience with exercise training should be of low-to-moderate intensity and slow-to-moderate progression that allows for gradual adaptation.[1-5] On the basis of much experience with adult programs, the abrupt approach can result in discouraging future motivation for participation in endurance or other activities. Improper advice or prescription also can lead to undue muscle or joint strain or soreness, other orthopedic problems, excessive fatigue, and risk of precipitating a heart attack. The last-mentioned is rare and occurs mainly with middle-aged and older participants. Most incidents have occurred because of the lack of appropriate previous medical evaluation and clearance, incorrect exercise prescription, inadequate supervision, or an extreme climatic condition such as excess heat and humidity or severe cold.[6-10] Although many of the suggestions and guidelines for exercise prescription are similar for both apparently healthy and diseased patients, this chapter will focus on exercise programs for the apparently healthy. Chapter 8 will be devoted to exercise prescription for the diseased patient.

The following guidelines are suggested in the exercise prescription process.

PRELIMINARY SUGGESTIONS

1. Have adequate medical information available to assess health status properly. This would include a medical history and risk factor analysis and possibly a physical examination and laboratory tests. See Chapter 6 for more details.

2. Have information concerning the present status of physical fitness and exercise habits.

3. Know the individual's needs, interests, and objectives for being in an exercise program.

4. Set realistic short-term and long-term goals.

5. Give advice on proper attire and equipment for an exercise program (see Chapter 10).

SUGGESTIONS FOR INITIAL PHASES OF AN EXERCISE PROGRAM

1. Properly educate the participant in the principles of exercise, exercise prescription, and methods of monitoring and recording exercise experiences.

2. Give adequate leadership and direction in the early stages of the exercise program to insure proper implementation and progress.

3. Remember that education, motivation, and leadership are the keys to a successful exercise program.

LONG-TERM SUGGESTIONS

1. Re-evaluations are desirable for reassessing individual status, functional physical fitness, and exercise prescription.

2. Re-evaluations are also important in the education and motivation processes.

The program is prescribed as soon as the health and fitness status and needs and objectives of the participants are determined. From this information, as well as from knowledge of the participants' activity interests and available time, the desired type and quantity of exercise may be determined. It is important for the initial exercise experience to be enjoyable, refreshing, and not too demanding either physiologically or in terms of time. The slow, gradual approach to initiating an exercise program will help cultivate a more positive attitude toward physical activity and enhance the probability of long-term adherence. In addition, as discussed in Chapter 3, if the prescribed program is too demanding, adherence is not as likely.[5-11] More details regarding program adherence will be discussed in Chapter 9.

The importance of a well-rounded exercise program should be emphasized. The well-rounded program will include aerobic activities for developing and maintaining cardiorespiratory fitness and proper weight control, strength and muscular endurance activities, and flexibility exercises. Specificity of exercise is an important concept to consider when prescribing exercise. As emphasized in Chapters 3 and 5, no one activity will give a participant total fitness. Strength and muscular endurance exercises are recommended to help maintain proper muscle tone and to protect against injury and low back pain. Flexibility exercises are important for developing and maintaining joint range of motion and should be practiced often. Reduced flexibility can lead to poor posture, fatigue, and injury. An endurance activity such as jogging can reduce the flexibility of the extensor muscles of the hip, leg, and ankle and flexor muscles of the leg. Thus, avoiding proper stretching exercises for these areas could lead to low back, hamstring, or calf muscle (Achilles tendon) problems.

Our experience has been that once individuals get started in a program, if strength, muscular endurance, and flexibility activities are not stressed, they tend to be forgotten. In addition, with the emphasis placed on the aerobic phase of the program, the participant may get the impression that the other activities are secondary and only necessary if there is enough time. For example, a few years ago, one of the authors integrated the Cooper point system into his adult fitness program. Cooper[2] had set up an elaborate point system that gave participants points for doing aerobic exercises. Points were based on the intensity and duration of the activity. In essence, an individual received points for expending kilocalories. Because little or no points were awarded for doing strength (calisthenics and weight training) and flexibility exercises, participants began to equate this with the lack of importance. Cooper himself feels that a well-rounded program is vital and that it is unfortunate if some have misinterpreted this fact from his books.[2,12] The significant factor is that the practitioner continues to practice with emphasis on a well-rounded program.

An adequate program stressing the various components of physical fitness can be designed for a 60-minute period. For most individuals, a program lasting more than 60 minutes may become a deterrent for long-term continuation. The four main components of an exercise program would include warm-up, muscle-conditioning, aerobic, and cool-down periods. Table 7-1 gives a suggested time frame for each component. The variability of each time frame—in particular, the muscle-conditioning and aerobic periods—depends on health and fitness status and individual needs and goals. For example, if the program was being designed for police officers or fire fighters, the muscle-conditioning component would become more important, and a minimum of 20 minutes would be recommended.[13] Depending on intensity, the aerobic period would be 20 to 30 minutes in duration. In contrast, a healthy but overweight 48-year-old executive would probably start out with 5 to 10 minutes of strength activities and an aerobic period of 30 to 45 minutes. Initially, the sedentary executive will emphasize

TABLE 7–1. COMPONENTS OF A TRAINING PROGRAM

COMPONENTS	ACTIVITIES	RECOMMENDED TIME
Warm-up	Stretching, low-level calisthenics, walking	10 minutes
Muscular conditioning	Calisthenics, weight training, pulley weights	10–20 minutes
Aerobics	Fast walk, jog/run, swim, bicycle, cross-country skiing, vigorous games, dancing	20–40 minutes
Cool-down	Walking, stretching	5–10 minutes

TABLE 7–2. RECOMMENDATIONS FOR
EXERCISE PRESCRIPTION

1. Frequency	3 to 5 days per week
2. Intensity	60 to 90 per cent of maximum heart rate (HR max) reserve
	50 to 80 per cent of maximum oxygen uptake
3. Duration	15 to 60 minutes (continuous)
4. Mode-activity	Run, jog, walk, bicycle, swim, or endurance sport and dance activities
5. Initial level of fitness	High = higher work load
	Low = lower work load

Reprinted with permission from American College of Sports Medicine: Position statement on the recommended quantity and quality of exercise for developing and maintaining fitness in healthy adults. Med. Sci. Sports *10*:vii–x, 1978.

stretching and low level muscle-conditioning exercises. The aerobic activity would be of low-to-moderate intensity, probably of an interval type stressing a combination of walking and jogging or slow and fast walking.

EXERCISE PRESCRIPTION FOR CARDIORESPIRATORY ENDURANCE AND WEIGHT REDUCTION

The research findings reported in Chapters 3 and 4 described the amount of work considered necessary to develop and maintain an optimal level of cardiorespiratory endurance and an optimal weight. Within certain limits, the total energy cost of a training regimen is the most important factor in the development of cardiorespiratory endurance and in weight reduction and control. For most people, this energy cost amounts to approximately 900 to 1,500 Kcal per week or 300 to 500 Kcal per exercise session. Table 7–2 summarizes the optimal frequency, intensity, and duration of training needed to attain a certain level of energy expenditure and gives general recommendations for exercise prescription.[14,15] These recommendations are designed for the general population and not for highly trained endurance athletes or persons in poor health.

FREQUENCY

Exercise should be performed on a regular basis from 3 to 5 days per week. Although programs of sufficient intensity and duration show some cardiorespiratory improvements with a frequency of fewer than 3 days per week, little or no loss of body weight or fat is found.[16] In addition, improvement in cardiorespiratory endurance is only minimal to modest in programs of fewer than 3 days per week (usually less than 10 per cent). Participants in 1- or 2-day-per-week programs often complain that the workout sessions are too intermittent and break the continuity of the training regimen. Another commonly heard complaint is the following: "It seemed as though I was starting anew each time I came out." Our experience has shown that feelings such as these often lead to dropping out of a program. Under unusual conditions, if time and available facilities are important considerations, then 1- or 2-day-per-week regimens may be acceptable and may serve a temporary purpose.[15]

Conditioning every other day is most frequently recommended when an endurance exercise regimen is initiated. Daily, vigorous exercise often becomes too demanding initially and does not allow enough rest time between workouts for the musculoskeletal system to adapt properly. This is particularly true with activities that have a running component.[11] This nonadaptive state generally leads to undesirable muscle soreness, fatigue, and possible injury. This guideline may seem to contradict the research findings reported in Chapter 3. However, the data from young men running 30 minutes, 5 days per week, or 45 minutes, 3 days per week, showed that they incurred injuries at a significantly higher rate than when they were on 3-day-per-week programs of 15- and 30-minute durations.[11] In fact, the men in the 3-day-per-week programs had little or no injury problems. Most of the injuries that did occur concerned problems of the knee, skin, ankle, or foot.

Persons who are at a low level of fitness and whose initial programs are restricted to 5 to 15 minutes per session may want to exercise twice each day and often every day.[17] An example of this special condition is a person who is placed into a walking program of low-to-moderate intensity and short duration. In this case, a person may adapt better to shorter but more frequent exercise sessions. Another substitute for exercising every other day is to alternate the regular exercise session with days of milder activity. For persons who are initiating a jog-walk program, stretching and moderate warm-up exercises (calisthenics) for 10 to 15 minutes followed by a continuous walk for 20 to 30 minutes on alternate days are recommended.

Participants can begin to increase their frequency of training to a daily basis after several weeks or months of conditioning. The point in time at which this increase in frequency can be accommodated properly is an individual matter and is dependent upon age, initial level of fitness, intensity of training, and freedom from excessive soreness or injury. Generally, persons who are older, overweight, and lower in fitness are more prone to musculoskeletal problems. For weight reduction programs, 5 days per week of training are generally better than 3.[18] The key is to alternate high-and low-intensity training sessions to allow time for adaptation. Generally, persons who are out of shape and overweight will be involved in lower intensity programs, so the added frequency and duration will be necessary to expend enough kilocalories.

INTENSITY AND DURATION

Although intensity and duration are separate entities, it is difficult to discuss intensity without mentioning its interaction with duration. As noted in Chapter 3, exercise regimens of lower intensity (less kilocaloric expenditure) but with a longer duration produced improvements similar to those of the higher intensity and shorter duration regimens; the total kilocaloric expenditures were approximately equal for both programs. The caloric difference between running a mile in 8 minutes and running a mile in 9 minutes is minimal; therefore, running a little extra time or distance at a slower pace will offset the extra kilocalories burned at the faster pace.[15,19] The important concept is that as long as the intensity is above the minimal threshold level, and a certain amount of total work is completed in an exercise session, the manner in which the end result is accomplished can vary.[12,15,19,20]

The above-mentioned concept has important implications for exercise prescription for adults, and it should be remembered that low-to-moderate intensity, longer duration types of programs are generally recommended for beginners. This recommendation is particularly true for those showing a poor performance or presence of heart disease on their initial evaluation. The important point is to prescribe a regimen at a low-to-moderate intensity so that the participant can accomplish a sufficient amount of work. Initially, the prescription may call for a moderate-to-brisk walk for 20 to 30 minutes.

Table 7–2 outlines a certain minimal threshold of intensity that is necessary for improving cardiorespiratory function. As was mentioned in Chapter 3, programs of an intensity of less than 60 per cent of maximum heart rate (HR max) reserve will often produce improvement in persons with low initial levels of fitness. These persons generally will qualify for fitness classifications 1 to 3, as listed in Table 6–3. Special starter programs of less than 60 per cent intensity may be recommended for these individuals. In addition, for weight control purposes, all expended kilocalories are important. Whether they are above or below the minimal threshold does not matter.

The training duration will vary from day to day and from activity to activity. The important factor is to design a program that meets the criteria for improving and maintaining a sufficient level of physical fitness, i.e., enjoyable (tolerable), and that will fit into the participant's time demands. It should be rewarding to the participant—preferably, it should be fun.

The level of training intensity that can be tolerated will vary greatly, depending on status of fitness and health, age, experience, and general ability. Long distance runners may tolerate 2 to 3 hours of continuous running at 80 to 90 per cent of maximum capacity, but most beginners cannot perform a continuous effort at this level for than a few minutes. For beginners to accomplish 20 to 30 minutes of continuous training, they must choose the proper intensity level. The proper intensity level for beginners will range from 60 to 75 per cent of HR max reserve (brisk walking programs) to 75 to 85 per cent of HR max reserve for jogging (the latter program is generally interspersed with bouts of walking, with peak intensity occurring during jogging). Most persons in fitness categories 1 and 2 (Table 6–3) will start with a walking program, and those in categories 3 and above will begin with a combination walk-jog routine.

The walk-jog routine, or low-intensity, moderate-intensity periods of work if another mode of activity is being performed, will have a peak intensity of 85 to 90 per cent of maximum and a low intensity of 50 to 65 per cent. The average intensity level will range between 70 and 80 per cent of HR max reserve. Experience has shown that an intensity level of 50 to 60 per cent of maximum can be tolerated comfortably for 20 to 30 minutes by most persons and can be classified as low-to-moderate training. Intensity levels ranging from 70 to 85 per cent are considered as moderate and those above 90 per cent of HR max reserve as high-intensity training. The results of the initial graded exercise test are important in placing the participant at a correct and safe level of intensity.

Upon initiating an endurance training regimen, most participants notice the training effect rather quickly. They usually experience the ability to perform more total work in subsequent exercise sessions. The increased total work is a result of the ability of the participant to increase the training duration or to tolerate a greater training intensity or both. The raised average intensity is a function of a higher peak intensity level or an elevation in the ratio of high to low bouts of work or both. For example, a participant in a walk-jog routine can tolerate longer periods of jogging interspersed with shorter periods of walking. As these adaptations to training occur, changes in the exercise prescription are recommended. Periodic re-evaluations will help in determining a new status of physical fitness, in enhancing motivation, and in facilitating proper exercise prescription.

ESTIMATION OF EXERCISE INTENSITY. How is a participant's exercise intensity determined and how can it be estimated during an exercise session? The three most popular ways in which training intensity is being estimated are as follows: metabolic (Kcal/min—METs),[4,21] HR (beats/min),[4,22,23] and rating of perceived exertion (RPE).[24-26] Metabolic determination of training intensity is accomplished by measuring the participant's

TABLE 7-3. RECOMMENDED TRAINING ZONE
FOR EXERCISE PRESCRIPTION

Oxygen uptake	50% ⟶	85%
Heart rate	60% ⟶	90%
RPE*	12 ⟶	16
	Somewhat hard	Hard

* Rating of Perceived Exertion, Borg Scale.[24]

$\dot{V}O_2$ max (aerobic capacity) during a graded exercise test (GXT) or some other indirect method as described in Chapter 6. The training intensity is usually calculated between 50 and 85 per cent of maximum aerobic capacity (METs).[4,23] As mentioned earlier, 50 per cent of maximum ($\dot{V}O_2$ max—METs) relates to the minimal threshold for improving cardiorespiratory fitness, and 85 per cent represents the upper limit at which most participants tolerate aerobic training.[15,27] A specified percentage of maximum limit recommended for training is called "target rate," and when an upper and lower limit range is specified, it is called the "training zone."

As shown in Figure 3-8, HR and oxygen uptake have a linear relationship.[28] Because of the impracticality of routinely measuring oxygen uptake and the ease with which HR can be measured, the HR standard is recommended for general use. Maximum HR can be determined (1) by using the highest HR found on a GXT,[26] (2) after a difficult bout of endurance exercise (for example, an all-out run), (3) by subtracting current age in years from 220,[28] or (4) by referring to the population-, sex-, age-specific norms shown in Appendix A, Tables A-1 to A-10. The first method of estimating HR max is preferred because there is considerable individual variation even for the same sex and age.[29,30] In addition, HR is usually attained while qualified personnel are evaluating the performance of a participant. The second method is to count the HR after an all-out 12-minute run or similar endurance field test (1.5-mile run). This type of test is not recommended for beginners or persons at a high risk of coronary heart disease.[2,12] The third and fourth methods of determining HR max are the least accurate but may be used as a rough approximation. The inaccuracy of the third and fourth methods stems from a variability of HR max at any given age (standard deviation = ± 12 beats/min).[29,30] For example, the HR max of a man 50 years of age averages approximately 170 beats/min, but presumably healthy individuals may have rates ranging from below 140 to over 200 beats/min.

The RPE scale that was described in Figure 6-11 also relates well to oxygen uptake and HR.[24] The training zone for RPE and how it relates to oxygen uptake and per cent of HR max reserve is shown in Table 7-3.

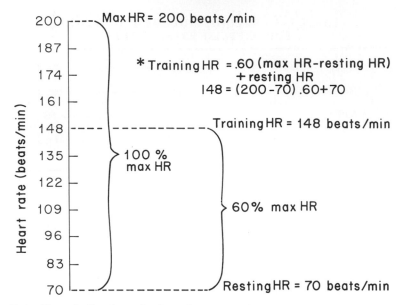

Figure 7–1. Formula for determination of per cent of maximum heart rate reserve. Also shown is an example of the calculation of target heart rate of 60 per cent of maximum. *Karvonen et al.[22] (Reprinted with permission from Pollock, M.L., Wilmore, J.H., and Fox, S.M.: Health and Fitness Through Physical Activity. New York, copyright © John Wiley and Sons, 1978.)

More precisely, 60 per cent of the HR max reserve corresponds to an RPE of 12 to 13 and 90 per cent corresponds to a rating of 16.[26,31]

There are three primary methods for calculating target HR. Method I represents the per cent of the maximum HR calculated from zero to peak HR (per cent HR max). Method II represents the per cent difference between resting and maximum HR added to the resting HR. As mentioned earlier, this technique was first described by Karvonen et al.[22] and is called per cent of HR max reserve. See Figure 7–1 for an example of calculating the target HR at 60 per cent of HR max reserve. Method III represents the HR at a specified per cent of maximum METs ($\dot{V}O_2$ max) (per cent of maximum METs).

Method I, per cent of HR max, is easier to use than the per cent of HRmax reserve method. All three techniques are acceptable for use in determining the target HR or training zone or both. Table 7–4 compares the training HRs calculated according to these three most used methods.[17] Data from 10 healthy adults and 10 cardiac patients were used to make these calculations. The table shows that the target HRs for both healthy adults and cardiac patients, calculated at 70 and 85 per cent of HR max reserve and maximum METs achieved on the GXT, are in close agreement. The target HR of healthy adults calculated by the per cent of HR max method was approximately 25 and 13 beats/min lower than that calculated by the other two methods at 70 and 85 per cent of maximum, respectively. For cardiac patients, the difference in HR is approximately 20 and 11 beats/min, respec-

TABLE 7-4. COMPARISON OF TRAINING HEART RATE CALCULATED
AS A PERCENTAGE OF MAXIMUM HEART RATE, PERCENTAGE OF
MAXIMUM HEART RATE RESERVE, AND HEART RATE AT
A PERCENTAGE OF MAXIMUM METs

		METHODS		
GROUP	INTENSITY (%)	% HR Max	% HR Max Reserve	% Max METs (HR)
Healthy adults[a] (N = 10)	70	130.1 ±7.5	154.0 ±8.6	158.9 ±9.0
	85	158.3 ±9.1	170.2 ±9.6	174.3 ±11.4
Cardiac patients[b] (N = 10)	70	106.9 ±14.8	131.2 ±19.0	126.1 +20.5
	85	129.8 ±18.2	141.8 ±20.3	139.9 ±22.8

[a] Data calculated on men 36.2 years (±3.2), standing resting heart rate, 78.7 beats/min (±12.6); maximum heart rate, 186.2 beats/min (±11.0); and maximum capacity of 11.9 METs (±1.5).

[b] Data calculated on cardiac patients (seven CABG and three MI) nine weeks postevent. Age, 50.8 years (+8.3); standing resting heart rate, 81.0 beats/min (±17.7); maximum heart rate, 152.7 beats/min (±21.5); and maximum capacity of 9.8 METs (±2.4).

(Reprinted with permission from Pollock, M.L., Foster, C., and Ward, A.: Exercise prescription for rehabilitation of the cardiac patient. In Pollock, M.L., and Schmidt, D.H., editors: Heart Disease and Rehabilitation. New York, copyright © John Wiley and Sons, 1979, pp. 413-445.)

tively. The difference between these methods has been discussed by Davis and Convertino[21] (young, healthy adults) and Kaufmann and Kasch (unpublished data [middle-aged adults] 1975, San Diego State University), who showed that per cent of HRmax reserve correlated closely with actual METs determined on a GXT. Our experience with a few coronary artery bypass surgery patients with high resting HRs has shown a target HR lower than resting HR when calculated by the per cent HR max method. The matter of simplicity is important, however, and the technique could be brought more in line with the other two methods by increasing the training HR by approximately 10 per cent.

Because of the large disparity between the two HR techniques in determining training intensity, both methods were compared using the RPE scale.[26]. Three diverse groups were tested: young, healthy adults ($\bar{x} = 28$ years), $n = 51$; healthy adults older than 40 years of age ($\bar{x} = 54$ years), $n = 42$; and cardiac patients ($\bar{x} = 54$ years), $n = 48$. Figure 7-2 plots the HR results calculated by the per cent of HR max and per cent of HR max reserve techniques at 60, 70, and 85 per cent of maximum versus the RPE rating. Method II, per cent of HR max reserve, clearly shows a more consistent pattern among groups and makes more sense relative to the RPE scale. Because most patients in an inpatient exercise setting rate ambulatory training at 11 to 12 and outpatients rate it at 12 to 13 on the RPE scale, the per cent of HR max method seems too conservative.[32-34]

How and when should HR be counted? Resting HR is less variable in

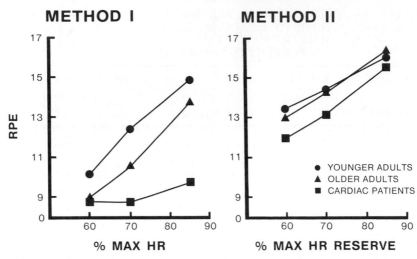

Figure 7–2. Relationship between heart rate (HR) and perceived exertion (RPE) with two methods of calculating training heart rate.[26] Per cent max HR (method I) was calculated on the basis of the percentage of the difference between zero and peak HR attained. Per cent HRmax reserve (method II) was calculated according to Karvonen et al.[22] and represents the per cent difference between the resting and maximal HR added to the resting HR. (Reprinted with permission from Pollock, M.L., Foster, C., Rod, J.L., and Wible, G.: Comparison of methods for determining exercise training intensity for cardiac patients and healthy adults. *In* Kellerman, editor: Comprehensive Cardiac Rehabilitation. Basel, S. Karger, 1982, pp. 129–133.)

the morning before rising.[35] Change in posture from lying to standing, smoking, eating, emotional stress, and so on will significantly increase resting and submaximal HR.[35] Maximal HR is not affected by these factors.[35] In order to estimate the target HR, resting HR should be counted for 30 seconds while the subject is in a comfortable, quiet, standing position. Although care should be taken in getting a reliable measure, minor fluctuations in resting heart rate (± 5 beats/min) have little effect on the calculated training HR. Because resting HR decreases with training, it should be periodically re-evaluated. Taking the average HR on two or three mornings is the best way to estimate resting HR.

Beta-adrenergic–blocking drugs significantly lower both resting and maximal HR.[36,37] Thus, when medications are changed, both resting and maximal HR should be re-evaluated under the same conditions in which the participant will be exercising.

Estimating exercise HR during training is usually accomplished by counting the pulse rate immediately after exercise is stopped by means of the palpation technique.[38,39] This is performed by placing the tips of the first two fingers lightly on the carotid artery, or on the radial artery, or by placing the heel of the hand over the left side of the chest (at the apex of the heart) and by counting the pulsations.[5] If the carotid artery is used, caution must be taken not to apply too much pressure. Excessive pressure on the carotid artery may cause the HR to slow down by reflex action.[40] Pulsations at the apex of the heart are normally felt only after vigorous exercise. Participants should experiment to see which technique is best for them. A few persons will not be able to count the pulse at any site and will need to revert to the use of a stethoscope.

White[41] found that counting the pulse by the carotid artery technique significantly reduced the immediate postexercise HR. He questioned its use for estimating training intensity. These results have not been replicated in subsequent investigations.[42-44] Thus, the use of the immediate postexercise carotid pulse for estimating training HR has been shown to be valid for both cardiac patients and healthy subjects. Its use with those few patients who are hypersensitive to the baroreceptor response is not recommended.

Heart rate begins to decelerate soon after cessation of exercise (usually after only 15 seconds); therefore, the count should begin as soon as possible.[38,45] It is recommended that one count the pulse for 10 seconds and complete it within 15 seconds after cessation of exercise. Only 2 to 4 seconds are needed to position the hand or fingers properly and to feel the heartbeat rhythm. Thus, by counting beats per 10 seconds, it is possible to complete the count within 15 seconds and to avoid errors resulting from the deceleration of the heartbeat.[39]

A wrist watch, wall clock, or stopwatch can be used for determining HR; however, a stopwatch will be the most accurate. The stopwatch facilitates starting the count more quickly as well as enhances general counting accuracy. After establishing the HR rhythm, the count can start on a full beat, with the first count being zero (it can start this way only when a stopwatch is being used). If the count does not end on an even beat, then one half a beat is added to the last fall count. This counting detail is important with the 10-second technique because each one-beat error in counting results in a 6 beat/min error.

Another HR counting procedure that can be used satisfactorily is to count beats per 15 seconds. This method has some advantages: Counting the heart rate over a longer time span can reduce the errors in counting, and multiplying the counted value by four to get beats per minute is easier for the beginners. The disadvantage is the possible 5 to 10 per cent error that may occur with the added counting time.[38,45]

Each of the techniques requires some experimentation and practice to ensure proficiency. Table 7–5 is a conversion chart for transforming raw HR data to beats per minute.

USE OF RATING OF PERCEIVED EXERTION AS AN ADJUNCT TO HEART RATE IN MONITORING TRAINING

The validity and use of the RPE scale for GXT were described in Chapter 6. The use of the scale is an important adjunct to HR for monitoring intensity of training.[25,26] As mentioned in Chapter 6, RPE correlates highly with HR, pulmonary ventilation, and lactic acid build-up.[24] Thus, like

TABLE 7-5. CONVERSION CHART FOR TRANSFORMING HEART RATE COUNTED FOR 10 or 15 SECONDS TO BEATS/MIN

HEART RATE

Beats/10 Sec	Beats/Min	Beats/15 Sec	Beats/Min
15	90	23	92
16	96	24	96
17	102	25	100
18	108	26	104
19	114	27	108
20	120	28	112
21	126	29	116
22	132	30	120
23	138	31	124
24	144	32	128
25	150	33	132
26	156	34	136
27	162	35	140
28	168	36	144
29	174	37	148
30	180	38	152
31	186	39	156
32	192	40	160
33	198	41	164
34	204	42	168
		43	172
		44	176
		45	180
		46	184
		47	188
		48	192
		49	196
		50	200
		51	204

Reprinted with permission from Pollock, M.L., Wilmore, J.H., and Fox, S.M.: Health and Fitness Through Physical Activity. New York, copyright © John Wiley and Sons, 1978.

HR, RPE will increase at standard work loads under hot environmental conditions or when going uphill and will decrease under cooler climatic conditions or when going downhill. It also decreases in proportion to HR when adaptation to training occurs.

For participants who do not have heart disease, the use of HR for monitoring training intensity may become laborious and unnecessary. When a training program is initiated, the use of both HR and RPE is recommended. The use of HR will illustrate to the participants where they are relative to the training zone. Knowledge of both HR and RPE will allow the exerciser to develop a more precise individual relationship between the two indicators. Once this individual relationship is determined, a participant can usually estimate training HR rather accurately by knowing RPE.[46] The obvious advantage of RPE at this stage of training is that training intensity can be accurately and continuously monitored throughout the total session without stopping. Knowledge of RPE informs the exercise leader of how the participant is adjusting to the exercise program and when further progression in training should occur.

Because RPE is a good general indicator of fatigue, it can be used to estimate the intensity of non–steady-state training sessions. This would include many of the game type of activities listed in Table 7–6. For example, the kilocalorie per minute expenditure for racquetball is listed at 10 to 15 (8 to 12 METs). How would a participant determine what value to use? We recommend that for a moderate, a moderate-to-hard, and a very hard workout, the RPEs of 12 to 13, 14 to 15, and 16 to 17, respectively, be used to estimate the severity of a training session. In this case, 12 to 13 would represent 10 Kcal/min, 14 to 15 would represent 12.5 Kcal/min, and 16 to 17 would represent 15 Kcal/min. The estimation of severity of training may vary depending on the participant's level of fitness.

MODE OF ACTIVITY

Many types of activities can provide adequate stimulation for improving cardiorespiratory function. Chapter 3 emphasized that the total energy cost of a program is important and that as long as various activities are of sufficient intensity and duration, the training effect will occur. In addition, activities of similar energy requirements will provide similar training effects.[19,20,47,48] In choosing the proper mode of training, the participant should be familiar with the variety of activities that are available. Table 7–6 categorizes activities by their kilocalorie cost (METs). An activity will vary in intensity depending on the enthusiasm and skill level of the participant as well as on the type of activity. For example, tennis singles would be significantly more demanding than doubles; thus, a range of energy costs is listed in the table.

Generally, an activity that expends fewer than 5 Kcal/min ($\sim$ 3.5 METs) is classified as "low" intensity and is not recommended for use in exercise regimens that are designed to develop cardiorespiratory fitness and reduce body weight. An exception to this would be for a person with a functional capacity below 6 METs. These persons can often improve their functional capacity with low-intensity work but should be encouraged to increase the duration of effort. Except for persons of extremely high or low functional capacities, activities that expend 5 to 10 Kcal/min (4 to 8 METs) are considered of moderate intensity; activities from 10 to 14 Kcal/min (8 to 12 METs), moderate-to-high intensity; and activities greater than 14 Kcal/min (12 METs), high intensity. These classifications are based upon exercising continuously for up to 60 minutes and for participants of average fitness.

When choosing the proper activity, the participant should take into account level of fitness, health status, physical activity interests, availability of equipment and facilities, geographical location, and climate.[5,49] The deconditioned adult should be involved initially in several weeks or months

TABLE 7-6. ENERGY COST OF VARIOUS ACTIVITIES[a]

ACTIVITY	KILOCALORIES[b] (Kcal/min)	METs[c]	OXYGEN UPTAKE (ml/kg·min^{-1})
Archery	3.7–5	3–4	10.5–14
Backpacking	6–13.5	5–11	17.5–38.5
Badminton	5–11	4–9	14–31.5
Basketball			
Nongame	3.7–11	3–9	10.5–31.5
Game	8.5–15	7–12	24.5–42
Bed exercise (arm movement, supine or sitting)	1.1–2.5	1–2	3.5–7
Bench stepping (see Table 6–5)			
Bicycling			
Recreation/transportation	3.7–10	3–8	10.5–28
Stationary (see Table 6–4)			
Bowling	2.5–5	2–4	7–14
Canoeing (rowing and kayaking)	3.7–10	3–8	10.5–28
Calisthenics	3.7–10	3–8	10.5–28
Dancing			
Social and square	3.7–8.5	3–7	10.5–24.5
Aerobic	7.5–11	6–9	21–31.5
Fencing	7.5–12	6–10	21–35
Fishing			
Bank, boat, or ice	2.5–5	2–4	7–14
Stream, wading	6–7.5	5–6	17.5–21
Football (touch)	7.5–12	6–10	21–35
Golf			
Using power cart	2.5–3.7	2–3	7–10.5
Walking, carrying bag, or pulling cart	5–8.5	4–7	14–24.5
Handball	10–15	8–12	28–42
Hiking (cross-country)	3.7–8.5	3–7	10.5–24.5
Horseback riding	3.7–10	3–8	10.5–28
Horseshoe pitching	2.5–3.7	2–3	7–10.5
Hunting, walking			
Small game	3.7–8.5	3–7	10.5–24.5
Big game	3.7–17	3–14	10.5–49
Jogging (see Table 7–7)			
Mountain climbing	6–12	5–10	17.5–35
Paddleball/racquet	10–15	8–12	28–42
Rope skipping	10–14	8–12	28–42
Sailing	2.5–6	2–5	7–17.5
Scuba diving	6–12	5–10	17.5–35
Shuffleboard	2.5–3.7	2–3	7–10.5
Skating (ice or roller)	6–10	5–8	17.5–28

TABLE 7-6. ENERGY COST OF VARIOUS ACTIVITIES[a] *(Continued)*

ACTIVITY	KILOCALORIES[b] (Kcal/min)	METs[c]	OXYGEN UPTAKE (ml/kg·min^{-1})
Skiing (snow)			
Downhill	6–10	5–8	17.5–28
Cross-country	7.5–15	6–12	21–42
Skiing (water)	6–8.5	5–7	17.5–24.5
Snow shoeing	8.5–17	7–14	24.5–49
Squash	10–15	8–12	28–42
Soccer	6–15	5–12	17.5–42
Softball	3.7–7.5	3–6	10.5–21
Stair-climbing	5–10	4–8	14–28
Swimming	5–10	4–8	14–28
Table tennis	3.7–6	3–5	10.5–17.5
Tennis	5–11	4–9	14–31.5
Volleyball	3.7–7.5	3–6	10.5–21
Walking (see Table 7–7)			
Weight training			
Circuit	10	8.2	28

[a] Energy cost values based on an individual of 154 pounds of body weight (70 kg).

[b] Kcal: a unit of measure based upon heat production. One Kcal equals approximately 200 ml of oxygen consumed.

[c] MET: basal oxygen requirement of the body sitting quietly. One MET equals 3.5 ml/kg·min^{-1} of oxygen consumed.

(Modified with permission from Pollock, M.L., Wilmore, J.H., and Fox, S.M.: Health and Fitness Through Physical Activity. New York, copyright © John Wiley and Sons, 1978.)

of moderate activity that does not require competition or extreme starting and stopping movements.[49] Under the latter conditions, many participants tend to overdo it and become unduly stiff and sore, fatigued, or injured. Since the joints and muscular system are not adequately developed in a beginner to handle such demands, the participant is vulnerable to injury. The need to get in shape to play games is true in most cases. Persons whose screening tests have indicated cardiovascular problems should avoid highly competitive activities. It is important not to exceed the safe limit of exercise. The starter programs outlined later in the chapter are recommended for beginners. (For more specific information concerning cardiac rehabilitation, see Chapter 8.)

Participation in a variety of activities is recommended and can be accomplished by interchanging some of the various activities listed in Table 7–6. Choosing different activities may keep a participant interested in endurance exercise over a long-term period. For example, one might jog 30 minutes on Monday and Thursday and play handball or basketball on Tuesday and Friday. The important factor is for the person to participate in these activities frequently and with sufficient intensity and duration.[15]

Although this discussion emphasized the variety of activities available for developing and maintaining cardiorespiratory endurance, this type of activity is only part of a total, well-rounded program.[5,49] Endurance activities are of paramount importance, but adequate flexibility and muscular strength and endurance add to a balanced physical fitness program.[1,5,49]

PROGRAMS FOR CARDIORESPIRATORY FITNESS AND WEIGHT CONTROL

Endurance exercises develop cardiorespiratory fitness and help individuals to reduce their body weight and fat.[15] Endurance exercises require a sustained effort, such as in jogging, walking, bicycling, swimming, and vigorous game types of activities.

EXERCISE PRESCRIPTION FOR CARDIORESPIRATORY ENDURANCE AND WEIGHT CONTROL

As mentioned earlier, in order to prescribe exercise properly, it is necessary to know something about the person's health status and physical fitness level. After undergoing the physical fitness examination, a participant may be classified into one of eight categories of cardiorespiratory fitness. Table 6–3 shows the fitness classification scores achieved on various tests. In order to be classified at the good level of cardiorespiratory fitness, a person should have a functional capacity of approximately 40 to 45 ml/ kg · min^{-1} of oxygen uptake (12 to 13 METs). Therefore, knowing the initial level of cardiorespiratory fitness will help guide the participant into the correct program.

The exercise prescription usually has three stages of progression: starter, slow progression, and maintenance (see Fig. 7–3). The initial stage of training is classified as a starter program. In this phase, the exercise intensity is low and includes a lot of stretching and light calisthenics followed by aerobic exercise of low-to-moderate intensity. The purpose at this stage of the program is to introduce one to exercise at a low level and to allow time for proper adaptation to the intitial weeks of training. If this phase is introduced correctly, the participant will experience a minimum of muscle soreness and can avoid debilitating injuries or discomfort of the knee, shin, ankle, or foot. The latter injuries are common in the initial stages of a jogging program but can be avoided if the participant takes some preliminary precautions, e.g., a good starter program, use of good training shoes, and proper warm-up and conditioning of the legs. Avoiding sharp turns and extremely hard running surfaces is also an important safeguard (see Chapter 10 for more detail).

The duration of the starter program is usually from 2 to 6 weeks but is dependent on the adaptation of the participant to the program. For

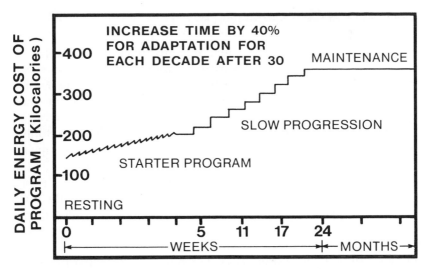

Figure .Schematic illustration for average participants in regard to progression in an aerobic training program.

Figure 7–3. Schematic illustration for average participants of a normal progression in an aerobic training program. (Modified with permission from Pollock, M.L., Wilmore, J.H., and Fox, S.M.: Health and Fitness Through Physical Activity. New York, copyright © John Wiley and Sons, 1978.)

example, a person who is classified at a poor or fair fitness level may spend as many as 4 to 6 weeks in a starter program, but for a participant scoring in the good or excellent categories, a starter program may not be necessary.

The slow progression stage of training differs from the starter phase in that the participant progresses at a more rapid rate. During this stage, the duration and intensity are increased rather consistently every 1 to 3 weeks. How well an individual adapts to the present level of training dictates the frequency and magnitude of progression. As a general rule, the older the participant and the lower the initial fitness level, the longer one takes to adapt and progress in a training regimen. It is estimated that the adaptation to the training load takes approximately 40 per cent longer for each decade in life after age 30.[5] That is, if the progression in distance run is every 2 weeks for men of 30 to 39 years, then the interval may be 3 weeks for those of 40 to 49 years and 4 weeks for those who are 50 to 59 years old.

The maintenance stage of prescription usually occurs after 6 months to 1 year of training.[5,12] At this stage, the participant has reached a satisfactory level of cardiorespiratory fitness and may be no longer interested in increasing the training load. At this point, further improvement is usually minimal, but continuing the same workout schedule (the number of miles or minutes trained per week) enables one to maintain fitness.

GENERAL GUIDELINES FOR GETTING STARTED

In designing an exercise regimen, one must select activities that can be performed on a regular basis. Generally, game types of activities are not recommended in the early stages of training. Before becoming involved in game types of activities in which running occurs, fast walking or walk-jog programs are recommended.

Table 7–6 lists the energy cost of a variety of activities commonly used in recreation and endurance fitness programs. The activities are quantified in terms of kilocalories per minute, METs, and oxygen uptake. As mentioned earlier, these values indicate the relative intensity of the effort. To achieve the total effect of the programs, one must determine the intensity level and multiply this by the total number of minutes of participation. Because games are not played continuously with an even amount of effort, some approximation will have to be made to estimate the intensity level for game types of activities. Intensity is dependent on how hard the game is played. As mentioned earlier, the use of the RPE scale will help in determining intensity. If the intensity is in doubt, use the average value listed in Table 7–6. For example, if handball is played for 60 minutes, then the intensity in kilocalories (12.5 Kcal/min) would be multiplied by the minutes played (60) to get the total kilocaloric expenditure (750). The important point here is that the participant counts only the time that was used in participation. Rest breaks and standing around do not count. For sports such as handball or racquetball, tennis singles, and so on, cutting the total time by one half usually approximates the proper kilocaloric expenditure. Therefore, in the preceding example, 60 minutes of handball would be calculated at 12.5 Kcal X 30 minutes = 375 Kcal.

The energy cost of running and walking is listed in Table 7–7. An endurance training program can be designed from Table 7–7, but because of the difficulty of knowing the proper pace or sequence of progression, several programs are outlined in Tables 7–9 to 7–19. The programs include walking and running routines and are designed relative to various levels of fitness.

Although walking and running can be done in a variety of settings—e.g. running tracks, roads, parks, and so on—the course should be a measured distance. This can be accomplished by the use of an odometer from an automobile or bicycle or by the use of a measured track. Training on an oval track can get boring over a long period of time but, if available, is a good way of getting started. Tracks generally have a smooth running surface and are of a known distance.

Table 7–8 will help in determining pace for walking and running programs. Speeds range from a moderate walk (2.9 mph) to a fast run (12.5 mph). To aid in pacing, reference points of 110 or 440 yards are helpful. If a stopwatch or wristwatch with a 60-second sweep hand is carried the pace can be kept very accurately during the entire training program. Monitoring of the program by pace, HR response, and RPE will help as a guide to proper initiation and progression of the training regimen.

TABLE 7-7. ENERGY COST OF WALKING AND RUNNING[a]

ACTIVITY	SPEED Mph	Min/Mile (min:sec)	GRADE (%)	KILOCALORIES[b] (Kcal/min)	METs[c]	OXYGEN COST (ml/kg·min^{-1})
Walking	2.0	30:00	0	2.5	2.0	7
	2.5	24:00	0	3.0	2.5	8.7
	3.0	20:00	0	3.7	3.0	10.5
	3.0	20:00	5	6.0	5.0	17.5
	3.0	20:00	10	8.5	7.0	24.5
	3.0	20:00	15	11.0	9.0	31.5
	3.5	17:08	0	4.2	3.5	12.3
	3.5	17:08	5	7.5	5.9	21
	3.5	17:08	10	10.0	8.3	29
	3.5	17:08	15	13.0	10.7	37.5
	3.75	16:00	0	4.9	4.0	14
	4.0	15:00	0	5.5	4.6	16.1
	4.0	15:00	5	9.0	7.3	25.6
	4.0	15:00	10	12.0	10.0	35
	4.0	15:00	15	15.6	12.8	44.8
	4.5	13:20	0	7.0	5.7	20
	5.0	12:00	0	8.3	6.9	24
Running	5.5	10:55	0	10.1	8.3	29
	6.0	10:00	0	12.0	10.0	35
	7.0	8:35	0	14.0	11.5	40.3
	8.0	7:30	0	15.6	12.8	44.8
	9.0	6:40	0	17.5	14.2	49.7
	10.0	6:00	0	19.6	16.0	56
	11.0	5:30	0	21.7	17.7	62
	12.0	5:00	0	24.5	20.0	70

[a] Energy cost values based on an individual of 154 pounds of body weight (70 kg).

[b] Kilocalorie: a unit of measure based upon heat production. One kilocalorie equals 200 ml of oxygen consumed.

[c] MET: basal oxygen requirement of the body sitting quietly. One MET equals 3.5 ml/kg· min^{-1} of oxygen consumed.

(Reprinted with permission from Pollock, M.L., Wilmore, J.H., and Fox, S.M.: Health and Fitness Through Physical Activity. New York, copyright © John Wiley and Sons, 1978.)

Generally, persons scoring in fitness categories 1 and 2 should begin their endurance training by walking. The walk should be at a comfortable but brisk pace. The initial speed may range from 3.0 to 4.0 mph. Distance (or time) will be approximately 1½ to 2 miles (30 to 40 minutes). The reason behind this combination of walking speed and distance is to get the participant started at a comfortable pace and at the same time to keep the distance long enough so that an endurance training effect can begin to occur.

Even though the kilocaloric cost of this regimen is low (150 to 200 Kcal), it will allow time for adaptation of most bodily systems. Do not be concerned about not working hard enough. Time, with proper progression and adaptation, will eventually lead to the higher, more demanding levels of training. Table 7–9 outlines two examples of 6-week starter programs for walking, with Program A being recommended for persons in fitness category 1 and Program B for persons in fitness category 2. See Table 6–3 for guidelines on placement into the proper fitness category.

TABLE 7–8. PACING CHART FOR WALKING AND RUNNING PROGRAM CONDUCTED ON TRACK MEASURED IN 110-YARD INCREMENTS

110 Yd (sec)	440 Yd (min:sec)	Mph	110 Yd (sec)	440 Yd (min:sec)	Mph	110 Yd (sec)	440 Yd (min:sec)	Mph
	PACE			PACE			PACE	
18	1:12	12.5	38	2:32	5.9	58	3:52	3.9
19	1:16	11.8	39	2:36	5.8	59	3:56	3.8
20	1:20	11.2	40	2:40	5.6	60	4:00	3.7
21	1:24	10.7	41	2:44	5.5	61	4:04	3.7
22	1:28	10.2	42	2:48	5.4	62	4:08	3.6
23	1:32	9.8	43	2:52	5.2	63	4:12	3.6
24	1:36	9.4	44	2:56	5.1	64	4:16	3.5
25	1:40	9.0	45	3:00	5.0	65	4:20	3.5
26	1:44	8.6	46	3:04	4.9	66	4:24	3.4
27	1:48	8.3	47	3:08	4.8	67	4:28	3.4
28	1:52	8.0	48	3:12	4.7	68	4:32	3.3
29	1:56	7.7	49	3:16	4.6	69	4:36	3.3
30	2:00	7.5	50	3:20	4.5	70	4:40	3.2
31	2:04	7.3	51	3:24	4.4	71	4:44	3.2
32	2:08	7.0	52	3:28	4.3	72	4:48	3.1
33	2:12	6.8	53	3:32	4.2	73	4:52	3.1
34	2:16	6.6	54	3:36	4.2	74	4:56	3.0
35	2:20	6.4	55	3:40	4.1	75	5:00	3.0
36	2:24	6.2	56	3:44	4.0	76	5:04	2.9
37	2:28	6.1	57	3:48	3.9	77	5:08	2.9

Reprinted with permission from Pollock, M.L., Wilmore, J.H., and Fox, S.M.: Health and Fitness Through Physical Activity. New York, copyright © John Wiley and Sons, 1978.

TABLE 7–9. SIX-WEEK STARTER PROGRAMS FOR PERSONS IN FITNESS CATEGORIES 1 AND 2[a]

PROGRAM	WEEK	PACE (mph)	DISTANCE (miles)	TIME (min:sec)	KILOCALORIES
A	1	3.0	1.5	36:00	133
	2	3.5	1.5	25:42	107
	3	3.5	2.0	34:16	143
	4	3.5	2.0	34:16	143
	5	3.5	2.5	42:50	179
	6	3.5	2.5	42:50	179
B	1	3.5	2.0	34:16	143
	2	3.5	2.0	34:16	143
	3	4.0	2.0	30:00	165
	4	4.0	2.0	30:00	165
	5	4.0	2.5	37:50	206
	6	4.0	2.5	37:50	206

[a] Programs based upon level walking at sea level and in an average climatic condition (temperature and humidity).

(Reprinted with permission from Pollock, M.L., Wilmore, J.H., and Fox, S.M.: Health and Fitness Through Physical Activity. New York, copyright © John Wiley and Sons, 1978.)

If one of the two examples of starter programs listed in Table 7–9 is too easy or difficult, then make an on-the-spot change in the program. Remember, the exercise prescription should be individualized. A satisfactory modification can usually be made by changing the speed or distance slightly (Tables 7–7 and 7–8). Walking programs for cardiac patients are shown in Chapter 8.

The programs listed here are based upon running or walking on a relatively flat surface, at sea level, and in an average climatic condition (temperature and humidity). Further program modifications will have to be taken into account when persons are exercising in moderate-to-extreme environmental conditions. Chapter 9 will discuss these modifications in more detail. Running or walking hills will also dramatically alter training pace. The use of the RPE scale will help a participant in adjusting to the proper training speed.

Once the participant has completed the 6-week starter program, then the walking program listed in Tables 7–13 and 7–14 or the combination walk-jog program outlined in Table 7–10 can be initiated. The starter program outlined in Table 7–10 is recommended for persons scoring in fitness category 3. Tables 7–11 and 7–12 show suggested starter programs for persons scoring in fitness categories 4 and 5. Normally, participants scoring in fitness categories above 50 ml/kg · min^{-1} of oxygen uptake (14 METs) are considered in excellent cardiorespiratory fitness and do not require a special starter program. Persons scoring in the excellent categories of fitness who have not been exercising on a regular basis should begin with the program outlined in Table 7–19.

MAINTENANCE PROGRAMS FOR CARDIORESPIRATORY FITNESS AND WEIGHT CONTROL

Upon completion of the 6-week starter and 20-week training programs outlined in Tables 7–9 to 7–19, a substantial improvement in fitness should have been attained. To maintain fitness, a specific program should be designed that will be similar in caloric cost to the initial program and that will also satisfy the needs of the participant over a long time span. For many, walking and jogging may become boring, and thus variety should be introduced into their programs. Participation in enjoyable activities is more likely to be continued.

The instructor should check over the list of activities in Table 7–6 to see which ones best meet the interests of the participants and can still give the necessary kilocalorie consumption. Fitness is not stored but must be practiced continually.[12,15] The guidelines for frequency, intensity, and duration of training do not change and should be taken into consideration when selecting activities for participation.

If goals have not been met or if further development is required, then added kilocaloric expenditure is needed. For example, since ideal (desired)

TABLE 7-10. SIX-WEEK STARTER PROGRAM FOR PERSONS IN FITNESS CATEGORY 3[a]

PROGRAM	WEEK	WALK			RUN			REPETITIONS				
		Pace (mph)	Distance (yd)	Time (sec)	Pace (mph)	Distance (yd)	Time (min:sec)	Walk	Run	Time (min:sec)	Kilocalories	Total Miles
A	1	3.75	110	60	5.5	110	:41	16	16	26:56	188.8	2.0
	2	3.75	110	60	5.5	110	:41	16	16	26:56	188.8	2.0
	3	3.75	110	60	5.5	220	1:22	11	11	26:02	205.7	2.0
	4	3.75	110	60	5.5	220	1:22	11	11	26:02	205.7	2.0
	5	3.75	110	60	5.5	330	2:03	8	8	24:24	204.8	2.0
	6	3.75	110	60	5.5	330	2:03	8	8	24:24	204.8	2.0
B	1	3.75	110	60	6.4	110	:35	16	16	25:20	197.8	2.0
	2	3.75	110	60	6.4	110	:35	16	16	25:20	197.8	2.0
	3	3.75	110	60	6.4	220	1:10	11	11	23:50	218.0	2.0
	4	3.75	110	60	6.4	220	1:10	12	12	26:00	238.0	2.25
	5	3.75	110	60	6.4	330	1:45	9	9	24:45	245.7	2.25
	6	3.75	110	60	6.4	330	1:45	9	9	24:45	245.7	2.25

[a] Programs based upon level walking at sea level and in an average climatic condition (temperature and humidity).
(Reprinted with permission from Pollock, M.L., Wilmore, J.H., and Fox, S.M.: Health and Fitness Through Physical Activity. New York, copyright © John Wiley and Sons, 1978.)

TABLE 7–11. SIX-WEEK STARTER PROGRAM FOR PERSONS IN FITNESS CATEGORY 4[a]

PROGRAM	WEEK	WALK			RUN			REPETITIONS		Time (min:sec)	Kilocalories	Total Miles
		Pace (mph)	Distance (yd)	Time (sec)	Pace (mph)	Distance (yd)	Time (min:sec)	Walk	Run			
A	1	3.75	110	60	6.8	220	1:06	11	11	23:06	218.5	2.0
	2	3.75	110	60	6.8	220	1:06	11	11	23:06	218.5	2.0
	3	3.75	110	60	6.8	330	1:39	8	8	22:12	218.7	2.0
	4	3.75	110	60	6.8	330	1:39	9	9	23:51	246.1	2.25
	5	3.75	110	60	6.8	440	2:12	8	8	23:24	248.6	2.25
	6	3.75	110	60	6.8	440	2:12	8	8	25:36	278.6	2.25
B	1	3.75	110	60	7.5	220	1:00	12	12	24:00	236.4	2.25
	2	3.75	110	60	7.5	220	1:00	12	12	24:00	236.4	2.25
	3	3.75	110	60	7.5	330	1:30	9	9	22:30	243.9	2.25
	4	3.75	110	60	7.5	330	1:30	10	10	25:00	271.0	2.25
	5	3.75	110	60	7.5	440	2:00	8	8	24:00	276.0	2.25
	6	3.75	110	60	7.5	440	2:00	8	8	24:00	276.0	2.25

[a]Programs based upon level walking at sea level and in an average climatic condition (temperature and humidity).
(Reprinted with permission from Pollock, M.L., Wilmore, J.H., and Fox, S.M.: Health and Fitness Through Physical Activity. New York, copyright © John Wiley and Sons, 1978.)

TABLE 7-12. SIX-WEEK STARTER PROGRAM FOR PERSONS IN FITNESS CATEGORY 5[a]

| PROGRAM | WEEK | WALK | | | RUN | | | REPETITIONS | | Time (min:sec) | Kilocalories | Total Miles |
		Pace (mph)	Distance (yd)	Time (sec)	Pace (mph)	Distance (yd)	Time (min:sec)	Walk	Run			
A	1	3.75	110	60	7.5	330	1:30	9	9	22:30	243.9	2.25
	2	3.75	110	60	7.5	330	1:30	9	9	22:30	243.9	2.25
	3	3.75	110	60	7.5	440	2:00	8	8	24:00	276.0	2.5
	4	3.75	110	60	7.5	550	2:30	7	7	24:30	293.3	2.63
	5	3.75	110	60	7.5	660	3:00	6	6	24:00	295.8	2.65
	6	3.75	110	60	7.5	880	4:00	5	5	25:00	320.5	2.81
B	1	3.75	110	60	8.0	330	1:24	9	9	21:36	240.7	2.25
	2	3.75	110	60	8.0	330	1:24	9	9	21:36	240.7	2.25
	3	3.75	110	60	8.0	440	1:52	8	8	22:56	272.1	2.5
	4	3.75	110	60	8.0	550	2:20	7	7	23:20	289.1	2.63
	5	3.75	110	60	8.0	660	2:48	6	6	22:48	291.5	2.63
	6	3.75	110	60	8.0	880	3:16	6	6	24:37	330.5	3.3

[a]Programs based upon level walking at sea level and in an average climatic condition (temperature and humidity).
(Reprinted with permission from Pollock, M.L., Wilmore, J.H., and Fox, S.M.: Health and Fitness Through Physical Activity. New York, copyright © John Wiley and Sons, 1978.)

TABLE 7–13.   TWENTY-WEEK WALKING PROGRAM
FOR FITNESS CATEGORY 1[a]

WEEK	PACE (mph)	DISTANCE (miles)	TIME (min:sec)	KILOCALORIES
1, 2	3.75	2.5	40:00	196
3–5	3.75	2.75	44:00	215.6
6–8	4.0	2.75	41:15	226.9
9–12	4.0	3.0	45:00	247.5
13–16	4.25	3.0	42.21	262.0
17–20	4.25	3.25	45:53	285.4

[a]Programs based upon level walking at sea level and in an average climatic condition (temperature and humidity.)

(Reprinted with permission from Pollock, M.L., Wilmore, J.H., and Fox, S.M.: Health and Fitness Through Physical Activity. New York, copyright © John Wiley and Sons, 1978.)

weight may not be attained in a 20-week program, the program design should increase kilocaloric output. Usually, added frequency of training of up to 5 or 6 days per week will greatly increase the total energy expenditure. The addition of one extra 400-Kcal workout per week to the training regimen should remove 1 pound of fat every 9 weeks. If this is matched by a similar reduction in food intake, it will amount to a reduction of 12 pounds in a year.

PROGRAMS FOR MUSCULAR STRENGTH AND ENDURANCE AND FOR FLEXIBILITY

As described in Chapter 5, muscular strength and endurance are developed by using the overload principle, i.e., by applying more tension on the muscle than is normally used.[30,50,51] Muscular strength is best developed by using heavy weights (maximum or nearly maximum tension applied) with few repetitions, and muscular endurance is promoted by using lighter loads, along with a greater number of repetitions.[52] To some extent, both strength and endurance can be developed under each condition, but each system favors a more specific type of development.[50,51]

Muscular strength and endurance can be developed by means of isometric (static), isotonic (going through the full range of motion), or isokinetic exercise (see Chapter 5 for further explanation). Although each type of training has its strong and weak points, isotonic and isokinetic exercises are recommended for the development and maintenance of muscular strength and endurance. Exercises should be rhythmical, should follow through the full range of motion, and should not impede normal forced breathing. Lifting heavy weights impedes blood circulation and breathing, increases blood pressure dramatically, and can be potentially dangerous for persons with high blood pressure, coronary heart disease, and other circula-

TABLE 7-14. TWENTY-WEEK WALKING-JOGGING PROGRAM FOR FITNESS CATEGORY 2[a]

WEEK	WALK Pace (mph)	Distance	Time (min:sec)	RUN Pace (mph)	Distance (yd)	Time (min:sec)	REPETITIONS	TOTAL TIME (min:sec)	KILOCALORIES	TOTAL MILES
1, 2	4.0	2.75 mi	41:15				1	41:15	226.9	
3, 4	4.25	2.75 mi	38:50				1	38:50	241.5	
5, 6	4.25	3.0 mi	42:21				1	42:21	262.0	
7, 8	4.5	3.0 mi	40:00				1	40:00	280.0	
9, 10	4.5	3.25 mi	43:20				1	43:20	303.2	
11, 12	4.0	110 yd	1:00	4.75	220	1:35	18	46:26	316.6	3.375
13, 14	4.0	110 yd	1:00	4.75	330	2:22	13	43:49	307.2	3.25
15, 16	4.0	110 yd	1:00	4.75	440	3:10	10/11[b]	44:50	321.4	3.375
17, 18	4.0	110 yd	1:00	5.0	330	2:15	13	42:15	314.3	3.25
19, 20	4.0	110 yd	1:00	5.0	440	3:00	10/11[b]	43:00	328.9	3.375

[a]Programs based upon level walking at sea level and in an average climatic condition (temperature and humidity).
[b]Ten walk, 11 run.
(Reprinted with permission from Pollock, M.L., Wilmore, J.H., and Fox, S.M.: Health and Fitness Through Physical Activity. New York, copyright © John Wiley and Sons, 1978.)

TABLE 7-15. TWENTY-WEEK WALK-JOG, JOGGING PROGRAM FOR FITNESS CATEGORY 3A[a]

WEEK	WALK Pace (mph)	Distance (yd)	Time (sec)	RUN Pace (mph)	Distance (yd:mi)	Time (min:sec)	REPETITIONS	TOTAL TIME (min:sec)	KILOCALORIES	TOTAL MILES
1, 2	3.75	110	60	5.6	440:¼	2:41	8	29:26	259.9	2.5
3, 4	3.75	110	60	5.6	660:	4:01	6	30:06	277.6	2.63
5, 6	3.75	110	60	5.6	880:½	5:22	5	31:47	300.4	2.81
7, 8	3.75	110	60	5.6	1320:¾	8:02	3	30:27	297.2	2.75
					550:	3:20	1			
9, 10	3.75	110	60	5.6	1760:1	10:42	3	35:08	345.7	3.19
11, 12	3.75	110	60	5.6	:1½	13:20	2	34:08	340.6	3.13
					:½	5:22	1			
13, 14	3.75	110	60	5.6	:1½	16:04	2	34:08	340.8	3.13
15, 16	3.75	110	60	5.6	:2	21:24	1	33:08	335.5	3.06
					:1	10:42	1			
17, 18	3.75	110	60	5.6	:2½	26:47	1	33:09	336.0	3.06
					:½	5:22	1			
19, 20				5.6	:3	32:08	1	32:08	331.0	3.00

[a] Programs based upon level walking at sea level and in an average climatic condition (temperature and humidity).
(Reprinted with permission from Pollock, M.L., Wilmore, J.H., and Fox, S.M.: Health and Fitness Through Physical Activity. New York, copyright © John Wiley and Sons, 1978.)

TABLE 7-16. TWENTY-WEEK WALK-JOG, JOGGING PROGRAM FOR FITNESS CATEGORY 3B[a]

WEEK	WALK			RUN			REPETITIONS	TOTAL TIME (min:sec)	KILOCALORIES	TOTAL MILES
	Pace (mph)	Distance (yd)	Time (sec)	Pace (mph)	Distance (yd:mi)	Time (min:sec)				
1, 2	3.75	110	60	6.4	440:¼	2:20	8	26:40	278.2	2.5
3, 4	3.75	110	60	6.4	660:	3:30	6	27:00	298.2	2.63
5, 6	3.75	110	60	6.4	880:½	4:20	5	26:40	301.7	2.81
7, 8	3.75	110	60	6.4	1320:¾	7:00	3	26:55	320.7	2.75
					550:	2:55	1			
9, 10	3.75	110	60	6.4	1760:1	9:24	3	29:12	365.8	3.19
11, 12	3.75	110	60	6.4	:1¼	11:44	2	28:48	360.7	3.13
					:½	4:20	1			
13, 14	3.75	110	60	6.4	:1½	13:44	2	28:28	356.5	3.13
15, 16	3.75	110	60	6.4	:2	18:48	1	29:12	365.8	3.06
					:1	9:24	1			
17, 18	3.75	110	60	6.4	:2½	23:08	1	28:28	356.4	3.06
					:½	4:20	1			
19, 20				6.4	:3	28:12	1	28:12	361.0	3.00

[a] Programs based upon level walking at sea level and in an average climatic condition (temperature and humidity).
(Reprinted with permission from Pollock, M.L., Wilmore, J.H., and Fox, S.M.: Health and Fitness Through Physical Activity. New York, copyright © John Wiley and Sons, 1978.)

TABLE 7-17. TWENTY-WEEK WALK-JOG, JOGGING PROGRAM FOR FITNESS CATEGORY 4A[a]

WEEK	WALK			RUN			REPETITIONS	TOTAL TIME (min:sec)	KILOCALORIES	TOTAL MILES
	Pace (mph)	Distance (yd)	Time (sec)	Pace (mph)	Distance (yd:mi)	Time (min:sec)				
1, 2	3.75	110	60	6.8	660:	3:18	6	25:48	298.7	2.63
3, 4	3.75	110	60	6.8	880:½	4:24	5	27:00	323.7	2.81
5, 6	3.75	110	60	6.8	1320:¾	6:36	3	25:33	321.4	2.75
					550:	2:45	1			
7, 8	3.75	110	60	6.8	1760:1	8:48	3	29:24	373.7	3.19
9, 10	3.75	110	60	6.8	:1¼	11:00	2	28:24	368.8	3.13
					:½	4:24	1			
11, 12	3.75	110	60	6.8	:1½	13:12	2	28:24	368.8	3.13
13, 14	3.75	110	60	6.8	:2	17:36	1	29:36	393.9	3.31
					:1¼	11:00	1			
15, 16	3.75	110	60	6.8	:2½	22:00	1	29:36	393.9	3.31
					:¾	6:36	1			
17, 18	3.75	110	60	6.8	:2¼	28:36	1	28:36	389.0	3.25
19, 20	3.75	110	60	6.8	:2½	30:48	1	30:48	418.9	3.5

[a]Programs based upon level walking at sea level and in an average climatic condition (temperature and humidity).

(Reprinted with permission from Pollock, M.L., Wilmore, J.H., and Fox, S.M.: Health and Fitness Through Physical Activity. New York, copyright © John Wiley and Sons, 1978.)

TABLE 7-18. TWENTY-WEEK WALK-JOG, JOGGING PROGRAM FOR FITNESS CATEGORY 4B[a]

WEEK	WALK			RUN			REPETITIONS	TOTAL TIME (min:sec)	KILOCALORIES	TOTAL MILES
	Pace (mph)	Distance (yd)	Time (sec)	Pace (mph)	Distance (yd:mi)	Time (min:sec)				
1, 2	3.75	110	60	7.5	660:	3:00	6	24:00	295.8	2.63
3, 4	3.75	110	60	7.5	880:½	4:00	5	25:00	320.5	2.81
5, 6	3.75	110	60	7.5	1320:¾	6:00	3	23:00	318.1	2.75
					550:	2:30	1			
7, 8	3.75	110	60	7.5	1760:1	8:00	3	27:00	369.9	3.19
9, 10	3.75	110	60	7.5	:1¼	10:00	2	26:00	365.0	3.13
					:½	4:00	1			
11, 12	3.75	110	60	7.5	:1½	12:00	2	26:00	365.0	3.13
13, 14	3.75	110	60	7.5	:2	16:00	1	27:00	389.7	3.31
					:1¼	10:00	1			
15, 16	3.75	110	60	7.5	:2½	20:00	1	27:00	389.7	3.31
					:¾	6:00	1			
17, 18				7.5	:3¾	26:00	1	26:00	384.8	3.25
19, 20				7.5	:3½	28:00	1	28:00	414.4	3.50

[a]Programs based upon level walking at sea level and in an average climatic condition (temperature and humidity). (Reprinted with permission from Pollock, M.L., Wilmore, J.H., and Fox, S.M.: Health and Fitness Through Physical Activity. New York, copyright © John Wiley and Sons, 1978.)

TABLE 7-19. TWENTY-WEEK WALK-JOG, JOGGING PROGRAM FOR FITNESS CATEGORY 5[a]

WEEK	WALK			RUN			REPETITIONS	TOTAL TIME (min:sec)	KILOCALORIES	TOTAL MILES
	Pace (mph)	Distance (yd)	Time (sec)	Pace (mph)	Distance (yd:mi)	Time (min:sec)				
1, 2	3.75	110	60	7.5	880:½	4:00	6	30:00	384.6	3.38
3, 4	3.75	110	60	7.5	1320:¾	6:00	4	28:00	374.8	3.25
5, 6	3.75	110	60	7.5	1760:1	8:00	3	31:00	429.1	3.69
					880:½	4:00	1			
7, 8	3.75	110	60	7.5	:1½	12:00	2	30:00	424.2	3.63
					:½	4:00	1			
9, 10	3.75	110	60	7.5	:2	16:00	1	30:00	424.2	3.56
					:1½	12:00	1			
11, 12				7.5	:3	24:00	1	24:00	355.0	3.0
13, 14				7.5	:3½	28:00	1	28:00	414.8	3.3
15, 16				7.5	:4	32:00	1	32:00	473.6	4.0
17, 18				7.7	:4	31:10	1	31:10	470.6	4.0
19, 20				8.0	:4	30:00	1	30:00	468.0	4.0

[a] Programs based upon level walking at sea level and in an average climatic condition (temperature and humidity).
(Reprinted with permission from Pollock, M.L., Wilmore J.H., and Fox, S.M.: Health and Fitness Through Physical Activity. New York, copyright © John Wiley and Sons, 1978.)

tory problems.[53] Therefore, the use of light-to-moderate weights is recommended.

It has already been stated that the exercise prescription should include a balanced training program that comprises activities for the development and maintenance of muscular strength and endurance and of flexibility, as well as aerobic training.[1,5,49] It is felt that this type of training program best meets the interests and needs of the adult population.[49] Therefore, as an adjunct to the previously described aerobics program, a series of exercises to develop and maintain muscular strength, endurance, and flexibility for most of the major muscle groups of the body is outlined.

UPPER BODY, TRUNK, AND LOWER BACK STRETCHING EXERCISES*

1. TRUNK ROTATION

Purpose: To stretch muscles in the back, sides, and shoulder girdle.
Starting Position: Stand astride with feet pointed forward; raise arms to shoulder level. May use bar to increase stretch to the deltoid muscle and waist.
Movement: Twist trunk to the right; avoid lifting heels. Repeat 3 to 4 times before twisting to left side.
Repetitions: 10

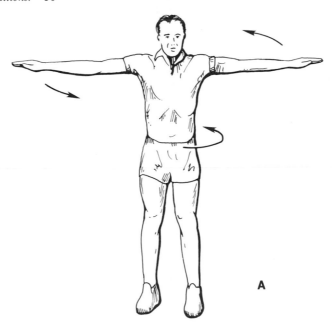

A

2. DOUBLE ARM CIRCLES AND TOE RAISES

Purpose: To stretch muscles of the shoulder girdle and to strengthen muscles of the feet.

*Reprinted with permission from Pollock, M.L., Wilmore, J.H., and Fox, S.M.: Health and Fitness Through Physical Activity. New York, copyright © John Wiley and Sons, 1978.

Starting Position: Stand with feet about 12 inches apart and arms at sides.
Movement: Swing arms upward and around, making large circles. As arms are raised and crossed overhead, rise on toes.
Repetitions: 10 to 15

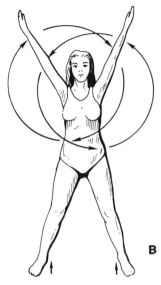

B

3a. FORWARD BEND

Purpose: To stretch muscles of the buttocks and posterior leg.
Starting Position: Stand astride with hands on hips.
Movement: Slowly bend forward to a 90-degree angle; return slowly to starting position; keep back flat.
Repetitions: 10

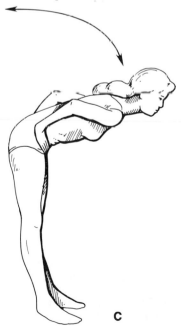

C

3b. ABDOMINAL CHURN

Purpose: To stretch muscles of the buttocks, abdomen, and posterior leg.

Starting Position: Stand astride with hands on hips.

Movement: Lower trunk sideward to left; rotate to forward position and to right; return to upright position. Repeat and reverse direction after two rotations.

Repetitions: 5 to 8

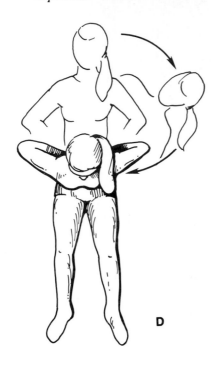

D

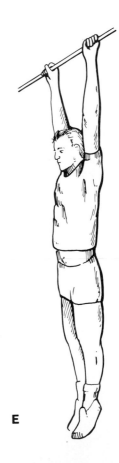

E

3c. BAR HANG

Purpose: To stretch muscles of arms, shoulders, back, trunk, hips, and pelvic regions. Good general body stretcher.

Starting Position: Hang from bar with arms straight.

Repetitions: 1 for up to 60 seconds

4. SHOULDER AND CHEST STRETCH

Purpose: To stretch muscles of the chest and shoulders.
Starting Position: Stand astride or kneel with arms at shoulder level and elbows bent.
Movement: Slowly force elbows backward and return to starting position.
Repetitions: 10 to 15

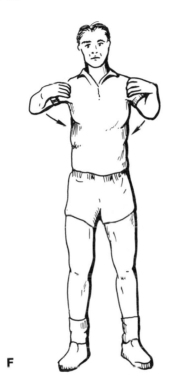

F

5a. LOWER BACK STRETCH

Purpose: To stretch muscles in the lower back.
Starting Position: Crouch on hands and knees.
Movement: Slowly rock back until buttocks touch heels; emphasize rounding back; return to starting position.
Repetitions: 10

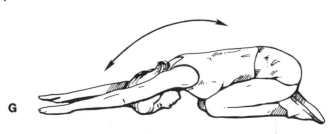

G

5b. ALTERNATE LOWER BACK STRETCH

Purpose: To stretch muscles in the lower back and buttocks.
Starting Position: Lie on back with the legs extended or stand erect.
Movement: Lift and bend one leg; grasp the knee and keep the opposite leg flat; pull knee to chest. Repeat with alternate leg.
Repetitions: 10

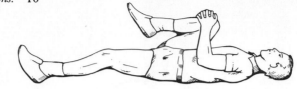

H

5c. ADVANCED LOWER BACK AND HAMSTRING STRETCH

Purpose: To stretch muscles of the lower back and hamstring muscles.
Starting Position: Lie on back with legs bent.
Movement: Keep knees together and slowly bring them over the head; straighten the legs and touch the toes to the floor; return to starting position.
Repetitions: 5 to 10

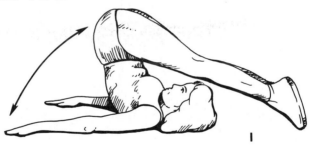

I

6. INVERTED STRETCH

Purpose: To stretch and strengthen the anterior hip, buttocks, and abdominal muscles.
Starting Position: Sit with arms at side.
Movement: Support body with heels and arms and raise trunk as high as possible.
Repetitions: 10

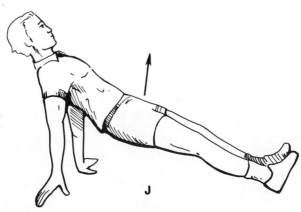

J

7a. FRONT LEG STRETCH

Purpose: To stretch the muscles in the anterior thigh and leg. Persons with knee problems should avoid this exercise.

Starting Position: Kneel with tops of ankles and feet flat on the ground.

Movement: Lean backward slowly; keep the back straight; maintain tension on muscles for 30 to 60 seconds.

Repetitions: 1 to 2

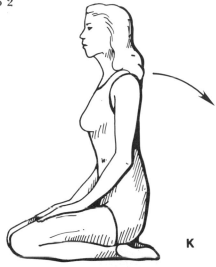

K

7b. FRONT LEG STRETCH

Purpose: To stretch the muscles of the anterior thigh and leg.

Starting Position: Kneel with feet turned outward.

Movement: Lean backward slowly; put constant tension on muscles; use arms to control the movement; hold backward position for 30 to 60 seconds.

Repetitions: 1 to 2

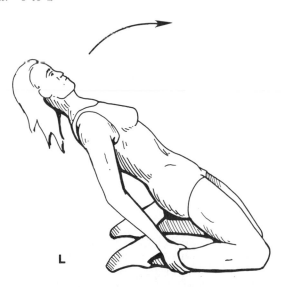

L

7c. ADVANCED FRONT LEG STRETCH

Purpose: To stretch the muscles of the anterior thigh and hip.

Starting Position: Lie on the ground with face down or stand erect.

Movement: Pull the ankle to the hip slowly; hold for 20–30 seconds and release the ankle. Use same procedure for the other side.

Note: If difficulty is encountered in assuming starting position, ask for assistance.

Repetitions: 1 to 2

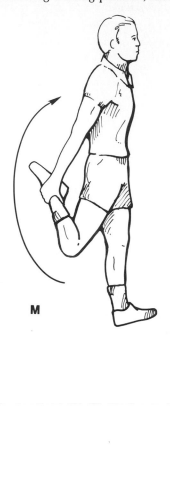

M

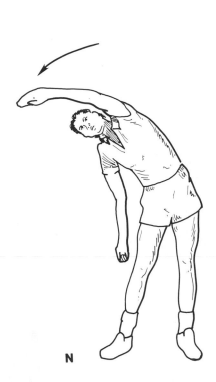

N

8. SIDE STRETCH

Purpose: To stretch the medial muscles of the thigh and the lateral muscles of the trunk and thorax.

Starting Position: Stand erect with one arm extended upward and the other relaxed at the side; place feet apart at more than shoulder width.

Movement: Bend trunk directly to the right with the left arm stretching overhead; keep both feet flat. Use same procedure for other side.

Repetitions: 5 to 10

9. GROIN STRETCH

Purpose: To stretch the groin muscles.
Starting Position: Sit with knees bent outward and the bottoms of feet together.
Movement: Grasp ankles and pull the upper body as close as possible to the feet. Hold stretch for 30 to 60 seconds.
Repetitions: 1 to 2

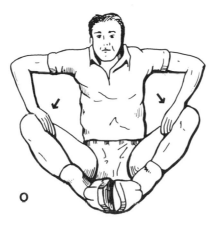

10. HAMSTRING STRETCH

Purpose: To stretch the muscles in the posterior leg and thigh.
Starting Position: Sit on ground with one leg extended straight forward; place the other leg forward with the knee bent and the sole touching the inner thigh of the extended leg.
Movement: Bend forward and attempt to touch the head to the knee; hold stretch for 30 to 60 seconds. Repeat with other leg.
Repetitions: 1 to 2

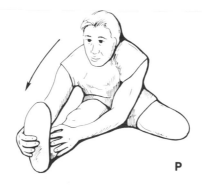

11a. CALF STRETCHER

Purpose: To stretch the posterior leg and ankle muscles.

Starting position: Stand in forward stride position with the forward knee partially flexed and the rear leg fully extended; keep feet pointed forward and heels flat on the ground.

Movement: Lean trunk forward until a continuous stretch occurs in the rear calf; hold stretch for 30 to 60 seconds. Repeat with other leg.

Repetitions: 1 to 2

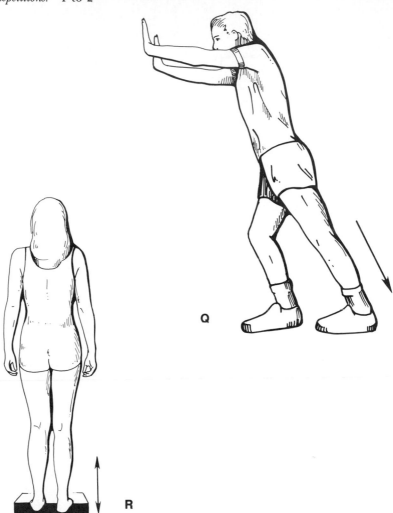

Q

R

11b. CALF STRETCHER

Purpose: To stretch the posterior leg muscles.

Starting Position: Stand in upright position with the balls of the feet on the edge of a step.

Movement: Slowly lower heels and hold for 30 to 60 seconds; raise heels and rise on toes.

Repetitions: 1 to 2

MUSCULAR STRENGTH AND ENDURANCE EXERCISES

Two options will be illustrated for each of the following routines. The first option (*a*) will utilize weights; the second (*b*) stresses the same muscle group, but without utilizing weights.

12a. WEIGHT TRAINING WARM-UP

Purpose: To utilize all of the major muscle groups in a warm-up routine prior to concentrating on specific muscle groups.

Starting Position: Place feet astride; bend knees; keep back straight; hold a bar with an overhand grip (Position A).

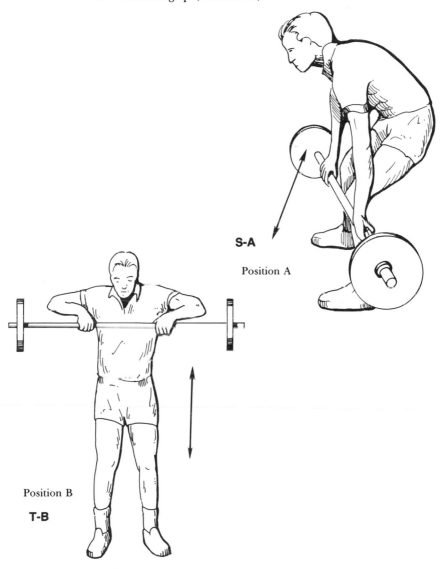

S-A

Position A

Position B

T-B

Movement: Straighten legs with back still straight; raise elbows to shoulder height or higher (Position B); lower elbows next to the trunk and keep the weight at chest level; press the weight over the head and fully extend arms (Position C); return weight to floor.

Repetitions: 8 to 10

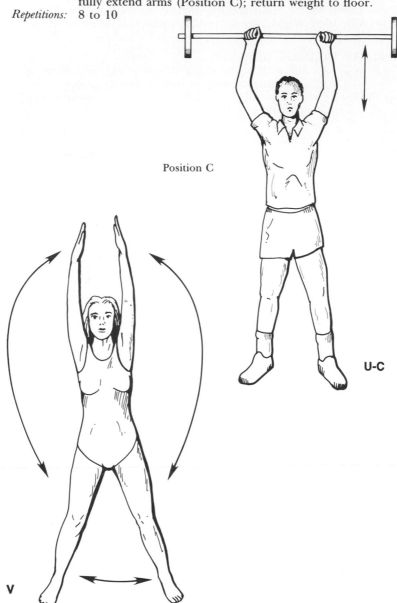

Position C

U-C

V

12b. JUMPING JACKS

Purpose: To utilize all of the major muscle groups in a warm-up routine prior to concentrating on specific muscle groups.

Starting Position: Stand erect with feet together and arms at the side.

Movement: Swing arms upward until over head and spread feet apart in one movement; in second movement, return to starting position.

Repetitions: 10 to 20

13. MILITARY PRESS

    Purpose: To strengthen the shoulder, upper back, and arm muscles.
Starting Position: Support weight at shoulder level with an overhand grip.
  Movement: Push weight directly overhead; keep the back and knees straight;
    return the weight slowly to starting position.
  Repetitions: 10 to 12

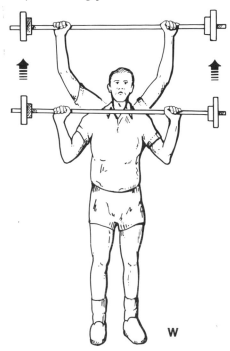

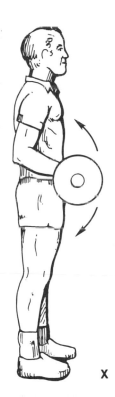

14a. CURL

    Purpose: To strengthen the anterior arm muscles.
Starting Position: Hold weight with a palms-up grip; keep arms straight.
  Movement: Bend arms and bring weight up to chest; return slowly.
  Repetitions: 10 to 12

14b. PULL-UP

Purpose: To strengthen the anterior arm, upper back, and shoulder muscles.

Starting Position: Place hands about 18 inches apart on overhead bar with either a palms-in or a palms-out grip; keep arms straight in order to support the body.

Movement: Pull body up so chin comes above the bar; slowly lower the body to starting position.

Repetitions: Progress to 10 to 15

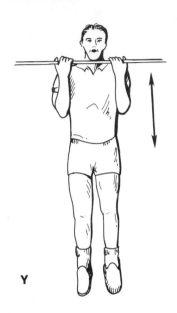

Y

15a. SIT-UP

Purpose: To strengthen the abdominal and hip flexor muscles.

Starting Position: Lie on back with knees bent and hands clasped behind neck or holding weight on chest.

Movement: Raise head and trunk to an upright position; hold position for one count; slowly return to starting position. Emphasize a roll-up type movement.

Repetitions: 15 to 20

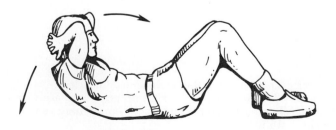

Z

15b. LEG PULL-UP

Purpose: To strengthen the abdominal and hip flexor muscles.
Starting Position: Hang from bar with body straight.
Movement: Bend knees slowly; bring knees to chest; return slowly to starting position.
Repetitions: Progress to 10 to 15

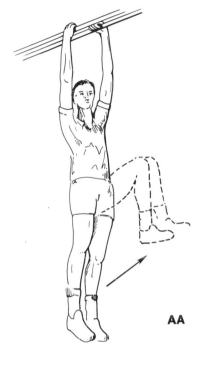

AA

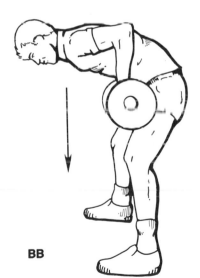

BB

16a. BENT-OVER ROWING

Purpose: To strengthen the mid to upper back and posterior arm muscles.
Starting Position: Stand with feet apart slightly more than shoulder width; bend forward at waist with back straight and legs slightly bent; keep arms straight to support the weight.
Movement: Raise weight to chest and return it slowly to starting position.
Repetitions: 10 to 12

16b. PULL-UP, WIDE GRIP

Purpose: To strengthen the mid to upper back and the posterior and anterior arm muscles.

Starting Position: Place hands about 24 inches apart on overhead bar with either a palms-in or palms-out grip; hang from the bar with arms straight to support the body.

Movement: Pull body up so chin comes above the bar; slowly lower the body to starting position.

Repetitions: Progress to 10 to 15

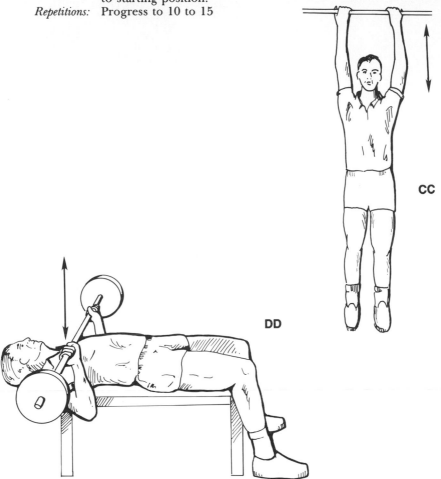

CC

DD

17a. SUPINE PRESS (BENCH PRESS)

Purpose: To strengthen the chest, anterior shoulder, and posterior arm muscles.

Starting Position: Lie on back on a bench 10 to 14 inches wide; use an overhand grip on a weight supported on standards or held by two assistants; keep arms straight.

Movement: Slowly lower weight to touch the chest; raise weight until arms are straight.

Repetitions: 10 to 12

17b. PUSHUPS

Purpose: To strengthen the chest, anterior shoulder, and posterior arm muscles.

Starting Position: Lie on stomach with hands flat on floor and positioned beneath the shoulders.

Movement: Push entire body except feet and hands off the floor until the arms are straight; lower body until chest touches floor.

Note: Positioning the hands beyond the shoulders or putting blocks beneath the hands increases the stretch and overload of the pectoral muscles.

Repetitions: Progress to 20 to 30

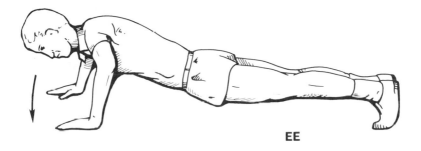

EE

18a. BACK EXTENSION

Purpose: To strengthen the lower back muscles.

Starting Position: Lie on a bench with the face down; extend the body from above the waist over the edge of the bench; strap or hold the feet to the other end of the bench

Movement: Lift head and trunk; slowly lower head and trunk.

Note: Do not hyperextend.

Repetitions: Progress to 10 to 15

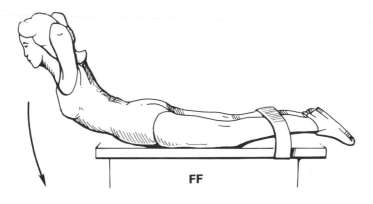

FF

18b. BACK TIGHTENER

Purpose:	To strengthen the lower back muscles.
Starting Position:	Lie on floor with face down; fold hands over lower back area.
Movement:	Raise head and chest and tense the gluteal and lower back muscles.
Caution:	Do not hyperextend; just raise head and chest slightly off the floor; concentrate mainly on tensing gluteal muscles.
Repetitions:	10 to 15

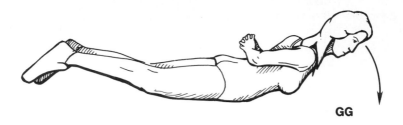

GG

19. SQUAT

Purpose:	To strengthen the anterior thigh and buttock muscles.
Starting Position:	Stand erect with feet astride and support weight on shoulders with palms-up grip.
Movement:	Keep the back straight and bend knees into a squat position; return to the standing position.
Note:	Do half squat if knees are weak.
Repetitions:	10 to 12

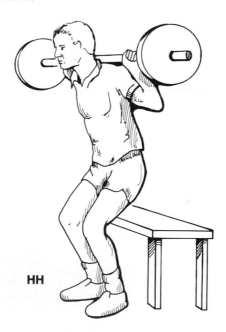

HH

20a. HEEL RAISES (WITH WEIGHTS)

Purpose: To strengthen the calf muscles.

Starting Position: Place feet astride and hold weight on shoulders with a palms-up grip.

Movement: Raise to a toe position; lower body.

Note: A board may be placed under the toes to increase the range of motion.

Repetition: 10 to 15

20b. HEEL RAISES

Purpose: To strengthen the calf muscles.

Starting Position: Place feet astride and use arms for balance if necessary.

Movement: Raise to a toe position; lower body.

Note: A board may be placed under the toes to increase the range of motion.

Repetitions: 10 to 15

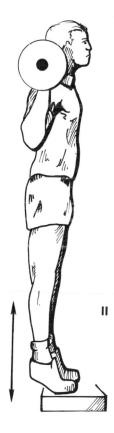
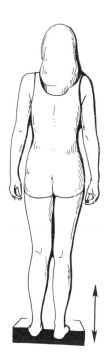

The exercise routines are divided into the following categories: upper body, trunk, and lower back stretching (1–6, pp. 276–280); leg stretching (7–11, pp. 281–284); and muscular strength and endurance (12–20, pp. 285–293). Many of the exercises have several options. In the first two categories (stretching exercises), some of the alternate exercises are more advanced and should be used only after the initial starter exercise has been mastered. The muscular strength and endurance exercises offer options depending on the availability of weight training equipment. Although not shown here, newer strength-training apparatus, e.g., Nautilus equipment, are popular and improve the safety with which strength training can be performed. These newer apparatus also appear to be able to integrate certain aspects of accommodating (variable) resistance into the weight-training program (see Chapter 5).

The stretching exercises should be included as part of the warm-up routine before starting the aerobics phase of the program. If time permits, they can be repeated during the cool-down period. The muscular strength and endurance routine can be used either after the stretching routine or after the aerobic phase.

Before beginning the aforementioned routines, the participants should be familiar with the described starting position, movement, and suggested repetitions. The training load has been designed to give the participant a moderate amount of muscular strength and endurance. We feel that this is the safest and most sensible manner to approach flexibility and muscular strength and endurance training.

To help avoid muscle soreness in weight-training exercises, the starting weight should be light (approximately 50 per cent of the maximum that can be lifted in one repetition). After a few weeks of training, 60 to 70 per cent of maximum can be attained. As soon as the required number of repetitions can be easily managed, more weight can be added. This is usually accomplished by adding 5 to 10 pounds of weight for arm exercises and 10 to 20 pounds for leg exercises. For those participants who want to place more emphasis on strength development, an increased training load and added sets would be necessary. The texts by Wilmore,[50] Berger,[52] Riley,[54] and Darden[55] are recommended for more advance weight training programs.

EXERCISE FOR THE BACK

Because lower back problems are considered among the most debilitating health problems for the middle-aged and elderly, special emphasis should be placed on including exercise for the development and maintenance of a healthy back.[56] The use of these special programs has been shown to relieve most lower back problems associated with muscular weakness and poor flexibility.[56]

What exercises should be included in a back routine? First of all, if serious organic problems are suspected, the participant should get medical clearance before starting the regimen. Lower back problems are usually precipitated by an imbalance of strength and flexibility of the lower back and abdominal areas, lifting or bending from an improper position, or just plain overdoing it. The following weaknesses and imbalances are generally present: tight hamstring, lower back muscle groups; tight hip flexor muscles; and weak abdominal and lower back muscles. Exercises that emphasize these special areas of concern include 5a, b, or c; 7a, b, or c; 10; 15a or b; and 18a or b. The *Y's Way to a Healthy Back*[57] is an excellent resource book and describes an extensive and progressive low back routine.

SUMMARY

General guidelines for exercise prescription have been discussed. The exercise prescription is based upon the results from the participant's medical screening and fitness examination. A specially individualized exercise prescription based on the participant's need, interest, and physical health status has been proposed. Special recommendations concerning frequency, intensity, and duration of training have been given for beginners and advanced exercisers. Individualized 6-week starter programs and 20-week training programs for walking and jogging have also been outlined.

The total energy cost of the exercise program is the important factor in exercise prescription and that kilocalories can be expended through a variety of physical activities has been emphasized. Thus, participants should choose an activity or activities that they enjoy. The notion that exercise should be done on a regular basis has been discussed. The need for a balanced, well-rounded program has been stressed; i.e., the training regimen should include exercises for the development of muscular strength and endurance and of flexibility, as well as of aerobic capacity.

Special exercises that can be used for developing and maintaining muscular strength and endurance, and flexibility were described. The exercises have been categorized in terms of the specific areas of the body that they affect and have been grouped in order of complexity. Both calisthenic exercises that need no special equipment and weight training exercises are listed.

REFERENCES

1. Cureton, T. K.: The Physiological Effects of Exercise Programs upon Adults. Springfield, IL, Charles C Thomas, 1969.
2. Cooper, K. H.: The New Aerobics. New York, J. B. Lippincott, 1970.
3. Wilmore, J.: Individual exercise prescription. Am. J. Cardiol. *33:*757–759, 1974.
4. Balke, B.: Prescribing physical activity. *In* Larson, L., editor: Sports Medicine. New York, Academic Press, 1974, pp. 505–523.
5. Pollock, M. L., Wilmore, J. H., and Fox, S. M.: Health and Fitness Through Physical Activity. New York, John Wiley & Sons, 1978.
6. Opie, L. H.: Sudden death and sport. Lancet *1:*263–266, 1975.
7. Gibbons, L. W., Cooper, K. H., Meyer, B. M., and Ellison, R. C.: The acute cardiac risk of strenuous exercise. J.A.M.A. *244:*1799–1801, 1980.
8. Thompson, P. D., Funk, E. J., Carleton, R. A., and Sturner, W. Q.: Incidence of death during jogging in Rhode Island from 1975 through 1980. J.A.M.A. *247:*2535–2538, 1982.

9. Vander, L., Franklin, B., and Rubenfire, M.: Cardiovascular complications of recreational physical activity. Phys. Sportsmed. *10:*89–97, 1982.
10. Hossack, K. F., and Hartwig, R.: Cardiac arrest associated with supervised cardiac rehabilitation. J. Cardiac Rehab. *2:*402–408, 1982.
11. Pollock, M. L., Gettman, L. R., Mileses, C. A., Bah, M. D., Durstine, J. L., and Johnson, R. B.: Effects of frequency and duration of training on attrition and incidence of injury. Med. Sci. Sports *9:*31–36, 1977.
12. Cooper, K. H.: The Aerobics Way. New York, M. Evans and Company, 1977.
13. Price, C. S., Pollock, M. L., Gettman, L. R., and Kent, D. A.: Physical Fitness Programs for Law Enforcement Officers: A Manual for Police Administrators. Washington, D.C., U.S. Government Printing Office, 1977.
14. Pollock, M. L.: How much exercise is enough? Phys. Sportsmed. *6:*50–64, 1978.
15. American College of Sports Medicine.: Position statement on the recommended quantity and quality of exercise for developing and maintaining fitness in healthy adults. Med. Sci. Sports *10:*vii–x, 1978.
16. Pollock, M. L., Miller, H. S., Linnerud, A. C., and Cooper, K. H.: Frequency of training as a determinant for improvement in cardiovascular function and body composition of middle-aged men. Arch. Phys. Med. Rehab. *58:*141–145, 1975.
17. Pollock, M. L., Foster, C., and Ward, A.: Exercise prescription for rehabilitation of the cardiac patient. *In* Pollock, M. L., and Schmidt, D. H., editors: Heart Disease and Rehabilitation. New York, John Wiley and Sons, 1979, pp. 413–445.
18. American College of Sports Medicine: Position statement on proper and improper weight loss programs. Med. Sci. Sports Exer. *15:*ix–xiii, 1983.
19. Pollock, M. L., Broida, J., Kendrick, Z., Miller, H. S., Janeway, R., and Linnerud, A. C.: Effects of training two days per week at different intensities on middle-aged men. Med. Sci. Sports *4:*192–197, 1972.
20. Pollock, M. L., Gettman, L. R., Raven, P. B., Ayres, J., Bah, M., and Ward, A.: Physiological comparisons of the effects of aerobic and anaerobic training. Presented to the American College of Sports Medicine. Washington, D.C., May 26, 1978.
21. Davis, J. A., Convertino, V. A.: A comparison of heart rate methods for predicting endurance training intensity. Med. Sci. Sports *7:*295–298, 1975.
22. Karvonen, M., Kentala, K., and Musta, O.: The effects of training heart rate: a longitudinal study. Ann. Med. Exptl. Biol. Fenn. *35:*307–315, 1957.
23. Fox, S. M., Naughton, J. P., and Gorman, P. A.: Physical activity and cardiovascular health II. The exercise prescription: intensity and duration. Mod. Concepts Cardiovasc. Dis. *16:* 21–24, 1972.
24. Borg, G. A. V.: Psychophysical bases of perceived exertion. Med. Sci. Sports Exer. *14:* 377–381, 1982.
25. Noble, B. J.: Clinical applications of perceived exertion. Med Sci. Sports Exer. *14:*406–411, 1982.
26. Pollock, M. L., Foster, C., Rod, J. L., and Wible, G.: Comparison of methods for determining exercise training intensity for cardiac patients and healthy adults. *In* Kellerman, J. J., editor: Comprehensive Cardiac Rehabilitation. Basel, S. Karger, 1982, pp. 129–133.
27. Åstrand, P. O.: Measurement of maximal aerobic capacity. Can. Med. Assoc. J. *96:* 732–735, 1967.
28. Taylor, H. L., Haskell, W., Fox, S. M., and Blackburn, H.: Exercise tests: a summary of procedures and concepts of stress testing for cardiovascular diagnosis and function evaluation. *In* Blackburn, H., editor: Measurement in Exercise Electrocardiography. Springfield, IL: Charles C Thomas, 1969, pp. 259–305.
29. Cooper, K. H., Purdy, J. G., White, S. R., Pollock, M. L., and Linnerud, A.C.: Age-fitness adjusted maximal heart rates. *In* Brunner, D., and Jokl, E., editors: Medicine and Sport, Vol. 10. The Role of Exercise in Internal Medicine. Basel, S. Karger, 1977, pp. 78–88.
30. Åstrand, P. O., and Rodahl, K.: Textbook of Work Physiology, 2nd ed. New York, McGraw-Hill, 1977.
31. Pollock, M. L., and Foster, C.: Exercise prescription for participants on propranolol. J. Am. Coll. Cardiol. (abstract) *2:*624, 1983.
32. Faraher Dion, W., Grevenow, P., Pollock, M. L., Squires, R. W., Foster, C., Johnson, W. D., and Schmidt, D. H.: Medical problems and physiologic responses during supervised inpatient cardiac rehabilitation: the patient after coronary artery bypass grafting. Heart Lung *11:*248–255, 1982.
33. Silvidi, G. E., Squires, R. W., Pollock, M. L., and Foster, C.: Hemodynamic responses and

medical problems associated with early exercise and ambulation in coronary artery bypass graft surgery patients. J. Cardiac Rehab. 2:355–362, 1982.

34. Pollock, M. L., Foster, C., Knapp, D., and Schmidt, D. H.: Cardiac rehabilitation program at Mount Sinai Medical Center, Milwaukee. J. Cardiac Rehab. 2:458–463, 1982.

35. Taylor, H. L., Wang, Y., Rowell, L., and Blomqvist, G.: The standardization and interpretation of submaximal and maximal tests of work capacity. Pediatrics 32:703–722, 1963.

36. Hombach, V., Braun, V., Hopp, H.-W., Gil-Sanchez, D., Behrenbeck, D. W., Tauchert, M., and Hilger, H. H.: Electrophysiological effects of cardioselective and non-cardioselective beta-adrenoceptor blockers with and without ISA at rest and during exercise. Br. J. Clin. Pharmacol. 13:285S–293S, 1982.

37. Tesch, P. A., and Kaiser, P.: Effects of beta-adrenergic blockage on O_2 uptake during submaximal and maximal exercise. J. Appl. Physiol. 54:901–905, 1983.

38. Cotton, F. S., and Dill, D. B.: On the relationship between the heart rate during exercise and that of immediate postexercise period. Am. J. Physiol. 111.554–558, 1935.

39. Pollock, M. L., Broida, J., and Kendrick, Z.: Validity of the palpation technique of heart rate determination and its estimation of training heart rate. Res. Q. 43:77–81, 1972.

40. Bevegard, S., and Shephard, J. T.: Circulatory effects of stimulating the carotid arterial stretch receptors in man at rest and during exercise. J. Clin. Invest. 45:132–142, 1966.

41. White, J. R.: EKG changes using the carotid artery for heart rate monitoring. Med. Sci. Sports 9:88–94, 1977.

42. Gardner, G. W., Danks, D. I., and Scharfsiein, L.: Use of carotid pulse for heart rate monitoring. Med. Sci. Sports (abstract) 11:111, 1979.

43. Oldridge, N. B., Haskell, W. L., and Single, P.: Carotid palpation, coronary heart disease and exercise rehabilitation. Med. Sci. Sport Exer. 13:6–8, 1981.

44. Couldry, W., Corbin, C. B., and Wilcox, A.: Carotid vs radial pulse counts. Phys. Sportsmed. 10:67–72, 1982.

45. McArdale, W. D., Zwiren, L., and Magel, J. R.: Validity of the postexercise heart rate as a means of estimating heart rate during work of varying intensities. Res. Q. 40:523–528, 1969.

46. Chow John, R., and Wilmore, J. H.: The regulation of exercise intensity by ratings of perceived exertion and by the palpation technique of heart rate determination. J. Cardiac Rehab. (in press).

47. Sharkey, B. J.: Intensity and duration of training and the development of cardiorespiratory endurance. Med. Sci. Sports 2:197–202, 1970.

48. Pollock, M. L., Dimmick, J., Miller, H. S., Kendrick, Z., and Linnerud, A. C.: Effects of mode of training on cardiovascular function and body composition of middle-aged men. Med. Sci. Sports 7:139–145, 1975.

49. Kasch, F. W., and Boyer, J. L.: Adult Fitness Principles and Practices. San Diego, San Diego State College, 1968.

50. Wilmore, J. H.: Training for Sport and Activity: The Physiological Basis of the Conditioning Process, 2nd ed. Boston, Allyn and Bacon, 1982.

51. Berger, R. A.: Applied Exercise Physiology. Philadelphia, Lea and Febiger, 1982.

52. Rasch, P. J.: Weight Training. Dubuque, IA, William C. Brown, 1966.

53. Lind, A. R., Phil, D., and McNicol, G.: Muscular factors which determine the cardiovascular responses to sustained and rhythmic exercise. Can. Med. Assoc. J. 96:706–713, 1967.

54. Riley, D. P.: Strength Training for Football: the Penn State way. West Point, NY, Leisure Press, 1982.

55. Darden, E.: Strength-Training Principles. Winter Park, FL, Anna Publishing, 1977.

56. Kraus, H.: Clinical Treatment of Back and Neck Pain. New York, McGraw-Hill, 1970.

57. Melleby, A.: The Y's Way to a Healthy Back. Piscataway, NJ, New Century Publishers, 1982.

Chapter 8

PRESCRIBING EXERCISE FOR REHABILITATION OF THE CARDIAC PATIENT

Cardiac rehabilitation can be considered the process of restoring psychological, physical, and social functions to optimal levels in those individuals who have had prior manifestations of coronary artery disease (CAD). In the past 30 years, there has been a profound shift away from the conservative approach that discouraged anginal and heart attack patients from becoming as active as their symptoms and medical status might have permitted. Many were told to resign from the golf club and some were advised to stop driving their cars and climbing stairs. Six weeks of bed rest after a myocardial infarction (MI) was the common standard.[1] Fortunately, many cardiologists [2-7] questioned this pessimistic and conservative approach. They demonstrated the safety of activity for the anginal patient, the early use of a bedside chair for the stabilized heart attack victim, and progressive, endurance-stimulating exercises for those whose myocardial infarcts had healed.[2-7]

Chapter 1 outlines the many effects of physical activity on physiological function, risk factors associated with CAD, and morbidity and mortality. Although the benefits of cardiac rehabilitation with regard to morbidity and mortality are not fully proven but strongly suggested, the effect on quality of life is not disputed.[8-15] In addition, the concept of cardiac rehabilitation includes not only exercise but also a wide spectrum of medical, physical, and psychosocial behavioral changes. The multiple intervention approach (smoking cessation, proper diet, and exercise) to cardiac rehabilitation has been more supportive in favor of decreased morbidity and mortality.[16,17]

Strict bed rest has been shown to have a significant detrimental effect on physiological function.[18-20] After just a few days or weeks, the patient has significantly decreased cardiorespiratory fitness, blood volume, red blood cell count, nitrogen and protein balance, strength, flexibility, and increased problems of orthostatic hypotension and thromboembolism. In those patients who have undergone coronary artery bypass graft surgery (CABG), physical activity can help decrease postsurgical stiffness and prevent complications of postsurgical atelectasis. Other potential benefits of cardiac rehabilitation include a decrease in the incidence and severity of depression and anxiety,[21,22] and earlier hospital discharge.[23] See Kellerman,[15] Naughton, Hellerstein and Mohler,[10] Leon and Blackburn,[13] and Pollock and Schmidt[14] for reviews of the beneficial effects of early ambulation and other aspects of cardiac rehabilitation on various medical, physiological, psychological, and social factors.

RISKS AND MEDICAL PROBLEMS ASSOCIATED WITH CARDIAC REHABILITATION PROGRAMS

Although cardiac arrest and death have occurred in cardiac rehabilitation programs, they have been infrequent.[24,25] What is the risk of fatal and nonfatal events associated with cardiac rehabilitation programs? First, as a base of comparison, what is the risk in a generally noncardiac population? Gibbons et al.[26] reported the acute cardiac risk of strenuous exercise in 2,935 men and women 13 to 76 years of age ($\bar{x} = 37$). the 65-month follow-up period included 374,798 person-hours of exercise and 1,694,024 miles of walking and running (81 per cent running). During this period, only two nonfatal cardiac events occurred. One complication occurred in a 61-year-old executive who collapsed with ventricular fibrillation (VF) during a 2-mile competitive race for which he had not adequately prepared. The other event occurred in a 35-year-old man who suffered an acute inferior MI while showering after completing a fast-paced 3-mile run. Both men had not been running regularly for 6 months before their event, and both incidents were associated with a high-intensity exercise session. No cardiac events occurred with the 1,001 women who participated in the study.

Haskell[24] reported the occurrence of major cardiovascular complications during exercise training in 30 cardiac rehabilitation programs in North America. The questionnaire included data from medically supervised exercise classes conducted in 103 locations on 13,570 participants who accumulated 1,629,634 patient-hours of supervised exercise. Programs accepted patients 2 to 12 weeks after the event, included an average of three exercise sessions per week with walking, walk-jogging, running, calisthenics, and recreational games being the predominant activities. A total of 50 cardiac arrests were observed, 42 of which were successfully resuscitated and 8 of which were fatal. Seven MIs were reported—five nonfatal and two fatal.

Table 8–1 compares the complication rates for the noncardiac and cardiac exercise programs reported previously. The cardiac programs came from a variety of YMCA or YMHA, hospital, university, and independent medical clinics, but all were medically supervised. A physician or nurse was on site for each exercise session. Although data are not available, it stands to reason that fatal cardiac events would be significantly higher in nonsupervised programs.

In the cardiac programs, 44 of the 61 major complications occurred during warm-up or cool-down, with the type of facility used not affecting the

TABLE 8-1. CARDIOVASCULAR COMPLICATION RATES FOR
ADULT FITNESS (NONCARDIAC) AND MEDICALLY SUPERVISED
CARDIAC REHABILITATION PROGRAMS IN NORTH AMERICA

	EVENTS PER HOUR	
GROUP	*Nonfatal*	*Fatal*
Cardiac	1 per 34,673	1 per 116,402
Noncardiac	1 per 187,399	0 in 374,798

Data from Haskell, W.L.: Cardiovascular complications during training of cardiac patients. Circulation *57*:920–924, 1974; and Gibbons, L.W., Cooper, K.H., Meyer, B.M., and Ellison, R.C.: The acute cardiac risk of strenuous exercise. J.A.M.A. *244*:1799–1801, 1980.

results. These results strongly suggest the need for adequate supervision during rest breaks or stops to the rest room, and a minimum of 15 to 20 minutes postexercise surveillance is necessary. A higher incidence rate was reported before 1970 (1 in 116,000 versus 1 in 212,000); this suggests improved guidelines and standards and more appropriate supervision.[10,24,27-29]

Which patients are at the highest risk for having a cardiac arrest or MI? Graded exercise testing has shown the following factors to be related to higher risk: angina pectoris, significant ST-segment depression or elevation from resting values, inappropriate blood pressure response to exercise, significant arrhythmia, and poor effort tolerance (fewer than 3 METs).[30-35] The combination of low left ventricular function and significant arrhythmia greatly increases the risk of sudden cardiac death.[36,37] Hossack and Hartwig[27] recently reported results from 13 years of the CAPRI program in Seattle, Washington. During this period, 2,464 patients (80 per cent male) performed 374,616 hours of supervised exercise. Twenty-five male participants experienced VF during training, and all were successfully resuscitated. When compared with a control group of patients who did not have VF, those in the VF group had a higher aerobic capacity and more marked ST depression on a GXT (68 per cent and 21 per cent, respectively). The incidence of angina pectoris, exertional hypotension, and exercise-induced arrhythmias was not different between groups. Those in the VF group exceeded their upper limit prescribed training HR for 56 per cent of the training session compared with 24 per cent for the controls. Angiography was available on 17 of the VF patients, and all had significant left main or proximal left anterior descending disease, or both. In addition, most of these incidents occurred in patients who had been in the program for more than 1 year. Thus, these data show that exercise in the range of 60 to 85 per cent of HR max reserve can be safe for most patients. Certain abnormal responses on the GXT and exceeding one's recommended upper limit of the target HR range during training are associated with a higher risk of major cardiovascular complications.

What medical problems occur during in-hospital phase I programs? Although the trend is to begin exercise therapy in patients closer to the event and surgery, few major complications requiring resuscitation are reported. A survey of in-hospital cardiac rehabilitation programs showed that medical patients begin treatment 2 to 4 days after the event and CABG patients, 1 to 3 days after surgery.[38] The low incidence rate is most likely due to careful patient selection and the adoption of appropriate guidelines and contraindications to exercise that are in current use.[10,28,29] These guidelines will be discussed in subsequent sections of this chapter. Even though life-threatening complications are rare, other types of major complications seem to be prevalent.

Dion et al.[39] reported medical problems associated with cardiac rehabilitation in 521 CABG patients who were 24 to 76 years of age. Ambulation and upper extremity range-of-motion (ROM) exercise began as early as 12 to 24 hours after surgery for 65 per cent of the patients. Patients were treated twice daily and monitored for arrhythmia, ischemia, and blood pressure for an average of 11 days. During the rehabilitation program, a total of 555 serious complications occurred. These included angina pectoris (4 per cent), incisional pain (14 per cent—mainly leg incision), claudication (3 per cent), lightheadedness (14 per cent), hypotension (8 per cent), hypertension (1 per cent), ST-segment changes (2 per cent), and arrhythmia (supraventricular, 17 per cent, and ventricular, 44 per cent). Approximately 25 per cent of these complications were first noted by the cardiac rehabilitation staff. The study emphasized not only the significance of early surveillance for the detection of major medical problems, but also its importance in assisting primary physicians to manage their patients medically before hospital discharge.

Medical problems associated with rehabilitation of the MI patient show a greater incidence of angina pectoris and ischemia than for CABG patients and fewer problems associated with hypotension.

SUPERVISION AND MONITORING OF CARDIAC REHABILITATION PROGRAMS

In general, the need for cardiac rehabilitation programs and the supervision of cardiac patients in their training programs is apparent. Questions arise, though, regarding how much supervision and how much sophisticated monitoring are necessary and for how long. The exact answers to these questions are not known. It is the continuing concern of medical and health professionals, as well as third party carriers. States vary greatly from no coverage for cardiac rehabilitation programs to almost "carte blanche" long-term coverage for an organized program. It appears that most state carriers and Medicaid and Medicare plans will reimburse for inpatient and up to 3 months of a hospital-based outpatient program. Many states will also cover a medically supervised phase III community program for up to 6 additional months.

When does rehabilitation end and prevention begin? In addition, should all patients be treated equally, or should discrimination occur based on medical and physical status? Many insurance carriers are designating an arbitrary 12-week postdischarge period as the rehabilitation period. From a physical standpoint, some data support this notion and show aerobic capacity to be restored by this time.[40] This does not mean that a patient cannot continue to improve, but 8 to 12 weeks after discharge, most uncomplicated cardiac patients have improved their physical status enough to return to work and carry on a relatively normal lifestyle.

The American Heart Association, Wisconsin Affiliate, has approved recommendations for insurance coverage of supervised cardiac exercise rehabilitation programs from its Exercise and Cardiac Rehabilitation Committee. The committee made the following recommendations for third party carriers.[41]

> The response to exercise rehabilitation will vary with the severity of cardiovascular disease, clinical status of the patient, and coexisting medical problems. Components of total rehabilitation also include: patient education, risk factor modification and individual counseling to increase adherence. The committee suggests a total of *six to nine months* of rehabilitation as the optimum target for the majority of patients described above. The nine months may be partitioned between three clinical phases which are defined as follows:

> Phase I   Involves immediate inpatient exercise rehabilitation emphasizing patient education and risk factor modification combined with musculoskeletal range of motion, muscle tone, and activity of daily living exercise. This phase lasts approximately 12–21 days, and patients who are candidates for a continuing exercise rehabilitation program are referred at this point to Phase II.

> Phase II   Involves continuing outpatient exercise rehabilitation, usually within a medical center or clinic program. Exercise training includes progressive light to moderate endurance activities with approximately three *supervised* and *monitored* exercise sessions per week. Phase II generally extends two-three months depending on patient progress. Occasionally, patients may require four to six months in Phase II. After satisfactory completion of Phase II, patients are referred to Phase III. The transition to Phase III is based on clinical and physiological responses to exercise.

> Phase III   Is conducted within community level supervised exercise programs. . . . In Phase III there is continuing emphasis on patient education and risk factor modification combined with participation and prescribed endurance exercise. The objective of this phase is to achieve a state of self-regulated physical activity. A total of six months should be available for optimum results.

The committee also described the minimum criteria for a supervised phase III program.

> *Cardiovascular exercise programs* require the direction of a qualified physician who will assume medical responsibility for the program. For the purpose of rendering emergency medical care, in the absence of a physician, a qualified nurse with the appropriate cardiovascular training must be present. It is recommended that ideally, exercise sessions be directed by physical therapists, occupational therapists, nurses or allied health personnel with certification in exercise rehabilitation, as specified by the *American College of Sports Medicine.* [29]

> In smaller programs a nurse with cardiovascular training who is also trained in cardiac exercise and rehabilitation would be acceptable. In addition, all persons involved in the supervision of patient exercise must be certified in basic life support according to standards for cardiopulmonary resuscitation and emergency cardiac care.[42]

> *The physical setting* for supervised exercise programs may be outside the immediate domain of a medical center. In most instances, a YMCA, a high school or university gymnasium, or Jewish community center may be the best available setting. Programs must have emergency equipment and supplies available for potential medical problems. Guidelines for this equipment are outlined by the American Heart Association.[28]

Monitoring

> Patient exercise should be monitored by frequent determination of pulse rate, blood pressure and work intensity, as outlined in *American Heart Association* and *American College of Sports Medicine* guidelines cited above. These data should be maintained in a patient record and reviewed periodically to determine progress in the program.

The elaborately organized cardiac rehabilitation plan developed by North Carolina[43] has been accepted by both professionals and third party carriers and is recommended for 1 year. Fox[44] has suggested a 1-year graduated step-down program. The patient attends a supervised program 3 days per week for 6 months, followed by 2 days per week for 3 months and 1 day per week the final 3 months. The latter approach allows a transition period in which the patient begins to make the adjustment to a less supervised home or community noncardiac program.

In summary, it appears that most experts agree that medically supervised cardiac rehabilitation is recommended, but there is varying opinion on how long and how much monitoring is necessary. Until better research data are available, phase I and phase II of the Wisconsin Plan are recommended by the authors. In addition, a minimum of 3 months is advised for phase III. In the meantime, the cardiac rehabilitation staff should be aware of escalating health care costs and should listen to the concerns of insurance carriers. Patients should not be monitored indiscriminately with expensive monitoring devices. The goal should be for patients to progress to nontelemetry and less expensive community types of programs as rapidly as possible. In phase II, the transition could take place for some patients as early as 4 to 6 weeks. A selected few high-risk patients may have to have telemetry from 9 to 12 months.

The concern of many is whether cardiac patients should ever be allowed to train on their own. Again, we do not know, and because coronary disease continues to progress, we can never be certain. As mentioned earlier, many cardiac arrests occur after patients have been participating in the program for more than 1 year. Thus, supervised programs, whether denoted as cardiac or noncardiac, seem advisable for patients. If this is not practical, it would be advisable to train with someone who knows cardiopulmonary resuscitation (CPR).

EMERGENCY CARE AND PROCEDURES

Cardiac arrests and other major cardiovascular events are not common in cardiac rehabilitation programs. Even so, an adequate emergency plan is necessary for all programs. In a hospital program where emergency medical teams are available, the situation is less complex than for the out-of-hospital community setting.

A list of drugs, equipment, and supplies that are recommended for use in cardiac rehabilitation programs can be found in Appendix B, Tables B–1 and B–2. All staff members involved in the conduct of the cardiac rehabilitation program should have current certification in CPR. If possible, someone should be trained in advanced cardiac life support. A plan should be established for handling emergencies. For programs outside a hospital, the following should be taken into account: telephone communications with local physicians, hospitals, paramedics and emergency medical technicians; physician and nurse coverage; CPR; in the absence of a physician, standing orders for nurses (for example, see Appendix B, Figure B–1); and crowd control and the handling of other patients. The emergency plan should be reviewed and rehearsed on a regular basis.

To handle emergency situations, a minimum of one physician and one nurse or a team of two nurses who are trained in acute cardiac care is preferable. For non–hospital-based programs, telephone monitoring systems would be advantageous for emergency situations. For outdoor programs conducted away from the main headquarters, golf carts equipped with a "walkie talkie" or short-wave radio may be necessary for adequate communications. For in-hospital programs, emergency "stat" buttons placed on the walls take the place of a telephone and can hasten communications to emergency teams.

Other safety features for programs include a minimum 15-minute recovery and surveillance period after completion of the program and emergency call buttons located in the locker room, showers, and restrooms. In addition, it is wise not to allow patients to train alone or to leave the exercise area by themselves during class sessions. Table 8–2 lists the causes of exercise-related cardiovascular emergencies, their signs and symptoms, and recommended emergency procedures.[29]

A COMPREHENSIVE CARDIAC REHABILITATION PROGRAM

Cardiac rehabilitation programs should incorporate a multidimensional approach. Exercise should be a major part of the program, but the program should also include proper education and counseling regarding the control of risk factors associated with the development of CAD. In addition, particularly in the earlier stages of rehabilitation, many questions and concerns about medical status, medications, diet, activities of daily living, return to work, exercise prescription, sex, and so on arise and should be answered. Thus, to cope with the many needs of the patient best, a variety of staff expertise is recommended. Staff members may include a physician (medical director), one or more nurses (educators and cardiac rehabilitation specialists), physical and occupational therapists, exercise physiologist, clinical psychologist, exercise specialist–physical educator, social worker, vocational rehabilitation counselor, dietician, and pharmacologist.[44] The cardiac rehabilitation nurse should be trained and have experience in a critical coronary care unit. Obviously, small programs will not be able to provide many full-time staff members dealing only with cardiac rehabilitation, but a variety of staff members from other departments of the hospital and community could be available for patient or staff consultation and education. More details concerning organization and administration of cardiac rehabilitation programs and staff responsibilities can be found elsewhere.[14,45–48]

Even though many types of staff members are recommended for a comprehensive cardiac rehabilitation program, their role is only to assist the primary physician in the management of his or her patient. The primary physician can use the information attained through the cardiac rehabilitation staff to help assess patient status and make decisions about management. A strong patient education program will further assist the primary physician in reinforcing important health issues and habits.

EXERCISE PRESCRIPTION FOR THE CARDIAC PATIENT

Many of the principles of exercise prescription outlined for noncardiac patients in Chapter 7 are appropriate for use with the cardiac patient. The major differences in programs are related to the application of these principles to the patient and how they affect the regulation of frequency, intensity, and duration of training; the rate of progression; and the selection of mode

TABLE 8-2. CAUSES OF EXERCISE RELATED CARDIOVASCULAR
EMERGENCIES, THEIR SIGNS AND SYMPTOMS, AND
RECOMMENDED EMERGENCY PROCEDURES

BASIC CAUSES	SIGNS AND SYMPTOMS	EMERGENCY PROCEDURES
I. CARDIAC ARREST		
A. Ventricular Fibrillation	See Standards for CPR and ECC Supplement to JAMA (227), 833–868, February 18, 1974. Revised *Circulation* (61) 1980	Defibrillate
B. Cardiac Standstill (Ventricular Asystole)		Defibrillate
II. LOW CARDIAC OUTPUT STATES		
A. Inadequate Venous Return	Tachycardia, Low B.P., Pallor, Dizziness	Supine with legs elevated Isometric or low-level dynamic exercise I.V. and/or oral fluid vasopressor medication
B. Arrhythmias 1. Tachycardia	Must define by ECG	Stop exercise, supine position Watch B.P. closely I.V. medications D.C. countershock or defibrillation as indicated
2. Bradycardia 3. Premature ventricular and atrial contractions		Treat for inadequate venous return (i.e., Atropine, Isuprel) or specific treatment depending on ECG diagnosis
C. Myocardial Failure	Inordinate Dyspnea, Rales, Gallop Rhythm	Stop exercise, sitting position Oxygen administration Positive pressure breathing Drugs 1. Use of sublingual nitroglycerin should be considered 2. Morphine
D. Drug Induced Low Output 1. Beta Blockers 2. Diuretics 3. Antihypertensives	Slow Heart Rate Low Blood Pressure	Supine with legs elevated I.V. fluids if appropriate Drugs appropriate to counteract cause
III. ISCHEMIC STATUS		
A. Chest Pain, Unrelenting	ECG Evidence of Ischemia	Stop exercise, immediate O_2, nitroglycerin, possible Inderal, possible hospitalization
B. Myocardial Infarct	ECG Evidence of Infarct, Ischemia or Supporting Clinical Evidence	Hospitalize, treat arrhythmia and circulatory inadequacy

TABLE 8–2. CAUSES OF EXERCISE RELATED CARDIOVASCULAR
EMERGENCIES, THEIR SIGNS AND SYMPTOMS, AND
RECOMMENDED EMERGENCY PROCEDURES *(Continued)*

BASIC CAUSES	SIGNS AND SYMPTOMS	EMERGENCY PROCEDURES
III. ISCHEMIC STATUS *(continued)*		
C. Papillary Muscle Dysfunction	Loud Systolic Murmur	Sitting position Nitroglycerin Hospitalization if it persists
D. Cerebral	Ataxia, Dizziness, Impaired Consciousness	Stop exercise, supine rest, monitor B.P., I.V. fluids
E. Gastrointestinal	Nausea, Vomiting, Vasovagal Syncope	Stop exercise, supine rest, emesis basin

NOTE: Cardiovascular collapse: A general term applied to impairment of the cardiovascular system of such severity that the subject cannot stand or walk. This table does not include those symptoms/signs which may occur during exercise testing which result in cardiovascular collapse.
(Reprinted with permission from American College of Sports Medicine: Guidelines for Graded Exercise Testing and Exercise Prescription, 2nd ed. Philadelphia, Lea and Febiger, 1980.)

of training. In addition, because of potential medical and hemodynamic problems associated with the diseased heart and the time required for MI and postsurgical patients to heal properly, program modifications and avoidance of certain activities are generally necessary.

BASIC COMPONENTS OF A TRAINING SESSION: THE CARDIAC PATIENT

The basic components of a training session for cardiac patients are shown in Table 8–3. In contrast to the healthy adult, Table 7–1, the cardiac patient may need a longer warm-up period and may require modifications of the endurance (aerobic) phase of the session, depending on medical status and phase of training.

As a result of the low state of fitness and the adverse effects of bed rest and surgery on the musculoskeletal systems of the cardiac patient, the need for special stretching and joint readiness is apparent. Thus, warm-up usually takes longer during phases I and II. During phase III, the warm-up period for the cardiac patient may be similar to that of the normal adult.

Once patients enter the phase II program, they are generally ready for low-level muscle-conditioning activities. Emphasis is placed on dynamic and rhythmical exercise that does not impede normal breathing. Activities could include calisthenics, light weight training (1 to 15-pound weights), and various other low-resistance apparatus. More specific recommendations for weight training and progression will be discussed under phase II programs.

The aerobic phase of training starts with a short ambulation period, which is performed two to three times daily. The phase I patient is generally weak and cannot tolerate long bouts of physical activity. Thus, a program

TABLE 8–3. BASIC COMPONENTS OF A
TRAINING SESSION: CARDIAC PATIENTS

COMPONENT	DURATION (min)	PHASE
Warm-up	15–20	I
	10	II, III
Muscular conditioning	10	II, III
Aerobic exercise	5–30	I
	20–60	II
	30–60	III
Cool-down	5–10	I, II, III

of shorter bouts with greater frequency is the best initial approach. A second daily training period would also be recommended to the patient after discharge and before returning to work. More specific details about suggested duration of activity and rate of progression will be discussed under the various phases of the program. The 300-Kcal minimum daily dosage (1,000 Kcal per week) prescribed for normal adults is also recommended for the patient. Because cardiac patients generally train at lower intensities, they require training of longer duration, or greater frequency, or both to reach this goal. In addition, it usually takes the cardiac patient 3 to 6 months longer than the healthy adult to reach this goal.[38,49] Because of the lower intensity factor (Kcal/min), the minimum duration of a training session during phases II and III is 10 to 15 minutes longer for the cardiac patient than for the normal adult.

RATE OF PROGRESSION IN TRAINING

The initial training load is lower and the rate of progression slower in the cardiac patient than in the healthy adult. Figure 8–1 shows the general progression of cardiac and noncardiac groups. The figure shows average estimates of progression for each group, progression being dependent on the participant's age, level of fitness, and health status. As discussed in Chapter 7 (Fig. 7–3), normal participants generally start at 150 to 200 Kcal per exercise session and progress to the 300-Kcal level by 8 to 12 weeks. In contrast, the cardiac patient begins (phase I) at a level below 50 Kcal per session and requires several weeks to months longer to reach the 300-Kcal level.[38] The slightly slower rate of progression for the MI patient, compared with the CABG patient, results from a reluctance to have the patient progress until 6 to 8 weeks after the MI. Generally, by 6 to 8 weeks, scar tissue has adequately developed on the heart, and the healing process is nearly complete.[50] After this time, training intensity can increase, and the patient progresses at a faster rate. It must be re-emphasized that during the first 6 to 8 weeks of recovery, the MI patient is exercised more conservatively than the CABG patient. Patients with perioperative infarcts progress like MI patients. It also takes 6 to 8 weeks for the sternum to heal fully after surgery;

thus a 20- to 25-pound lifting restriction is recommended (only 10 pounds over the head). In addition, during this healing period, activities that place undue pressure on the sternum should be avoided. During the inpatient phase, activities are of a low intensity and a short-to-moderate duration and are designed to offset problems associated with bed rest.

The suggested rates and levels of progression for cardiac and noncardiac groups shown in Figure 8–1 are realistic estimates. Whether or not patients can progress faster without added risk of an event is not known at this time. Research by DeBusk et al.[51] suggests that during the first 12 weeks of rehabilitation, patients with no complications can progress at a rate faster than that shown in Figure 8–1, but more research is necessary to clarify this question. In the meantime, the slower, conservative approach seems appropriate.

The progression in Figure 8–1 stops at the 300- to 400-Kcal level per exercise session and does not take into account further increases (additional kilocaloric expenditure) in training or changes in intensity. For example, noncardiac participants entering a jogging program usually begin with short periods of jogging interspersed with equal distances of walking. As they progress, they will walk less and jog more. As they adapt, their total time and distance may also increase. An important point here is that the participant can reach the 300-Kcal level fairly rapidly and before reaching the maintenance phase of a training program.

As with noncardiac participants, the exercise prescription for cardiac patients involves three stages of progression: starter, slow-to-moderate progression, and maintenance. The starter phase is conducted at a low intensity and includes joint readiness, stretching and light calisthenics, and low-level aerobic activities. The purpose of this stage of the program is to introduce the participant to exercise at a low level and to allow the patient the time to adapt properly to the initial rigors of training. During this phase, the patient progresses by increasing frequency and duration of training first, then intensity. If this phase is properly introduced, the participant experiences a minimum of muscle soreness and avoids debilitating injuries or discomfort.

The slow progression phase differs from the starter phase in that the participant progresses at a more rapid rate. During this stage of training, the duration or intensity of training, or both, are increased consistently every 1 to 4 weeks. How well the exerciser adapts to the present level of training dictates the frequency and magnitude of progression. As a general rule, older and less fit participants require longer to adapt and to progress in a training regimen.[52-54]

A healthy adult usually reaches the maintenance stage of training after 6 to 12 months. At this stage, the participant has attained a satisfactory level of fitness and may no longer be interested in increasing the training load; further development is minimal, and the emphasis of the program becomes that of maintaining fitness rather than of seeking further development. Progression for the cardiac patient is slower and may take from 6 to 18

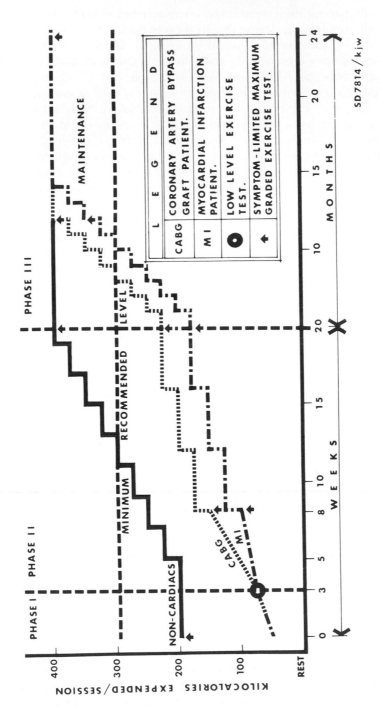

Figure 8–1. Progression in aerobic training in noncardiac and cardiac patients. (Reprinted with permission from Pollock, M.L., Foster, C., and Ward, A.: Exercise prescription for rehabilitation of the cardiac patient. *In* Pollock, M.L., and Schmidt, D.H., editors: Heart Disease and Rehabilitation. New York, copyright © John Wiley and Sons, 1979, pp. 413–445.)

months longer than for noncardiac subjects. Kavanagh et al.[49] have shown that younger cardiac patients improve their aerobic capacity for up to 2 years.

Table 8–4 lists guidelines for exercise prescription for cardiac patients.[55] Phases I and II of these guidelines show the slower progression and intensity levels for cardiac patients in their earlier stages of training and coincide with the kilocaloric progression shown in Figure 8–1. As the patient reaches phase III, the program begins to be comparable to the general guidelines recommended for noncardiac participants. The big difference in the exercise prescription guidelines for the phase III cardiac patient versus the noncardiac participant would be the greater frequency (5 days per week) and duration (30 to 60 minutes) of training for cardiac patients needed to compensate for their lower intensity. Further, many cardiac patients will never be capable of moderate- to high-intensity training; thus their program would always include a greater frequency and duration of training. More specific aspects of exercise prescription for cardiac patients will be described under the various phases of rehabilitation.

The starter program has a similar purpose for both cardiac and healthy participants. The starter program for the cardiac patient involves the first 6 to 8 weeks of training and encompasses phase I and the first part of phase II. As mentioned previously for MI patients, the scar tissue has developed and other aspects of the healing process are completed by this time. It also takes about 6 to 8 weeks for the sternum to heal, for hemoglobin to approach normal, and for other aspects related to surgery to normalize.[56] For example, data collected 2 weeks after CABG surgery show hemoglobin and hematocrit values to be 11 gm and 33 per cent, respectively.

At 6 to 8 weeks after MI or CABG surgery, a symptom-limited graded exercise test (SL-GXT) is recommended. The purpose of the test is to evaluate medical status and improvement (or regression) in the cardiac rehabilitation program and to refine the exercise prescription. If the test results are unremarkable, then a faster rate of training may begin.

INPATIENT CARDIAC REHABILITATION—PHASE I

The inpatient cardiac rehabilitation program should begin as soon as the patient is considered stable. Depending on the type of patient, it is usually within 2 to 4 days for an uncomplicated MI patient and 1 to 2 days for a postsurgical patient.[38] The following contraindications to exercise have been used as guidelines for the inpatient program at Mount Sinai Medical Center, Milwaukee, Wisconsin. The suggested contraindications to exercise have been modified for inpatients from recommendations of the American Heart Association[28] and the American College of Sports Medicine.[29]

TABLE 8–4. GUIDELINES FOR EXERCISE PRESCRIPTION FOR CARDIAC PATIENTS AS RECOMMENDED AND PRACTICED AT MOUNT SINAI MEDICAL CENTER, MILWAUKEE, WISCONSIN[a]

PRESCRIPTION	PHASE I (inpatient program)	PHASE II (discharge → 3 mo)	PHASE III (3 mo →)	HEALTHY ADULTS
Frequency	2–3 times/day	1–2 times/day	3–5 times/wk	3–5 times/wk
Intensity	MI: RHR + 20 CABG: RHR + 20	MI: RHR + 20[b], RPE 13 CABG: RHR + 20[b], RPE 13	70%–85% HR max reserve	60%–90% HR max reserve
Duration	MI: 5–20 min CABG: 10–30 min	MI: 20–60 min CABG: 30–60 min	30–60 min	15–60 min
Mode-activity	ROM, TDM, bike, 1 flight of stairs	ROM, TDM (walk, walk-jog), bike, arm erg, Wgt Trg	Walk, bike, jog, swim, cal, Wgt Trg, endurance sports	Walk, jog, run, bike, swim, endurance sports, Wgt Trg, cal

[a]Symbols and abbreviations. MI, myocardial infarction patient; CABG, coronary artery bypass graft surgery patient; HR, heart rate, beats/min; RHR, standing resting HR; ROM, range of motion exercise; TDM, treadmill; arm erg, arm ergometer; cal, calisthenics; Wgt Trg, weight training; RPE, rating of perceived exertion.

[b]Six to eight weeks after surgery or event, a symptom-limited exercise test is performed. Heart rate intensity is then based on 70 per cent maximum heart rate reserve.

(Reprinted with permission from Pollock, M.L., Foster, C., Knapp, D., and Schmidt, D.H.: Cardiac rehabilitation program at Mount Sinai Medical Center, Milwaukee, J. Cardiac Rehabil. 2: 458–463, 1982.)

A. Absolute Contraindications

1. Patients on bed rest with motion restrictions
2. Prolonged or unstable angina pectoris
3. Recent acute MI and unstable
4. Resting diastolic blood pressure over 120 mm Hg or resting systolic blood pressure over 200 mm Hg
5. Inappropriate blood pressure response: orthostatic or exercise-induced and patient symptomatic
6. Severe atrial or ventricular dysrhythmias
7. Second- or third-degree heart block
8. Recent embolism, either systemic or pulmonary
9. Thrombophlebitis
10. Dissecting aneurysm
11. Fever greater than 100°F; for the patient in the critical care area, 102°F
12. Excessive sternal movement—contraindication for upper extremity and trunk ROM exercises
13. Uncompensated heart failure
14. Active pericarditis (primary) or myocarditis
15. Severe aortic stenosis (> 50 mm Hg gradient)
16. Acute systemic illness

B. Relative Contraindications

1. Resting diastolic blood pressure over 110 mm Hg or resting systolic blood pressure over 180 mm Hg
2. Inappropriate increase in blood pressure with exercise
3. Hypotension (see comments in subsequent pages)
4. Moderate aortic stenosis (25 mm to 50 mm Hg gradient)
5. Compensated heart failure
6. Significant emotional stress
7. Pericarditis associated with myocardial revascularization surgery
8. Resting ST depression (≥ 3 mm)
9. Uncontrolled diabetes
10. Neuromuscular, musculoskeletal, or arthritic disorders that would prevent activity
11. Excessive incisional drainage
12. Sinus tachycardia greater than 120 beats/min at rest
13. New electrocardiographic (ECG) changes postoperative or post-MI indicative or suggestive of fresh infarct
14. Ventricular aneurysm
15. Symptomatic anemia (hematocrit < 30 per cent)

C. Conditions Requiring Special Consideration and/or Precautions

1. Conduction disturbances
    a. Left bundle branch block

      b. Wolff-Parkinson-White syndrome
      c. Lown-Ganong-Levine syndrome
      d. Bifascicular block
2. Controlled dysrhythmias
3. Fixed-rate pacemaker
4. Mitral valve prolapse
5. Angina pectoris and other manifestations of coronary insufficiency
6. Electrolyte disturbance
7. Cyanotic heart disease
8. Marked obesity (20 per cent above desirable body weight)
9. Renal, hepatic, and other metabolic insufficiency
10. Moderate-to-severe pulmonary disease
11. Intermittent claudication

Some of the above contraindications may seem somewhat vague and arbitrary. The reason for this is because it is difficult to get a consensus on many of the conditions considered. In most cases, clinical judgment takes precedence, and this may vary greatly among physicians. For example, a resting ST-segment depression of 3 mm or greater is the consensus of experts, but who is to say that 2 mm or 4 mm may be a better criterion? Another vague issue is what constitutes dangerous dysrhythmias. Clinical judgment about what individual medical directors and referring physicians are comfortable with is important. In addition, the competence of the staff and the extent of supervision, as well as whether the patient is being monitored for ECG rhythm, would make a difference. In many institutions, the monitored inpatient program is used in conjunction with other methods to evaluate drug therapy for dysrhythmias. In this situation, even ventricular tachycardia (VT) may not be a contraindication to exercise. In addition, patient records, including physical and mental status and medications, are reviewed by the medical director of the cardiac rehabilitation program and by the attending physician before acceptance into the program. An example of an important medical evaluation form can be found in Appendix B, Figure B–2.

Once the patient is accepted into the program, the activity schedule guidelines listed in Table 8–5 for MI patients and in Table 8–6 for CABG patients are initiated. The various exercises and stages of progression for the MI patient have been modified from the program outlined by Wenger.[57] The guidelines are designed in three parts: (1) the activity program when the cardiac rehabilitation staff is supervising the patient; (2) the ward activity when the primary nurse or patient supervises the program; and (3) patient education. These guidelines were designed so that at step 6 of the MI protocol and step 5 of the CABG protocol, the patient goes to an inpatient exercise center once a day for the activity part of the program.[55] This will be discussed further later, but if treadmills and stationary cycles are not available, the program would be continued in the patient's room and adjacent ward.

Generally, the patient progresses one step each day. The rate of progression is individualized and depends on how successfully the patient adapts to each stage of the program. The following guidelines are used either to modify (reduce) or to terminate the exercise routine:[29,38]

1. Fatigue
2. Failure of the monitoring equipment
3. Lightheadedness, confusion, ataxia, pallor, cyanosis, dyspnea, nausea, or any peripheral circulatory insufficiency
4. Onset of angina with exercise
5. Symptomatic supraventricular tachycardia
6. ST displacement ($\geq$ 3 mm horizontal or downsloping from rest)
7. Ventricular tachycardia
8. Exercise-induced left or right bundle branch block
9. Onset of second- and third-degree heart block
10. R on T PVCs (1)
11. Frequent unifocal PVCs ($>$ 10/min)
12. Frequent multifocal PVCs ($>$ 4/min)
13. Couplets ($>$ 2/min)
14. Increase in HR over 20 beats/min above standing resting HR for both MI and CABG patients
15. Inappropriate drop in resting (orthostatic) and exercise systolic blood pressure. See comments below.
16. Excessive blood pressure rise: systolic $\geq$ 220 or diastolic $\geq$ 120 mm Hg
17. Inappropriate bradycardia (drop in heart rate $\geq$ 10 beats/min) with increase or no change in work load

EARLY PHASE I PROGRAM

The early part of the phase I program is conducted in the critical care units and the intermediate critical care areas. As mentioned earlier, the program begins in the critical care unit as soon as the patient is considered stable. Although the guidelines listed in Tables 8–5 and 8–6 are geared for the MI and CABG surgery patients, they can be adapted for use with patients having varied diagnoses and symptomatology. Patients who appear to be at a higher risk or who are symptomatic with exercise are treated more conservatively. For example, patients who develop angina or severe dysrhythmia with exercise will usually train at a HR below the level at which signs or symptoms occur. Special precautions or management techniques used for patients with intermittent claudication, severe dysrhythmia, angina pectoris, arthritis, hypertension, excess fat, fixed rate pacemakers, pulmonary disease, other surgical procedures (valve, septal, or aneurysm repair), perioperative MIs, and percutaneous transluminal coronary angioplasty (PTCA) will be discussed later.

The programs for MI and CABG surgery patients differ in the following ways:

TABLE 8–5. POST MI INPATIENT (PHASE I) REHABILITATION PROGRAM GUIDELINES

Heart rates, blood pressures, and comments are recorded on Inpatient Data Record or Exercise Log.

STEP/DATE	CARDIAC REHAB/PHYSICAL THERAPY	WARD ACTIVITY*	PATIENT EDUCATION
1 1.5 METs _/_/_	WARD TX: Passive ROM to major joints, active ankle exercises, 5 Reps; deep breathing (supine) BID.	1. Bedrest. 2. May feed self.	Orient to CCU. Orientation to exercise component of rehabilitation program. Answer patient and family questions regarding progress, procedures, reason for activity limitation. Explain perceived exertion (RPE).
2 1.5 METs _/_/_	WARD TX: Active-assistive ROM to major muscle groups, active ankle exercises, 5 Reps; deep breathing (supine/sitting) BID.	1. Feeding self. 2. Partial AM care (washing hands and face, brushing teeth in bed). 3. Bedside commode.	
3 1.5 METs _/_/_	WARD TX: Active ROM to major muscle groups, active ankle exercises, 5 Reps; deep breathing (sitting) BID.	1. Begin sitting in chair for short periods as tolerated 2x/day. 2. Bathing self. 3. Bedside commode.	
4 1.5 METs _/_/_	WARD TX: Active exercises: shoulder: flexion, abduction; elbow flexion; hip flexion; knee extension; toe raises; ankle exercises; 5 Reps; deep breathing (standing) BID.	1. Bathroom privileges. 2. Sitting in chair 3x/day. 3. Up in chair for meals. 4. Bathing self, dressing, combing hair (sitting).	
5 1.5–2 METs _/_/_	WARD TX: Active exercises: shoulder: flexion, abduction, circumduction; elbow flexion; trunk lateral flexion; hip: flexion, abduction; knee extension; toe raises; ankle exercises; 5 Reps (standing); BID. Monitored ambulation of 100–200 ft, BID (refer to diagram on last page) with physician approval.	1. Bathroom privileges. 2. Up as tolerated in room. 3. Stand at sink to shave and comb hair. 4. Bathe self and dress. 5. Up in chair as tolerated.	Answer patient and family questions. Orient to ICCU phase of recovery. Present discharge booklet and other printed material (AHA). Encourage patient and family to attend group classes or do 1:1 sessions.

Step / METs	Ward TX / Exercise Center	Activity	Instructions
6 1.5–2 METs / /	WARD TX: STANDING: Exercises outlined in Step 5, 5–10 Reps; once daily. Monitored ambulation for 5 min (≤40 ft.) EXERCISE CENTER: Transport to Inpatient Exercise Center (IEC) for monitored ROM/strengthening exercises from Step 5, 5–10 Reps; leg stretching (posterior thigh muscles, gastrocnemius), 10 Reps; treadmill and/or bicycle 5 min; and stair-climbing (2–4 stairs) with physician approval.	1. Continue ward activity from Step 5. 2. Increase ambulation up to 1** Lap (440 ft) with assistance if appropriate, 2x/day. 3. Walk short distance in hall (room and quad area) as tolerated.	Instruction in pulse-taking and rationale. Explain value of exercise. Present T-shirt and activity log.
7 1.5–2.5 METs / /	WARD TX: STANDING: Exercises from Step 5 with 1 lb weight each extremity, 5–10 Reps; once daily. Monitored ambulation for 5–10 min (440–1100 ft) EXERCISE CENTER: Transport to IEC for monitoring ROM/strengthening exercises from Step 6 with 1 lb weight each extremity, 5–10 Reps; leg stretching, 10 Reps; treadmill and/or bicycle 5–10 min; and stair-climbing (4–8 stairs).	1. Continue ward activity from Step 6. 2. Sit up in chair most of the day. 3. Increase ambulation up to 3 Laps (up to 1100 ft) daily.	Begin discharge instructions with patient and family when appropriate. Encourage group class attendance or offer 1:1 as needed.
8 1.5–2.5 METs / /	WARD TX: STANDING: Exercises from Step 5 with 1 lb weight each extremity, 10 Reps, once daily. Monitored ambulation for 10 min (up to 1980 ft) if appropriate. EXERCISE CENTER: Ambulate to IEC for monitored ROM/strengthening exercises from Step 6 with 1 lb weight each extremity, 10 Reps; leg stretching, 10 Reps; treadmill and/or bicycle 10–20 min; and stair-climbing (10–12 stairs).	1. Continue ward activity from Step 7. 2. Increase ambulation up to 5 Laps (up to 1980 ft) daily.	
9 1.5–2.5 METs / /	WARD TX: STANDING: Exercises from Step 5 with 2 lb weight each extremity, 10 Reps; once daily. Monitored ambulation if appropriate. EXERCISE CENTER: Ambulate to IEC for monitored ROM/strengthening exercises from Step 6 with 2 lb weight each extremity, 10 Reps; leg stretching, 10 Reps; treadmill and/or bicycle 20–25 min; and stair-climbing (12–14 stairs).	1. Up as tolerated in room and quad area. 2. Increase ambulation up to 5 Laps (up to 2640 ft) daily.	Begin instruction in home exercise program. Initiate referral to Phase 2 if appropriate. Explain predischarge graded exercise test (PDGXT) and upper limit heart rate.

TABLE 8–5. POST MI INPATIENT (PHASE I) REHABILITATION PROGRAM GUIDELINES *(Continued)*

Heart rates, blood pressures, and comments are recorded in Inpatient Data Record or Exercise Log.

STEP/DATE	CARDIAC REHAB/PHYSICAL THERAPY	WARD ACTIVITY*	PATIENT EDUCATION
10	A predischarge graded exercise test is recommended at this time.	Continue previous ward activity.	Complete discharge instructions. Complete referral to Phase 2.

3 SOUTH ICCU CCU

SUN ROOM

3S DESK

ICCU DESK

1 LAP = 424 ft
12 LAPS = 1 mile*

NORTH

*Distance is 100 ft short of 1 mile.

ICU

CV-ICU

68 ft 100 ft

112 ft

CAST ROOM | GUEST LOUNGE

*Ward Activity = Activities performed alone, with family, or primary nurse.

**Lap = Distance of approximately 424 feet or once around the square.

(Courtesy of Cardiac Rehabilitation Program, Cardiovascular Disease Section, Mount Sinai Medical Center, Milwaukee, MI.)

TABLE 8–6. POST OPEN HEART SURGERY INPATIENT (PHASE I) REHABILITATION PROGRAM GUIDELINES

Heart rates, blood pressures, and comments are recorded in Inpatient Data Record or Exercise Log.

STEP/DATE	CARDIAC REHAB/PHYSICAL THERAPY	WARD ACTIVITY*	PATIENT EDUCATION
1 1.5 METs _/_/_	AM WARD TX: SITTING: with feet supported: active-assistive to active ROM to major muscle groups, active ankle exercises, active scapular elevation/depression, retraction/protraction, 3–5 Reps; deep breathing. Monitored ambulation of 100 ft as tolerated. PM WARD TX: SITTING with feet supported: Active ROM to major muscle groups, 5 Reps; deep breathing. Monitored ambulation 100–200 ft with assistance as tolerated.	1. Begin sitting in chair (when stable) several times/day for 10–30 min. 2. May ambulate 100–200 ft. with assistance, 1–2x daily.	Orient to CVICU. Reinforce purpose of physical therapy and deep breathing exercises. Orient to exercise component of rehabilitation program. Answer patient and family questions regarding progress.
2 1.5 METs _/_/_	WARD TX: SITTING: repeat exercises from Step 1 and increase repetitions to 5–10; deep breathing BID. Monitored ambulation of 200 ft with assistance as tolerated (stress correct posture) BID.	Continued activities from Step 1.	Continue above.
3 1.5–2 METs _/_/_	WARD TX: STANDING: Begin active upper extremity and trunk exercises bilaterally without resistance (shoulder flexion, abduction, internal/external rotation, hyperextension, circumduction backwards; elbow flexion; trunk lateral flexion, rotation); knee extension (if appropriate); ankle exercises; 5–10 Reps; BID. Monitored ambulation of 300 ft BID.	Increase ambulation to 300 ft or approximately 3 corridor lengths at slow pace with assistance, BID.	Begin pulse-taking instruction when appropriate and explain RPE scale. Answer questions of patient and family. Reorient patient and family to ICCU. Encourage family attendance at group classes.
4 1.5–2 METs _/_/_	WARD TX: STANDING: Active exercises from Step 3, 10–15 Reps; BID. Monitored ambulation of 424 ft BID.	Increase ambulation to 1 Lap** (424 ft or once around square) at slow pace with assistance BID.	

319

TABLE 8–6. POST OPEN HEART SURGERY INPATIENT (PHASE I) REHABILITATION PROGRAM GUIDELINES *(Continued)*

Heart rates, blood pressures, and comments are recorded in Inpatient Data Record or Exercise Log.

STEP/DATE	CARDIAC REHAB/PHYSICAL THERAPY	WARD ACTIVITY*	PATIENT EDUCATION
5 1.2–2.5 METs __/__/__	WARD TX: STANDING: Active exercises from Step 3, 15 Reps; once daily. Monitored ambulation for 5–10 min (424–848 ft) as tolerated. EXERCISE CENTER: Walk to Inpatient Exercise Center (IEC) for monitored ROM/strengthening exercises from Step 3, 15 Reps; leg stretching (posterior thigh muscles, gastrocnemius), 10 Reps; treadmill and/or bicycle 5–10 min (refer to treadmill/bicycle protocol) with physician approval.	1. Increase ambulation up to 3 Laps (up to 1320 ft) daily as tolerated. 2. Begin participating in daily ADL and personal care as tolerated. 3. Encourage chair sitting with legs elevated.	Orient to IEC. Continue instruction in pulse-taking and use of RPE scale. Explain value of exercise. Present T-shirt and activity log.
6 1.5–2.5 METs __/__/__	WARD TX: STANDING: Active exercises from Step 3 with 1 lb weight each upper extremity, 15 Reps; once daily. Monitored ambulation for 10–15 min (up to 1980 ft) if appropriate. EXERCISE CENTER: Walk to IEC for monitored ROM/strengthening exercises from Step 5 with 1 lb weight each upper extremity, 15 Reps; leg stretching, 10 Reps; treadmill and/or bicycle 15–20 min; and stair-climbing (6–12 stairs) with assistance.	1. Increase ambulation up to 5 Laps (up to 1980 ft) daily. 2. Encourage independence in ADL. 3. Encourage chair sitting with legs elevated.	Give discharge booklet and general discharge instructions to patient and family. Encourage group class attendance. Individual instruction by physical therapist, nutritionist, pharmacist.
7 2–3 METs __/__/__	WARD TX: STANDING: Active exercises from Step 3 with 1 lb weight each upper extremity, 15 Reps; once daily. Monitored ambulation for 15–20 min (up to 3300 ft) if appropriate. EXERCISE CENTER: Walk to IEC for monitored ROM/strengthening exercises from Step 5 with 1 lb weight each upper extremity, 15 Reps; leg stretching, 10 Reps; treadmill and/or bicycle 20–30 min; and stair-climbing (up to 14 stairs) with assistance.	1. Continue activities from Step 6. 2. Increase ambulation up to 8 Laps (up to 3300 ft) daily.	Discuss referral to Phase 2 program if appropriate.

Step / METs	Ward/Exercise Activity	Ambulation	Teaching
8 2–3 METs __/__	WARD TX: STANDING: Exercises from Step 3 with 2 lb weight each upper extremity, 15 Reps; once daily. Monitored ambulation if appropriate. EXERCISE CENTER: Walk to EC for monitored ROM/strengthening exercises from Step 5 with 2 lb weight each upper extremity, 15 Reps; leg stretching, 10 Reps; treadmill and/or bicycle 20–30 min; and stair-climbing (up to 16 stairs).	1. Continue activities from Step 7. 2. Increase ambulation up to 9 Laps (up to 3746 ft) daily.	Reinforce prior teaching. Explain pre-discharge graded exercise test (PDGXT) and upper limit heart rate. Continue with possible referral to Phase 2.
9 2–3 METs __/__	WARD TX: STANDING: Exercises from Step 3 with 2 lb weight each upper extremity, 15 Reps; once daily. Monitored ambulation is appropriate. EXERCISE CENTER: Walk to EC for monitored ROM/strengthening exercises from Step 5 with 2 lb weight each upper extremity, 15 Reps; leg stretching, 10 Reps; treadmill and/or bicycle 20–30 min; and stair-climbing (up to 18 stairs).	1. Continue activities from Step 8. 2. Increase ambulation up to 12 Laps (up to 5060 ft) daily.	Finalize discharge instructions. Complete referral to Phase 2.
10 2–3 METs __/__	WARD TX: STANDING: Exercises from Step 3 with 3 lb weight each upper extremity, 15 Reps; once daily. Monitored ambulation if appropriate. EXERCISE CENTER: Walk to EC for monitored ROM/strengthening exercises from Step 5 with 3 lb weight each upper extremity, 15 Reps; leg stretching, 10 Reps; treadmill and/or bicycle 20–30 min; and stair-climbing (up to 24 stairs).	1. Continue activities from Step 9. 2. Increase ambulation up to 14 Laps (up to 5940 ft) daily.	
11 __/__	A pre-discharge graded exercise test (PDGXT) is recommended at this time.		

*Ward Activity = Activities performed alone, with family, or primary nurse.

**Lap = Distance of approximately 424 feet or once around square. See diagram in Table 8.5 on page 318.

(Courtesy of Cardiac Rehabilitation Program, Cardiovascular Disease Section, Mount Sinai Medical Center, Milwaukee, WI.)

1. Surgical patients begin the program sooner and usually ambulate on the first treatment day.
2. Surgical patients progress at a slightly higher intensity (approximately 0.5 mph), and duration of ambulation is more accelerated.
3. Upper extremity ROM exercise is emphasized more with the surgical patient.

Although cardiac rehabilitation programs have many similar components, they often differ in their execution. Most inpatient programs include ROM exercise, ambulation, and stair-climbing activities. One exception is the reluctance of some surgeons to allow surgical patients to do upper extremity ROM activities. Since 1977, Mount Sinai Medical Center in Milwaukee, Wisconsin, has used active ROM exercise with surgical patients. Their experience shows that approximately 95 per cent of surgical patients can do upper extremity ROM exercises with no overt problems. Patients who experience sternal movement or who have postsurgical sternal wound complications will not perform these exercises.

Why are upper extremity ROM exercises important in the early recovery from open heart surgery? Significant soft tissue and bone damage of the chest wall and of the anterior and superior regions of the arms and shoulders occurs during surgery. If these areas (joints, muscles, and other supporting tissues) are not taken through a full range of motion, adhesions develop, and musculature becomes weaker and foreshortened. Patients will also favor these areas, which accentuates later problems of poor posture and difficulties in attaining their previous strength and full ROM. In addition, exercise increases blood flow to the damaged area and thus should accelerate tissue repair.[58] Thus, it appears that the longer the delay in receiving upper extremity ROM exercise, the more difficult it will be for the open heart surgery patient to reach full recovery.

Tables 8–5 and 8–6 outline the exercise prescription (ROM exercises, aerobic phase, and stair climbing) and patient education program for inpatient cardiac rehabilitation. The guidelines listed under the column entitled "Cardiac Rehabilitation/Physical Therapy" is performed by the cardiac rehabilitation staff. Ideally, the formal program will take place twice a day. Most treatments are performed in the patient's room or ward, but in the program outlined in Tables 8–5 and 8–6, patients begin receiving treatments once a day in an inpatient exercise center (step 6 for MIs and step 5 for CABG surgery patients). The diagram shown as a part of Table 8–5 illustrates how the cardiac ward can be measured for distance and used to provide a more precise progression in training.

Activities listed under "Ward Activities" are generally carried out by the patient under the supervision of the primary care nurse. The patient education program can be conducted by specialized educators, the primary nurse, or some combination thereof.

The education program usually involves both individual and group sessions. For the CABG patient, it includes presurgery assessment and instructions. The presurgery instructions contain an evaluation of ROM and strength. Knowing patient limitations and weaknesses before surgery often helps in the postsurgical assessment and recommendation of the exercise routine. If possible, the spouse is included in the education process. The main educational topics that can be covered include anatomy and physiology, risk factors, diet, pharmacology, stress reduction, return to sexual activity, exercise, getting ready to go home, and a general question-and-answer period. Special education booklets, films, and filmstrips have been developed for the MI and CABG patients and are available through several sources.[59-64]

The ROM exercises used in the cardiovascular intensive care unit for surgical patients typically include shoulder flexion, abduction, and internal and external rotation; elbow flexion; hip flexion, abduction, and internal and external rotation; and ankle plantar and dorsal flexion, inversion, and eversion for the surgery patients. The protocol for MI patient's in the critical care unit involves most of the same exercises as for surgical patients, excluding hip abduction and lower extremity internal and external rotation.

Before initiating the ROM exercises, each patient is evaluated by a physical therapist (exercise specialist). The position and type of exercise vary, depending upon the results of the evaluation. Tables 8–5 and 8–6 provide guidelines for the patient during this stage of their rehabilitation. Note the differences in patient position and progression of MI and surgical patients. Once patients leave the critical care areas, the ROM exercises described later in this chapter for surgical patients and for medical patients are used. Upper extremity ROM exercise with sticks or canes have been helpful with surgical patients. Initially, five repetitions of each exercise are performed with a progression to 10 to 15 repetitions. When patients can comfortably execute 10 to 15 repetitions, 1- to 3-pound weights can be added progressively.

Ambulatory activity and progression are described in Tables 8–5 and 8–6. Because hypotension is one of the major medical problems associated with early treatment of patients (particularly surgical),[39] the following guidelines may be recommended for use in patients first starting a cardiac rehabilitation program:

All patients will have orthostatic blood pressure measurements before beginning exercise. After obtaining a blood pressure on the patient in the sitting position, a second reading will be taken after the patient has been in a standing position for 30 seconds. Patients should be reminded to stand from a sitting position slowly to avoid lightheadedness. The systolic blood pressure should be at least 90 mm Hg before exercise. Typically, systolic blood pressure and heart rate rise with exercise. However, patients may be anxious initially, and resting blood pressure and HR may be higher than usual. During exercise, systolic blood pressure and HR may not increase over resting levels in this case.

The following procedure will be utilized to check for orthostatic and exercise-induced hypotension on the ward or later in the inpatient and outpatient exercise programs.

1. Symptomatic patients will not be exercised.
2. If the standing systolic blood pressure is below 90 mm Hg (without symptoms), the attending physician will be notified, and the patient will not be allowed to exercise until consulting with the medical director or attending physician.

3. If the patient exhibits a 10 to 20 mm Hg orthostatic drop in the systolic blood pressure (without symptoms), the medical director will be consulted before the patient exercises.
4. If the patient exhibits more than a 20 mm Hg orthostatic drop in the systolic blood pressure (without symptoms), the attending physician will be notified. If the attending physician wishes his or her patient to continue, the medical director will be consulted before the exercise session is begun.
5. Before the medical director or the attending physician is consulted regarding hypotension, blood pressure measurements will be taken in both arms by two staff members.

RANGE-OF-MOTION EXERCISES FOR THE SURGICAL PATIENT*

Upper Extremity Exercises

The purpose of these exercises is to stretch and strengthen muscles of the chest and shoulder girdle.

1. BEHIND HEAD PRESS

Starting Position: Stand erect with the feet shoulder-width apart, and hold the stick in front of body. Note that wrist weights are used only when a patient can satisfactorily complete 15 repetitions without weights.

Movement: Raise the stick straight out and up over the head. Lower the stick behind the head and then raise up over the head. Keeping the arms straight, return the stick to the starting position.

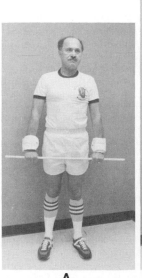 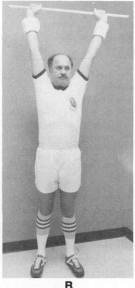 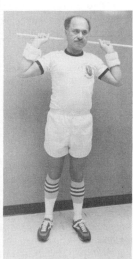

A   B   C

*Photographs from the Cardiac Rehabilitation Program, Mount Sinai Medical Center, Milwaukee, Wisconsin. Published with permission.

2. SWINGING STICK

Starting Position: Stand with the feet shoulder-width apart and hold the stick in front of the body, with the arms extended.

Movement: Using the stick, push one arm out to the side and up to ear level. Repeat to the other side.

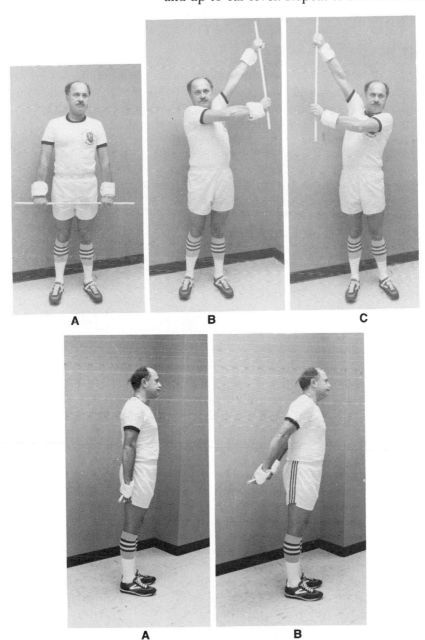

A   B   C

A   B

3. STICK BEHIND BACK (See bottom of page 325)

Starting Position: Stand erect with the feet shoulder-width apart; hold the stick behind the back, with hands shoulder-distance apart.

Movement: Move the stick backward, keeping the arms straight. All movement should come from the shoulders. Do not lean forward. Return to starting position.

4. STICK SLIDING UP BACK

Starting Position: Stand erect with the feet shoulder-width apart and the stick behind the back, with hands together and the arms extended.

Movement: Raise the elbows and slide the stick up the back as high as possible. Return to starting position.

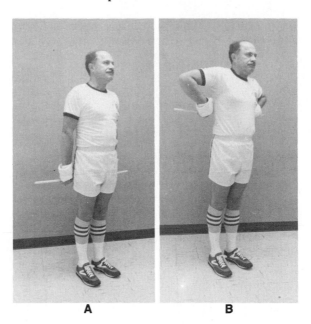

A   **B**

5. ARM CIRCLES

Starting Position: Stand erect with the fingertips touching shoulders.

Movement: Rotate elbows in large circles backward, emphasizing upward and outward movements of the shoulders.

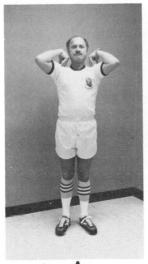 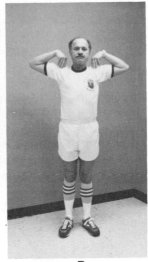

A   B

6. ADVANCED ARM CIRCLES

Starting Position: Stand erect with the arms extended sideways.

Movement: Rotate the arms backward in large circles. One- to 3-pound weights are ordinarily used with this exercise.

Note: Initially, completing this exercise with one arm at a time may be advisable with many patients.

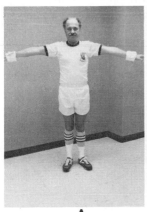 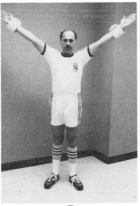 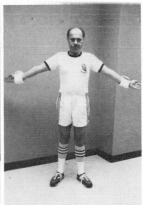

A   B   C

Trunk Exercises

The purpose of these exercises is to stretch the muscles of the trunk area.

7. SIDE BENDS

Starting Position: Stand erect with the feet shoulder-width apart and the hands on hips.

Movement: Without twisting the trunk or bending the knees, lean the trunk to the left as far as possible. Repeat to the right side. Keep the feet flat on the ground.

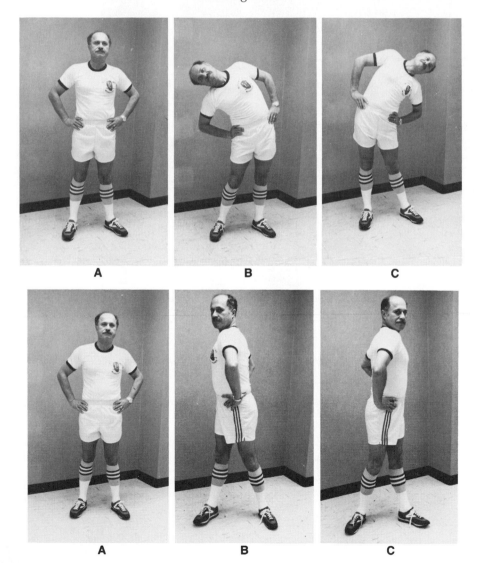

A   B   C

A   B   C

8. TRUNK ROTATION (See bottom of page 328)

Starting Position: Stand with the feet shoulder-width apart and the hands on hips.

Movement: Twist the trunk to the right. Repeat to the left. The head should be kept to the front.

Lower Extremity Exercises

The purpose of these exercises is to stretch the calf muscles and posterior thigh muscles.

9. CALF STRETCH

Starting Position: Stand an arm's length away from a wall with the feet less than shoulder-width apart and the toes turned slightly inward. Lean against the wall, with the head resting on the forearms. Relax the upper body.

Movement: Slowly move the hips forward, keeping the back straight, until stretch is felt in the back of the lower legs (calves). Hold for 30 to 60 seconds. Keep the heels on the floor.

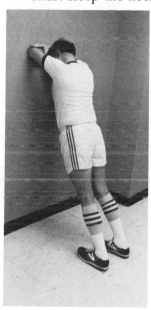

10. HAMSTRING STRETCHES (See top of page 330)

Starting Position: Sit on the floor with the legs extended in front.

Movement: Keeping the back of the knees against the floor, slowly reach the hands toward the feet and hold for 5 seconds. *Do not bounce or hold the breath.* Repeat 2 to 5 times.

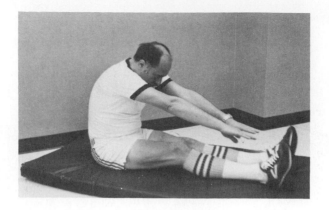

RANGE-OF-MOTION EXERCISES FOR MEDICAL PATIENTS*

Upper Extremity Exercises

    1. ARM RAISES

Starting Position: Stand erect, with the feet shoulder-width apart and the arms at the side. Note that wrist weights are used only when a patient can satisfactorily complete 10 repetitions without weights.

Movement: Raise both arms out straight and over the head. Return to the starting position.

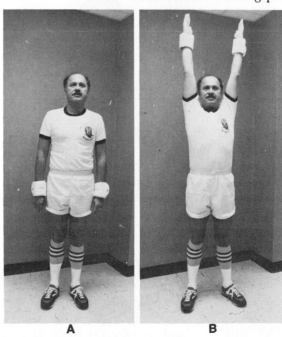

A   B

---

*Photographs from the Cardiac Rehabilitation Program, Mount Sinai Medical Center, Milwaukee, Wisconsin. Published with permission.

2. ARM RAISES TO SIDE

> *Starting Position:* Same as arm raises.
> *Movement:* Simultaneously raise arms to the side laterally and up overhead. Return to the starting position.

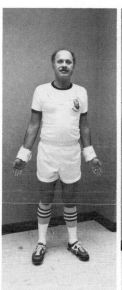 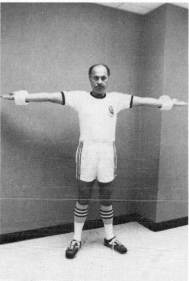 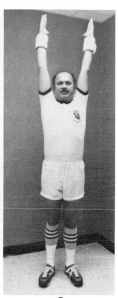

A   B   C

3. ARM CIRCLES

> Same as exercise number 5 for surgical patients.

4. ADVANCED ARM CIRCLES

> Same as exercise number 6 for surgical patients. Exercise both forward and backward.

5. ELBOW FLEXION (See top of page 332)

> *Starting Position:* Stand erect with the feet shoulder-width apart and with the arms at the side.
> *Movement:* Flex the elbows and bring the fingertips to the shoulders.

6. SIDE BENDS

> Same as exercise number 7 for surgical patients.

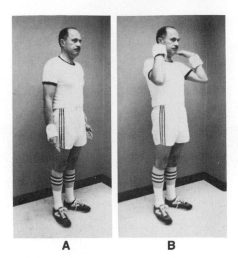

A   B

Lower Extremity Exercises

7. MARCHING IN PLACE

Starting Position: Stand erect (use the wall for balance purposes only), with the feet placed comfortably apart.

Movement: March in place, raising the leg to a comfortable height.

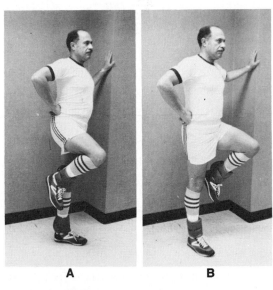

A   B

8. KNEE LIFT (may substitute for exercise number 7) (See top of page 333)

Starting Position: Sit in a chair with the feet flat on the floor.

Movement: Flex the hip and raise one knee upward. Return to the starting position. Repeat with the other leg.

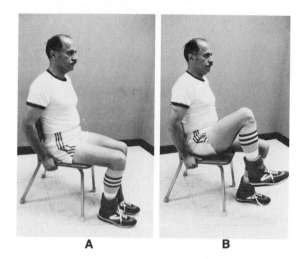

A   B

9. SIDE LEG LIFTS

Starting Position: Stand flat-footed, holding onto support.
Movement: Raise the right leg out to the side and return to the starting position. Repeat movement with the left leg.

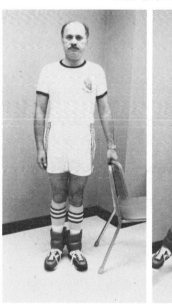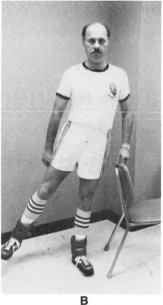

A   B

10. TOE RAISE   (See top of page 334)

Starting Position: Stand next to the table (for balance) with the feet 6 inches apart.
Movement: Raise up on the toes, bringing heels off the floor. Return to the starting position.

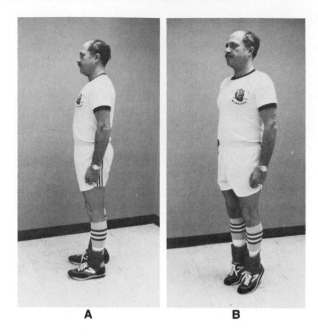

A   **B**

11. KNEE EXTENSION

Starting Position: Sit in a chair with the feet flat on the floor.
Movement: Fully extend the right leg. Return the leg to the initial position. Repeat with the left leg.

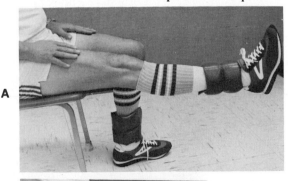

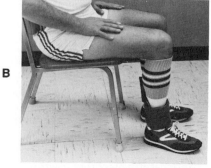

12. CALF STRETCH

Same as exercise number 9 for surgical patients.

13. ANKLE EXERCISE (may be substituted for number 12)

Starting Position: Sit in a chair with the feet flat on the floor.
Movement: Extend the leg and point the toes, first up and then down. Follow by rotating the feet in a circle, with motion occurring at the ankle. Repeat with the other ankle.

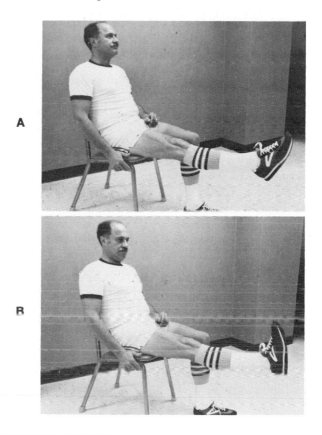

14. HAMSTRING STRETCHES

Same as exercise number 10 for surgical patient.

All early inpatient exercise is usually within a 2-MET level. Exercise HRs usually increase no more than 5 to 10 beats/min above resting levels for either ROM exercise or ambulation. Systolic blood pressure usually rises no more than 5 mm Hg for ROM exercise and 10 mm Hg for ambulation. Because of comprehension problems resulting from fatigue and medications associated with an MI or surgery, RPE is not determined until the third or fourth treatment day (see Chapter 6 for more details on RPE). The latter part of the early treatment phase is usually rated between 10 and 12 (fairly light) for both ROM exercise and ambulation.[39,65]

Two other important points to consider during the early rehabilitation phase are breathing exercises and how the patient sits on the side of the bed. When the patient begins to sit on the edge of the bed, the feet should be supported. Leg "dangling" is no longer permitted in most hospitals because the pressure of the mattress edge under the thighs tends to block venous blood return to the heart. This pressure promotes the same clotting tendency in static blood that the sitting up was intended to avoid. Therefore, a stool should be placed under the feet to lift the knees and thighs off the edge of the bed when the patient is sitting up. Diaphragmatic or "belly" breathing helps avoid atelectasis of the lower lobes of the lung near the diaphragm, i.e., the collapse of some air spaces of the lung that makes gas exchange impossible in the involved segments. A respiratory therapist or trained nurse or exercise specialist should initially provide instruction in these maneuvers. Some patients—most typically, those who have seen military service—have great difficulty in belly breathing when lying on their backs, since they are used to elevating the ribs and chest. The maneuver is often easier for these patients if they try it when lying on their side.

Much of the early phase I cardiac rehabilitation program should be monitored by direct or telemetered electrocardiographic units. A portable monitor can be used in the critical care areas, where direct monitors may be detached when the patient ambulates. Early ambulation in the critical care unit for surgery patients is supervised by a cardiac rehabilitation staff member with the assistance of the primary nurse. In the intermediate coronary care area, patients receive instruction on how to count HR. The palpation technique as described in Chapter 7 is used.

Figure 8–2 shows an example of a cardiac rehabilitation inpatient data record form. A special section entitled Cardiac Rehabilitation is recommended in the patient's chart. The availability of the inpatient daily record form, as well as the appropriate MI or surgical protocol inserted in the patient's chart, can be helpful to the attending or primary physician in patient assessment and in understanding at what level his or her patient is in the rehabilitation program.

LATER INPATIENT PHASE I PROGRAM

At this stage of rehabilitation, patients generally feel stronger; CABG patients are able to ambulate approximately 400 feet (usually the fifth or sixth postoperative day) and MI patients, 200 feet (usually the seventh or eighth day after the MI). In addition, they can complete 10 repetitions of the ROM exercises. At this stage, patients progress more rapidly in their ambulation program, and stair climbing can be introduced. ECG monitoring during training can become less frequent, and patients may become more independent in their ambulation program; i.e., during their regularly

Inpatient Data Record

Date of MI/Surgery ____________ Name ____________

Date	Time (0–2400)	Weight lb/kg	Step No.	Feet Amb	Heart Rate Rest	Heart Rate Immed. Post Ex.	Blood Pressures Rest	Blood Pressures Immed. Post Ex.	RPE*	Comments/Signature
/ /							/	/		
/ /							/	/		
/ /							/	/		
/ /							/	/		
/ /							/	/		
/ /							/	/		
/ /							/	/		
/ /							/	/		
/ /							/	/		
/ /							/	/		
/ /							/	/		
/ /							/	/		
/ /							/	/		
/ /							/	/		
/ /							/	/		

* Rating of Perceived Exertion.

Figure 8–2. The inpatient data record form is used to record vital information obtained during the inpatient cardiac rehabilitation. It is recommended that this record be included in the patient's chart. (Courtesy of the Cardiac Rehabilitation Program, Cardiovascular Disease Section, Mount Sinai Medical Center, Milwaukee, WI.)

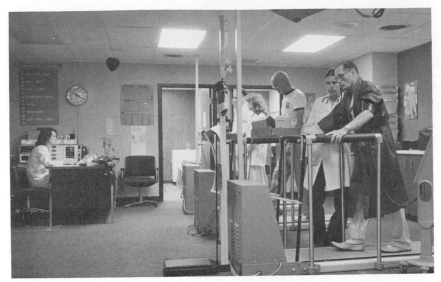

Figure 8–3. Inpatient Exercise Center.[55] Cardiac rehabilitation nurse station with four-channel ECG monitor at left with inpatient education classroom entrance in center background. Physical therapist is supervising patient during treadmill walking (right foot). (Courtesy of the Cardiac Rehabilitation Program, Mount Sinai Medical Center, Milwaukee, WI.)

scheduled exercise sessions, the cardiac rehabilitation staff may not find it necessary to spend the full time with the patient. As patients feel stronger, they should be encouraged to ambulate on their own in addition to the prescribed formal program.

As mentioned earlier and as outlined in Tables 8–5 and 8–6, much of the later inpatient phase I program can be conducted in a specially designed exercise room (step 5 of the CABG protocol and step 6 of the MI protocol). If an exercise room is used, it may be feasible to exercise a patient there only once a day. The second session would then be conducted in the ward. An example of an inpatient exercise center is shown in Figure 8–3.[55] In this example, the inpatient exercise center is located adjacent to the cardiology ward. It contains 4 treadmills, 1 cycle ergometer, a special set of stairs with a handrail for stair climbing, and a mat for ROM exercises. In the inpatient center, four patients can be monitored by telemetry at one time. A special inpatient exercise record has been developed for use in the inpatient exercise center (see example in Appendix B, Figure B–3). This additional record makes it easier to evaluate different activities separately.

In order to keep track of patient activity outside the formal program and to help reinforce certain monitoring techniques, activity logs may be used (see Appendix B, Fig. B–4). The log reminds patients of the need for keeping track of time and the distance ambulated or time and the resistance used for stationary cycling and for taking periodic determinations of HR and RPE. The back of the log has a conversion table for converting HR to beats per minute and an RPE scale.

Because most patients live in homes or visit facilities that require stair climbing, practice on stairs is recommended before hospital discharge. The practice of proper pacing gives the patient confidence in using stairs after discharge. Initially, all patients should be monitored for blood pressure before and immediately after stair climbing. Patients should climb stairs at a slow, comfortable pace, as tolerated. When taking the blood pressure reading after stair climbing, have the patient alternately shift weight from one leg to the other (step in place) to help prevent venous pooling and hypotension. A blood pressure reading should be taken before and immediately after climbing approximately 6 stairs. If there is less than a 10 to 20 mm Hg drop in the systolic blood pressure (without symptoms), the patient may climb six additional stairs, and a final blood pressure reading is taken. If the systolic blood pressure drops more than 20 mm Hg (without symptoms), no further stair climbing should be done that day, and the attending physician should be notified.

Does the sequence of activity make a difference in the patient's response to training? Usually not. Traditionally, patients begin their program with ROM exercise followed by either stair climbing or ambulation (stationary cycling). For asymptomatic patients who tend to develop hypotension during stair climbing, ambulating before stair climbing sometimes improves their response to subsequent stair climbing.

PROGRAMS FOR CARDIAC PATIENTS WITH SPECIAL MEDICAL PROBLEMS

There are specific problems associated with exercise prescription for cardiac patients with angina pectoris, diabetes mellitus, pacemaker implants, peripheral vascular disease (intermittent claudication), arthritis, amputations, paralysis, and pulmonary disease.

Angina pectoris is the squeeze or strangling in the chest first and best described by Heberden in 1772.[66] Although actual pain is present in moderately severe cases, angina is more frequently experienced as a severe discomfort or sense of constriction behind the breast bone.[67] Radiation of the discomfort up to the neck, jaw, individual teeth, or arms is typical. Since the appearance of anginal symptoms can be quite varied, upper abdominal discomfort without the chest component must be taken seriously. Palpation of the discomfort area may help to differentiate musculoskeletal pain from that of true angina.

The symptoms of angina can provide a warning to the individual approximately proportional to the electrocardiographic evidence of ischemia. Thus, the discomfort can be interpreted as a signal to ease up on either exertional intensity or psychological involvement. When the patient does recognize chest discomfort, it can be a useful guide to making the appropriate adjustments for such influences as cold, heat, humidity, previous meals, or continued psychological burden after a tense situation.

Because the perception of pain differs widely, attempts to grade the degree of discomfort on some simple scale have been extremely difficult. A rating from grade 1 to 4 has been useful, although more precise assessment would be preferable. A 1 to 4 grading system is advised by both the American Heart Association and the Canadian Cardiovascular Society.[67,68] The following descriptive comments listed by each grade is recommended for use by one of the authors of this text (SMF).

Grade 1 (light) is the discomfort that is established—but just established. Some patients speak of grade 1/2 discomfort as that premonitory sensation that precedes the grade 1 level as they walk, have sex, or get emotionally upset.

Grade 2 (light-moderate) discomfort is that from which one can be distracted by a noncataclysmic event. It can be "pain" but usually is not.

Grade 3 (moderate-severe) discomfort or pain prevents distraction by a pretty girl, handsome man, or TV show or other consuming interest. Only a tornado, earthquake, or explosion can distract one from grade 3 discomfort or pain. During exercise testing, it should rarely be permitted for long, even when no other evidence of danger exists. In an unsupervised situation, it should definitely be avoided.

Grade 4 (severe) is the most excruciating experienced or imaginable. It should be avoided completely.

Borg et al.[69] have used a 9-point scale to rate angina pectoris. The scale is as follows: 1, no discomfort; 2, extremely light; 3, very light; 4, rather light; 5, not so light, rather strong; 6, strong; 7, very strong; 8, extremely strong; and 9, maximum, unbearable.

ANGINA PATIENT. Nitroglycerin tablets should be available at all exercise classes. The anginal patient should carry nitroglycerin tablets in a light-resistant container. To insure freshness, they should be replaced at least every 6 months. Storage in the refrigerator may help preserve effectiveness. The nitroglycerin is sufficiently strong if it has a sharp, "bitey" taste and gives a pounding in the head, if not a brief (10 to 20 minute) headache.

The effective action of nitroglycerin should occur in 1 to 3 minutes and last for 10 to 30 minutes. If relief does not occur, one or two repeat tablets can be taken at 5-minute intervals. Pain for more than 15 minutes that persists after three rounds of active nitroglycerin tablets is usually considered sufficient cause to seek emergency medical treatment.

Two common ways for determining the upper limit training/target HR for anginal patients are (1) having patients exercise at a HR that is 5 to 10 beats/min below the onset of angina, or (2) calculating a HR that is 70 to 85 per cent of the anginal threshold. Some experimentation can be helpful. For example, sometimes a longer, slower warm-up period of 10 to 15 minutes may prevent or relieve symptoms or shift the anginal threshold upward. Although there is some controversy about allowing more stable patients to train with some anginal discomfort, it is generally not recommended to have patients attempt to walk through their angina when the discomfort level reaches 2 (4-point scale). If patients become proficient in detecting and rating their anginal discomfort, then they can be counseled to train at a level just below their threshold of discomfort (pain). The trial-and-error process should be accomplished in a supervised setting.

Taking nitroglycerin to help alleviate angina during training is an accepted practice. It is particularly useful for patients with a low angina threshold. Some institutions premedicate their angina patients prior to beginning their exercise routine.

DIABETES MELLITUS. For the patient with diabetes mellitus, two potential problems occur when exercising those who are insulin-dependent. The first problem is that lack of sufficient insulin may permit a hyperglycemic effect in the blood because cellular absorption of glucose is restricted. A second problem is the hypoglycemic effect, which can occur owing to an increased mobilization of depot insulin, particularly if the injection site was in the exercising muscle.[70–72] For this reason, it is strongly recommended that the injection site not be in the primary muscles involved in training.

Since physical activity has an insulin-like effect, the exercise program requires an insulin-dependent diabetic either to reduce insulin intake or to increase carbohydrate intake. To help regulate the dose response, the patient should be consistent in the amount of insulin taken and the time taken before the exercise session.[71] It is important to instruct the diabetic participant and the rehabilitation staff that during prolonged activities adequate nourishment must be available in the form of sugar, fruit juice, and/or other readily digestible carbohydrates.[70,71] The rehabilitation staff should be aware of any participants who are diabetic and their hypoglycemic symptoms. Special attention should be paid to patients taking insulin and beta blocker medication, as the hypoglycemic symptoms may be masked.

PACEMAKERS. For patients with new subclavicular permanent pacemaker implantation, no upper extremity movement with the affected arm is recommended for 24 to 48 hours. After 48 hours, upper extremity exercise is limited to that associated with normal daily activity. To prevent the pacemaker wire from dislodging, no additional ROM exercise should be performed for approximately the first 2 weeks. After this, upper extremity ROM exercises may commence. Patients with new abdominal permanent pacemaker implantation should not perform hamstring or gastrocnemius stretching for 2 weeks.

Patients with fixed-rate pacemakers who are 100 per cent dependent can still exercise.[73] The use of the RPE scale will be helpful in monitoring the training of these participants. Their systolic blood pressure should be monitored during training more frequently than for other patients. As long as systolic blood pressure makes the appropriate response and no signs or symptoms develop, then the heart should be adapting properly to the prescribed level of work.

INTERMITTENT CLAUDICATION. Patients with intermittent claudication are limited in their ambulation (cycling) program by their peripheral vascular disease rather than their heart condition. In this case, patients use an interval training method of exercise.[74] This will include 1- to 5-minute bouts of low-level aerobic exercise followed by 2 to 10 minutes of rest. This procedure may be repeated four to six times. As patients progress, longer periods of aerobic exercise should be introduced. Depending on where their blockage is located, some patients tolerate stationary cycling better than walking. In this case, at least 50 per cent of their aerobic program should be completed on the stationary cycle. Because walking will be a patient's major mode of transportation and walking training significantly improves walking performance,[74,75] some walking training is always recommended. Alternative exercises—e.g., swimming and rowing—should be considered as part of the training program for phases II and III.

In addition to using the RPE scale for monitoring the aerobic phase of training, it is also useful in rating peripheral discomfort (pain). Usually when the leg discomfort level reaches 13 to 15 (somewhat hard to hard), the rest period should commence.

ARTHRITIS—AMPUTEES. Arthritic or paralyzed patients or amputees are exercised in the activities that they can perform without undue symptomatology. Alternate aerobic activities may be substituted. For example, if lower extremity activities such as walking and stationary cycling cannot be performed or tolerated, arm ergometry with little or no resistance may be used. Patients with wheelchairs may be allowed to propel themselves slowly during this stage of their training program. Crutch walking is too strenuous at this phase of recovery and is not recommended. Caution should be taken with surgery patients so that little pressure is placed on the sternum. If sternal movement or clicking occurs, this type of activity should be discontinued. For phases II and III, other alternative activities—e.g., swimming, walking, or jogging in water—may be substituted.

PULMONARY PROBLEMS. Pulmonary patients (chronic obstructive pulmonary disease [COPD]) can be monitored and trained as described for patients with intermittent claudication. The main difference is that COPD patients usually are not able to progress as much in their training. Pulmonary patients should also have special education concerning pulmonary hygiene and breathing exercises.[76] Patients with severe COPD may need to train with an oxygen supplement. More detailed information about rehabilitation of the pulmonary patient is available.[77,78]

OTHER TYPES OF HEART OR RELATED PROCEDURES. Patients who have undergone open heart surgery for valve repair or replacement, aneurysm resection, or repair of septal defects can take part in the CABG surgery protocol as described in Table 8–6. What type of program is given to patients who have had percutaneous transluminal coronary angioplasty (PTCA)? Because the patients are discharged within 2 to 3 days after the procedure, there is little time to provide them with an inpatient program. Most hospitals who perform PTCA procedures routinely give pre- and post-procedure GXTs and other diagnostic tests. This would leave possibly 1 day for an evaluation from the cardiac rehabilitation staff. The exercise session should include the various components of a training program. The ROM exercises for MI patients are recommended. Usually, patients can complete the entire 10 repetitions of exercise, climb and descend one flight of stairs, and ambulate (stationary cycle) for 20 to 30 minutes. If the patients have had their GXT before their training session, the test results should be used as a guide for exercise prescription. A patient with a 5+ MET capacity should be able to complete the program previously mentioned, with ambulation being conducted at 2 to 3.0 mph for 30 minutes. After completion of the training session and GXT (if possible), a review of the principles of exercise and some instruction on counting HR and the use of the RPE scale are given. Then a 12-week home exercise program is designed and recommended for the patient. The program is individually designed, and PTCA patients usually can progress at a faster rate than MI and CABG patients.

At 2 weeks after discharge, PTCA patients usually return for a consultation with their cardiologist. If these patients are not involved in an organized outpatient program, it may be advisable to have them meet with someone from the cardiac rehabilitation staff for an exercise prescription update. Depending on time and facilities, the consultation can be simply a review and discussion of how the patients have progressed in their home programs. If time and facilities are available, the home program can be actually simulated in the outpatient clinic. The consultation would help clear up any questions and confusion that patients may have concerning their program, and, if necessary, their existing program can be modified.

PATIENT DISCHARGE

During the final couple of days in the hospital, patients should be primed in regard to continuing their program after discharge. If available, an organized outpatient program can be recommended. An organized program at this stage would be most important if patients are confused and apprehensive or are considered at high risk and if medical management is in transition—i.e., new medications are being used, or medications are being adjusted. For the latter reason, this type of surveillance can be important to the physician for patient management.

The predischarge plan includes dietary counseling, education on medications, and a home discharge consultation on exercise prescription. In addition, educational booklets designed to aid the patients in understanding their disease and how to cope with it are available and recommended.[59-64] These booklets often include a glossary of terms and a question-and-answer section on important issues.

The exercise plan for home use should include a list and description of the ROM, information on a walking or stationary cycling program, and recommendations for stair climbing and other potential activities. Basic guidelines on exercise prescription should be re-emphasized (warm-up, cool-down, progression, frequency, intensity, duration, modes, taking HR, and RPE). To help regulate intensity, patients should be given an upper limit target and training HR. A list of unfavorable symptoms to watch for may help make their program safer. If necessary, special instructions for exercising in a hot or cold environment should be included.

For inclement weather (hot, cold, or rain), indoor shopping malls are often available for walking. Maps of malls may be developed and given to patients for home use.

An important part of the discharge plan should include a summary progress report sent to the referring physician. The report may include information on progress in the various stages and activities of the inpatient program (including HR and blood pressure responses); medical problems associated with or observed during the program; ECG strips, if available; patient limitations; and recommended home program. An example of an inpatient progress report can be found in Appendix B, Figure B–5.

DETERMINATION OF THE DISCHARGE UPPER LIMIT TARGET/ TRAINING HEART RATE

There is no set answer as to the best manner in which to determine the target or training HR. A survey of experts in the field of cardiac rehabilitation from 18 inpatient centers showed that training intensity was kept low in all programs and below the patient's level of symptoms, but the means of determining an upper limit was quite varied.[38] There was 11 different ways in which the upper limit target and training HR was established. The two most common guidelines were (1) the use of fixed low-level HR (12 of 18) and (2) a certain HR above standing resting HR (5 of 18). In the former method, the upper limit HRs were usually between 110 and 120 beats/min. In the latter method, 10 to 20 beats/min above resting was most commonly used. One program used a HR of 140 beats/min as its upper limit of HR intensity. It must be noted that one director was reluctant to give an upper limit HR, indicating that the ultimate determination should be signs, symptoms, and perception of effort.

As mentioned earlier, the authors feel that in lieu of significant signs or symptoms, the upper limit target and training exercise HR for both medical and surgical patients should be approximately 20 beats/min above the standing resting heart rate for the inpatient. Unless a predischarge GXT is performed, this same standard is generally used until a symptom-limited GXT (SL-GXT) is performed at 6 to 8 weeks after the MI or surgery.

Why use 20 beats/min above standing resting and why not used a fixed low-level HR? Most inpatient activities are performed at a HR of 10 to 15 beats/min above standing rest (RPE is approximately 11 to 12).[39,65] In addition, because of the generally wide range of resting HRs in cardiac patients, 50 to 120 beats/min, a fixed HR seems inappropriate. For example, if a fixed HR of 110 or 120 beats/min were used, patients at one extreme would be allowed to double their resting HR, while at the other extreme would not be allowed to exercise because the resting HR was already at the fixed HR. Surgical patients are generally tachycardic, and many have resting HRs of 110 to 120 beats/min. In addition, SL-GXT data at hospital discharge have shown that 30 to 40 beats/min above standing

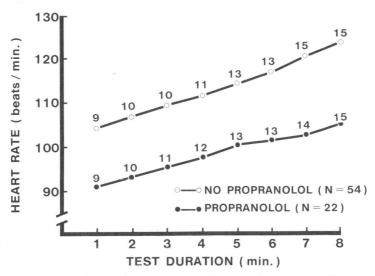

Figure 8–4. Increase in heart rate and rating of perceived exertion (RPE) during graded exercise testing in patients taking and not taking propranolol. Numbers above circles represent RPE. (Reprinted with permission from Squires, R.W., and Rod, J.L., Pollock, M.L., and Foster, C.: Effect of propranolol on perceived exertion soon after myocardial revascularization surgery. Med. Sci. Sports Exer. *14*:276–280, 1982.)

rest is nearly maximum for most patients, and 13 on the RPE scale is approximately 20 beats/min above standing rest.[79]

What about the patient on beta-adrenergic–blocking drugs? When these drugs are administered, the patient's HR is significantly depressed.[80,81] A dose-response relationship also exists between the quantity of the drug administered and HR reduction.[82] One study showed that early after CABG surgery, the average HR increment per MET increase in exercise intensity was 6 beats/min for patients not on propranolol therapy and 4 beats/min for patients using propranolol.[79] Thus, a chronotropic response is apparent after CABG surgery, whether the patient is on propranolol therapy or not. The same chronotropic response has been shown with MI patients.[83,84] This response seems to persist approximately 8 to 12 weeks after the MI or surgery.

Figure 8–4 shows the HR and RPE response to submaximal exercise using a modified Naughton protocol (2-minute stages) with patients who were administered propranolol and with ones who were not.[85] These data reveal that even though HR is significantly depressed at each work load with the propranolol group, RPE is the same. This is in agreement with similar studies conducted with noncardiac subjects. These findings, along with the data from Figure 7–2, are significant and give important information for exercise prescription. The data show that the guidelines used for determining target and training HR for patients not taking beta-adrenergic–blocking drugs can also be used for patients taking these drugs.[85,86]

Thus, as a result of the above-mentioned information, the following

TABLE 8–7. RESULTS FROM A PREDISCHARGE GRADED EXERCISE
TEST AND DETERMINATION OF UPPER-LIMIT TARGET AND
TRAINING HEART RATE, PATIENT NUMBER ONE*

PATIENT #1   AGE 44   HT 6′ 2″   WT 193 lb
SEX M   PREVIOUS MI YES   SURGERY 3 GRAFTS 7–23–80
MEDICATION COUMADIN
TYPE OF TEST PREDISCHARGE 8–7–80   PROTOCOL MODIFIED NAUGHTON

Time	METs	HR	BP	RPE
Rest	—	110	116/70	—
1		111		6
2	2	108	124/60	7
3		115		8
4	3	112	132/60	8
5		119		8
6	4	127	140/60	9
7		132		11
8	5	136	154/60	12
9		143		13
10	6	147	160/60	15
11		152		16
12	7	157	160/60	17

NORMAL RECOVERY   REASON FOR STOPPING: FATIGUE
• RECOMMENDED UPPER LIMIT HR 143
HIGHEST TRAINING HR INPATIENT CENTER 133, WORK LOAD 2.5–3 mph, 30 min

*Patient was recovering from CABG surgery and had an above-average MET capacity. See text for further information.

guidelines can be used for determining an upper limit target and training HR at hospital discharge.

1. Patients who *do* complete a GXT before hospital discharge.

    a. Medical status (signs and symptoms).
    b. Evaluation of patients' performance on the GXT and participation in the inpatient program.
    c. Heart rate that corresponds to an RPE of 13 (somewhat hard) on the predischarge GXT.
    d. Clinical judgment.

2. Patients who *do not* complete a GXT before hospital discharge. In lieu of medical problems, a HR of 20 beats/min above standing rest should be used.

3. If significant signs or symptoms can be identified, a HR of 5 to 10 beats/min below that value is often used.

Tables 8–7 and 8–8 give examples of the results from a predischarge GXT and subsequent determination of upper limit target and training HR of two patients without complications. The patients had no significant signs

TABLE 8-8. RESULTS FROM A PREDISCHARGE GRADED EXERCISE
TEST AND DETERMINATION OF UPPER-LIMIT TARGET AND
TRAINING HEART RATE, PATIENT NUMBER TWO*

PATIENT #2   AGE 51   HT 5' 10''   WT 210 lb
SEX M   PREVIOUS MI YES   SURGERY 5 GRAFTS 9-3-80
MEDICATION COUMADIN, ISORDIL, INDERAL
TYPE OF TEST PREDISCHARGE 9-12-80   PROTOCOL MODIFIED NAUGHTON

Time	METs	HR	BP	RPE
Rest	—	75	120/60	—
1		82		7
2	2	85	126/60	8
3		86		11
4	3	87	136/60	13
5		92		14
6	4	95	160/60	16
7	4.5	101	170/60	18

NORMAL RECOVERY   REASON FOR STOPPING: LEG FATIGUE-DYSPNEA
• RECOMMENDED UPPER LIMIT HR 92
HIGHEST TRAINING HR INPATIENT CENTER 90, WORK LOAD 2 mph, 30 min

*Patient was recovering from CABG surgery and had an average MET capacity. See text for
further information.

or symptoms and had normal HR, blood pressure, and RPE response to
exercise. The recommended upper limit HR of patient number one was set
at 143 beats/min. This was higher than the 133 beats/min HR achieved
during his last training session in the cardiac rehabilitation program. Since
his medical course was unremarkable and a HR of 143 was rated 13 on the
RPE scale, 143 was recommended. Patient number 2 was taking a beta-
adrenergic–blocking drug. Because the patient had ambulated for 30
minutes (2 mph) at a HR of 90 beats/min the previous day with no apparent
difficulty, a HR of 92 (RPE 14) was advised. As shown in both examples,
clinical judgment based on the factors listed under number 1, a to c, above,
was used in making the final HR designation.

Should patients attend cardiac rehabilitation sessions the same day they
receive a predischarge GXT? To prevent undue fatigue, the patient will be
advised to keep ambulation to a minimum on the day of the GXT. Undue
fatigue before taking the test will affect results. Other guidelines would
include the following:

1. Patients undergoing an exercise test (predischarge GXT or rest and
   exercise nuclear dynamic studies) in the afternoon may receive
   rehabilitation in the morning for ROM exercises.
2. Patients undergoing an exercise test in the morning may receive
   rehabilitation in the afternoon for ROM exercises. Depending on
   patient fatigue, ambulatory activity may have to be modified.

RESUMPTION OF SEXUAL ACTIVITY

One of the chief objectives of the predischarge exercise evaluation is to assess the risks of resuming sexual activity and to help compose a convincing presentation of the facts to both the patient and the spouse. Studies show that sexual intercourse with one's spouse approximates a 4 to 5 MET level of work and in most cases is associated with a HR lower than 130 beats/min.[87,88] Extramarital sexual relations are likely to cause a higher HR response.[89] Many physicians feel that if patients can climb two flights of stairs at a modrate rate without complications (HR of approximately 120 beats/min), then they are ready to resume sexual relations.[88]

Data suggest that there is a frequent reduction in sexual activity after an MI or CABG surgery.[87] Much of this reduction can be attributed to anxiety in the patient or spouse or both and apprehension of a recurring cardiac event. Thus, it is important that the cardiac rehabilitation team instruct the patient and spouse on how to achieve a healthy sex life through modifying the intensity and orchestrating the encounter with a light touch of low energy demand. Patient education materials that discuss the problem of resuming sexual activity and offer suggestions for coping with this situation are available.[59] If the evaluation suggests that sex can be undertaken at acceptably low risk, the patient needs to be reassured that he or she can resume sex and be an adequate partner. It is crucial, although not easy, to provide counsel in this area, even with the help of an early discharge evaluation. It is also important that the physician or other designated members of the rehabilitation staff initiate a discussion with and solicit questions from partners on this occasionally embarrassing topic. Usually, if the patient is medically stable and asymptomatic and has a MET capacity of at least 5 METs, sexual activity can be recommended as soon after hospital discharge as the patient desires.

OUTPATIENT CARDIAC REHABILITATION—PHASE II

Organized, supervised outpatient and nonsupervised home programs have become more established only in recent years. The earlier strategy was to send patients home to rest for a few weeks and then encourage them to participate in an organized phase III community program, some 2 to 3 months after discharge. A survey of experts in the field showed a lack of organized and supervised outpatient cardiac rehabilitation programs.[38] A review of exercise training in patients with CAD published by the American Heart Association emphasized the need in the early stages of rehabilitation for formal supervised classes with personnel trained in exercise prescription and cardiopulmonary resuscitation.[90] Although most of the experts surveyed agreed with this concept, only 6 of 17 programs had organized and supervised programs that commenced within 1 week of discharge. Of the six stations that had programs, two were not hospital-based and two were research programs.

Including home programs, 10 of 17 stations initiated their programs immediately after the patient had been discharged from the hospital; 4 of 17, within 2 to 4 weeks; and 3 of 17, within 6 to 12 weeks. Most experts agree that the first 6 to 8 weeks of rehabilitation are often the most critical for the patient. Because of the many anxieties and apprehensions that are apparent when the healing process is still incomplete and because medication dosage is often being altered to find the proper balance, it seems contradictory not to have well-planned and supervised outpatient programs soon after discharge. Therefore, the recent trend is to start patients earlier after hospital discharge and to give them more definitive guidelines and instruction before going home.

The outpatient program can begin when the patient is discharged from the hospital and is generally organized as a hospital-based or free-standing program, as a recommended home program, or as a program based in a community gymnasium type of facility. The outpatient phase of cardiac rehabilitation is the intermediate phase during which the patient progresses from a restricted low-level training program and a condition of unknown stability to a less restricted moderate-level training program and more stability. Programs conducted in hospitals and clinics usually include more telemetry monitoring of HR and ECG than those in the community setting. Details on the organization, administration, and facilities of various outpatient programs are available elsewhere.[14,46,47,91] Of particular interest would be the October 1982 issue of the *Journal of Cardiac Rehabilitation*.[91] This issue includes the description (programmatic and facilities) of 17 different well-established cardiac rehabilitation programs. An example of outpatient cardiac rehabilitation hospital-based programs is shown in Figures 8–5 to 8–8. Free-standing clinics may look similar. Thus depending upon available space, equipment, size of program, and so forth, the cardiac outpatient facility varies.

As mentioned previously, the patient should begin their home program as soon as possible. Keeping records of the home program on a log, as shown in Figure B–4 (Appendix B), is important. The information can be helpful to the patient's physician (or designate) on subsequent visits. Progress and improvement (or nonimprovement or regression) can be noted and problems resolved or modifications made. One study has shown that during their first 11 weeks after hospital discharge, patients who participated in a regular home exercise program had improved almost as much in aerobic capacity as patients who were in formal outpatient programs.[51] These data are encouraging, but for nonmotivated, apprehensive, and high-risk patients, the home program may not be preferable. Our experience has shown that during the first 12 weeks after hospital discharge, patients in nonsupervised home programs showed less progress (in duration and intensity) than patients in formal outpatient programs (unpublished data, Mount Sinai Medical Center, Milwaukee, Wisconsin).

Although more research is necessary to determine the optimal amount of supervision that is necessary or cost-effective for patient compliance with cardiac rehabilitation programs, most experts feel that 6 to 12 weeks may

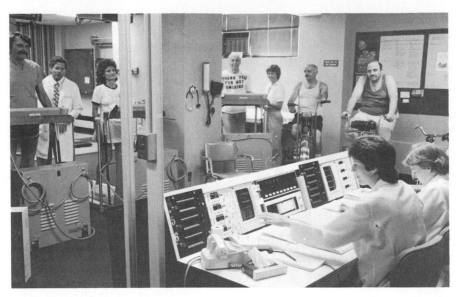

Figure 8–5. The figure shows a hospital-based outpatient exercise center. The nurses' station is shown in the foreground (eight-ECG telemetry monitoring units). The patient ROM/strengthening exercise area is in the background. Overhead monitors (upper left) can be rotated for observation in the ROM/strength training area. Exercise leaders are supervising patients on treadmills and cycle ergometers. Not shown are men's and women's locker rooms, education classroom, and lounge. (Courtesy of the Cardiac Rehabilitation Program, Mount Sinai Medical Center, Milwaukee, WI.)

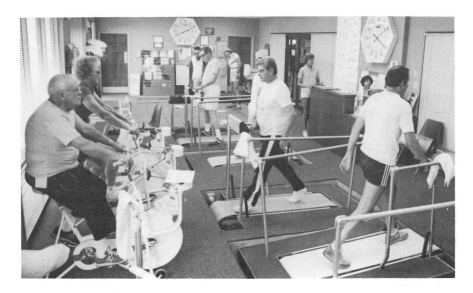

Figure 8–6. The figure shows an outpatient exercise center. The nurse's station is shown at the right (eight-ECG telemetry units are available), and the ROM/strength training area is in the background. (Courtesy of the Cardiac Rehabilitation Program, Arizona Heart Institute, Phoenix, AZ. From J. Cardiac Rehab. 2:453–456, 1982.)

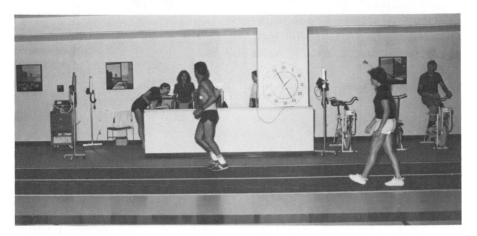

Figure 8–7. An outpatient exercise center with small indoor track and exercise facilities. The facility is used for both phase II and III programs. The nurse monitoring station is in the center. (Courtesy of the Cardiac Rehabilitation Program, Sid. W. Richardson Institute for Preventive Medicine, the Methodist Hospital, Houston, TX. From J. Cardiac Rehab. 2:453–456, 1982.)

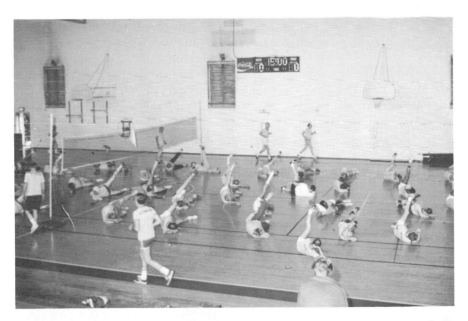

Figure 8–8. A combination community–hospital-based cardiac rehabilitation program facility. The gymnasium is connected to the Georgia Baptist Medical Center and houses a phase II and III program. (Courtesy of Cardiac Rehabilitation Program, Georgia Baptist Medical Center, Atlanta, GA. From J. Cardiac Rehab. 2:453–456, 1982.)

be a minimum. In programs in which patients live too far away from or do not have transportation to an outpatient facility, other methods of monitoring the home program are being used. For example, the Gunderson Clinic, La Crosse, Wisconsin, rents stationary cycle ergometers to their patients for home use and requires periodic but systematic visits to their center for progress checks. Patients who are at higher risk have telemetry by a telephonic system. In this way, a HR and ECG rhythm strip can be transmitted from the patient's home to the physician's office.

The formal outpatient program can begin as soon after discharge as the patient is referred. Having the referral forms signed before patient discharge can prevent unnecessary delays in program entrance. An example of an outpatient referral form is shown in Appendix B, Figure B–6. Upon entrance into the program, the program director or designate should explain the various aspects of the program to the patient. Realistic goals and expectations of the program should be covered. Patients should then be asked to read and sign an informed consent. An example of an outpatient informed consent is shown in Appendix B, Figure B–7.

The contraindications and guidelines used to modify or terminate the exercise routine listed for the inpatient program are also appropriate for the outpatient program. Exceptions to this should be mentioned in regard to ST-segment displacement and the systolic blood pressure rise during exercise. There is no exact standard of how much ST-segment displacement should be allowed during an exercise program. Most experts agree that 0.10 mV of horizontal or downsloping displacement from rest is significant, but depending on other medical factors concerning the patient's clinical status, opinions are varied with regard to the proper standard. The same variance of opinion exists with the upper limit for exercise systolic blood pressure. After the acute stage of recovery for CABG surgery or MI, many experts feel that the upper limit should be approximately 250 mm Hg. The upper limit target and training HR is calculated differently in the outpatient program and will be discussed in the following section.[38]

DETERMINATION OF INTENSITY OF TRAINING IN THE OUTPATIENT PROGRAM

The upper limit target and training HR standard used can vary significantly, depending on medical status, and number of weeks in the program, RPE, symptomatology, method of calculation, personal preference, and whether the patient had a GXT. [28,29,38,92] Table 8–4, under phase II program, describes the standards recommended for use in outpatient programs. The method of estimating the target and training HR described earlier for hospital discharge is used for the first 6 weeks of the outpatient program.

As in phase I, the philosophy is to keep the intensity low and to raise the work load by increasing duration of training. Table 8–9 shows a 12-step walking program that can be used in an outpatient program. The patients

TABLE 8–9. TWELVE-STEP WALKING PROGRAM FOR OUTPATIENTS

FUNCTIONAL CAPACITY (METs)	STEP	SPEED (mph)	ELEVATION (%)	DURATION (min)	METs	CALORIES (Kcal/min)
5 METs	1	1.5	0	20–30	2.0	2.0
	2	2.0	0	20–30	2.0	2.5
5–8 METs	3	2.0	0	5	2.0	2.5
		2.5	0	40–60	2.5	3,0
	4	2.5	0	5	2.5	3.0
		3.0	0	40–60	3.0	3.7
8 METs or greater	5	3.0	0	5	3.0	3.7
		3.5	0	40–60	3.5	4.2
	6	3.0	0	5	3.0	3.7
		3.5	0 (1 min)[a]	40–60	3.5	4.2
		3.5	2.5 (4 min)		4.2	5.9
	7	3.0	0	5	3.0	3.7
		3.5	0 (1 min)[a]	40–60	3.5	4.2
		3.5	2.5 (6 min)		4.2	5.9
	8	3.0	0	5	3.0	3.7
		3.5	0 (1 min)[a]	40–60	3.5	4.2
		3.5	2.5 (10 min)		4.2	5.9
	9	3.0	0	5	3.0	3.7
		3.5	0 (1 min)[a]	40–60	3.5	4.2
		3.5	2.5 (14 min)		4.2	5.9
	10	3.0	0	5	3.0	3.7
		3.5	2.5	40–60	4.2	5.9
	11	3.0	0	5	3.0	3.7
		3.5	0 (1 min)[a]	40–60	3.5	4.2
		3.5	5.0 (1 min)		6.9	7.5
	12	3.0	0	5	3.0	3.7
		3.5	0 (1 min)[a]	40–60	3.5	4.2
		3.5	5.0 (2 min)		6.9	7.5

[a] Two lines denote interval training; for example, in step six, the patient will alternate one minute at 0 per cent grade with four minutes at 2.5 per cent.

(Reprinted with permission from Pollock, M.L., Foster, C. and Ward A.: Exercise prescription for rehabilitation of the cardiac patient. *In* Pollock, M.L. and Schmidt, D.H., editors: Heart Disease and Rehabilitation. New York, John Wiley and Sons, 1979, pp. 413–445.)

progress from step to step as tolerated. Usually a patient should be stable at a step for a minimum of 1 to 2 weeks before progressing to a higher level. The duration of training varies and depends on the patient's level of tolerance and available time. As mentioned earlier, the ultimate goal is to have the patient progress in such a way that a minimum of 300 Kcal per session, or 1,000 Kcal per week, are expended. Therefore, at a slow-to-moderate walking speed, patients must eventually walk 45 to 60 minutes per session or increase the training frequency or both. Although patients are not necessarily expected to reach these kilocaloric levels during the outpatient program (many do), those patients who have a lower exercise tolerance or who are limited in time when visiting the outpatient exercise center may be encouraged to train twice a day, once at the center and once at home.

As mentioned in Table 8–4, 6 to 8 weeks after surgery or MI, a SL-GXT is recommended. Then the HR intensity is based on 70 per cent of HR

TABLE 8–10. RESULTS FROM 8-WEEK SYMPTOM-LIMITED GXT*

PATIENT #1 AGE 44 HT 6' 2" WT 193 lb
SEX M PREVIOUS MI YES SURGERY 3 GRAFTS 7–23–80
MEDICATION PRONESTYL
TYPE OF TEST SL MAX, 8 WEEKS 9–17–80 PROTOCOL MODIFIED NAUGHTON

Time	METs	HR	BP	RPE
Rest	—	100	116/70	—
1		99		6
2	2	100	134/70	6
3		103		6
4	3	104	134/70	7
5		109		8
6	4	112	136/70	10
7		120		10
8	5	126	146/70	11
9		133		12
10	6	138	160/70	12
11		142		13
12	7	145	166/70	14
13		152		14
14	8	158	170/70	15
15		163		16
16	9	167	172/70	16
17	9.5	173		17

NORMAL RECOVERY REASON FOR STOPPING: FATIGUE
BASED ON 70% OF MAXIMUM (KARVONEN)
• RECOMMENDED UPPER LIMIT HR 151

*Data shows improvement from the predischarge test (Table 8–7). New upper limit target and training heart rate is based on 70 per cent of the maximum heart rate reserve. See text for further information.

max reserve. This will usually increase the target and training HR by approximately 10 beats/min.[93] Examples of an SL-GXT 6 to 8 weeks after surgery and determination of upper limit target and training HR are shown in Table 8–10. Compare Table 8–7, predischarge GXT results, with Table 8–10 for differences in MET capacity and target and training HR. It should be noted that the target and training HR as described here (all phases) refers to an upper limit HR. Many programs use a lower HR limit as well as the upper limit. For example, the target and training HR could range from 60 to 75 per cent of HR max reserve. The idea would be to train the patient within that HR zone.

As patients improve, higher levels of intensity may be prescribed, depending on medical status. How soon can this higher intensity limit occur, and how does this relate to initiation of a jogging program? Although not generally recommended, a few programs allow patients to begin jogging in the early part of phase II. These few patients have had a discharge SL-GXT, have had no medical complications, and have an above-average fitness level.

TABLE 8-11. FIVE-STEP WALK-JOG PROGRAM FOR OUTPATIENTS

STEP	SPEED (mph)	ELEVATION (%)	DURATION (min)	METs	METs (avg/workout)	ENERGY COST[a] (Kcal/min)
1	3.0	0	5			3.7
	3.0 (1 min)[b]	0		3.0		3.7
	5.5 (1 min)	0	30–40	8.3	6.5	12.0
2	3.0	0	5			3.7
	3.0 (1 min)[b]	0		3.0		3.7
	5.5 (2 min)	0	30–40	8.3	7.24	12.0
3	3.0	0	5			3.7
	3.0 (1 min)[b]	0		3.0		3.7
	5.5 (4 min)	0	30–40	8.3	7.5	12.0
4	3.0	0	5			3.7
	3.0 (1 min)[b]	0		3.0		3.7
	5.5 (7 min)	0	30–40	8.3	7.7	12.0
5	3.0	0	5			3.7
	3.0 (1 min)[b]	0		3.0		3.7
	5.5 (10 min)	0	30–40	8.3	7.8	12.0

[a] Energy cost or kcal are based on an individual of 154 pounds of body weight (70 kg) walking 3.0 mph expending approximately 3.7 Kcal/min, and jogging 5.5 mph expending about 12.0 Kcal/min. To calculate the number of calories expended during a workout, multiply the number of calories expended per minute for each workload by the number of minutes at that workload.

[b] Two lines represent interval training program. For example, in step 1, after a 5 minute warm-up, the patient will alternate walking for 1 minute with jogging for 1 minute.

(Reprinted with permission from Pollock, M.L., Foster, C., and Ward, A.: Exercise prescription for rehabilitation of the cardiac patient. In Pollock, M.L., and Schmidt, D.H., editors: Heart Disease and Rehabilitation. New York, John Wiley and Sons, 1979, pp. 413–445.)

Philosophically, it does not seem necessary to accelerate the rehabilitation process until after the estimated 6- to 8-week healing period. After the 6- to 8-week SL-GXT, patients without complications who are above average in fitness may safely initiate a jog-walk program. These patients are usually younger than average (< 50 years of age) and have a MET capacity above 8. Our experience has shown that once a patient can walk at 3.5 mph, 5 per cent grade, they can jog. A five-step walk-jog program is shown in Table 8-11. The starting jogging speed may vary from 4.75 to 5.5 mph and walking from 3.0 to 4 mph. The speed of walking and jogging should be regulated to keep the HR at a level at which a training effect will occur. Thus, the walking HR should not be allowed to go below 50 to 60 per cent of HR max reserve. Initially, the jogging HR may reach 75 to 80 per cent of HR max reserve. Of those patients who continue in an outpatient program for 2 to 3 months, approximately 30 per cent are capable of initiating a jogging program. After several weeks of a walk-jog program, or on reaching step 8 (Table 8-9) of walking, a patient is encouraged to progress to a community-based program. Some patients who are considered stable and who do not wish to progress to step 8 of walking also are encouraged to graduate to a community-based program.

It should be noted that the 6- to 8-week SL-GXT results could be used to classify patients into a fitness category, as shown in Table 6–3. Then the suggested starter programs and 20-week walk or walk-jog programs listed in Chapter 7 may be used.

What did the survey of experts mentioned earlier have to stay about regulating intensity of training in a phase II program? Returns show that as in the inpatient program, training intensity was kept at a low level in all programs and maintained below the patient's level of symptoms.[38] The standard used for determining the upper limit of training intensity varied. The diversity in program organization and philosophy (structured versus unstructured, supervised versus unsupervised, monitored with telemetry versus unmonitored, and different policies regarding GXT determination) added to the variety of methods used in prescribing training intensity for the outpatient. In general, exercise intensity was more conservative in the unsupervised programs.

With regard to intensity of training, the survey dichotomized the phase II program into early and late stages. The early stage was 1 to 6 weeks after discharge and generally culminated with an SL-GXT. In many programs, the later stage (after the SL-GXT) marked the beginning of entrance into a phase III program. This was generally true with programs that had no organized phase II program.

In the early stage, the most common guidelines for estimating the upper limit of training intensity were 20 to 30 beats/min above standing resting HR; HR of 120 to 130; and 5 to 10 beats/min below symptoms or endpoint on discharge GXT. Five programs had no set HR standard and instructed their patients to train at low work levels and to slow down or stop if symptoms occurred.

In the later stage of phase II, the guidelines for intensity used were 5 to 10 beats/min below achieved HR on SL-GXT, and 60 to 85 per cent of HR calculated as a per cent from zero to peak or 70 to 75 of HR max reserve on a SL-GXT. One medical director had established different guidelines according to whether the patient was in a supervised or an unsupervised program; i.e., in the later stage of phase II, the patient would train at either 80 to 85 per cent (supervised) or 70 to 75 per cent of HR max (unsupervised). Before making a decision on what technique should be used to calculate target and training HR, refer to the section on Estimation of Exercise Intensity in Chapter 7.

FREQUENCY AND DURATION OF TRAINING

The recommended frequency and duration of training during phase II is shown in Table 8–4. A daily program is recommended. If a patient is active in an organized outpatient program, this would usually represent 3 days per week in the organized program and 4 days per week in a home program. For patients who are not considered stable and are at high risk, the home program (unsupervised) would not be recommended. This may necessitate the patient attending the outpatient center 5 days per week, In the early stages of rehabilitation when the kilocaloric expenditure of a program is low, and before the patient goes back to work, an extra session per day at home is recommended.

Table 8–4 shows the duration of aerobic training starting at where it left off in the inpatient program. This will vary greatly, depending on whether a patient was involved in an inpatient program, medical status, and time of entry into the outpatient program. The goal is to increase the time of aerobic training to 45 minutes as rapidly as the patient can adjust. This may take from 2 to 4 weeks.

MODE OF TRAINING

The modes of training recommended for phase II are listed in Table 8–4. Steps for a walking and jogging program have been outlined in Tables 8–9 and 8–11 (also see Chapter 7). Stationary cycling is of equal value, and the time components and progressive stages used for walking and walking-jogging in Tables 8–9 and 8–11 can be used by substituting resistance for speed. Usually, stationary cycling can be initially tolerated at 100 to 300 kpm/min. If one work load cannot be tolerated for the required time span, then the interval training method should be used. For patients with low fitness, this may include some zero-resistance pedaling.

Often patients have uncalibrated stationary cycles for home use, thus making it more difficult to regulate their home program. In this case, more trial and error is involved. The patients should use the same time components as they would with the calibrated cycle, but intensity will be estimated solely by HR and RPE. In essence, the program conducted on a calibrated cycle will be regulated in a similar manner as with the uncalibrated cycle, but because of the known work load settings, adjustments can be made more quickly with the calibrated cycle.

Although swimming can be introduced in the phase II program, it is not recommended until after the 6- to 8-week GXT. This allows sufficient time for healing of the sternum and leg incisions in the surgery patient and heart tissue in the MI patient.[50] In addition, patient stability is particularly important before entering a swimming program. The advantages of a swimming program are many: It is an aerobic activity involving both arms and legs; it puts the patient in a nongravity type of situation, thus helping venous return; it keeps the HR lower (may allow symptomatic patients to do more exercise); it causes fewer musculoskeletal injuries; and it can be therapeutic for patients with arthritis, intermittent claudication, limb amputations, or paralysis.[58,94,95] Swimming or other water activities, such as walking or jogging in water (using arms to paddle in combination with legs), can be the best alternative aerobic conditioner for the aforementioned patients.

The wide variation in skill level and energy cost of swimming among patients are major problems in regulating such programs.[94,96,97] For nonswimmers and those with poor skills, swimming would most likely be an anaerobic activity and is not recommended. Walking in waist- or chest-deep water while paddling backward with the arms and the use of flotation devices around the waist for swimming on the back are two excellent ways of introducing water activities to patients, and are of particular help for the non-swimmer and swimmer with poor skills. Initially, it is recommended that nonswimmers begin their program on the side or back using the side or elementary back strokes. Frequent stops at the side of the pool should be made to count the pulse. It is also important to have the patient avoid either entry chilling or later uncomfortable cooling in a pool in which the temperature is too cold.[97]

After patients have had a sufficient amount of time to adjust to their water activities, their program can be regulated in much the same way as other aerobic activities; i.e., pacing will be regulated by HR and RPE with total time of the exercise period being increased to 45 minutes. In regard to regulating intensity of training by HR, it has been shown that the HR in the water is lower for a given work load as measured on the treadmill.[95,96] Therefore, if the target and training HR for water activity is estimated by a treadmill or cycle GXT, then the calculated swimming HR should be reduced 5 to 10 beats/min.

Along with the ROM exercises previously mentioned, strength training can also be emphasized at this stage of recovery. These activities are integrated as part of a total fitness program and as a result of the need a patient may have in preparation for return to work or leisure activities. What is the safety of this type of training? Keep in mind that moderate-to-heavy static exercise significantly increases blood pressure.[58,98–100] In addition, the increase in blood pressure is inversely related to the size of the muscle group involved.[99,100] For example, using a similar weight for the muscles involved in palmar flexion of the hand compared with elbow flexion would produce a significantly higher increase in blood pressure with the former. Therefore, the strength training recommended should be dynamic, with as little an isometric component as possible, and should use large muscle groups, e.g., arms, legs, shoulders, and back. When possible, avoid hand-gripping activities. As far as safety is concerned, the use of rhythmical arm activity at HR levels similar to those used for leg work has not been associated with increased dysrhythmia, ischemia, or incidence of cardiac events.[101,102]

What strength exercises can be included? In general, activities such as push-ups and sit-ups that have a significant isometric component to them are not recommended. Some programs use a circuit training method of training.[38,46] This method incorporates a combination of leg stations (stationary cycling, treadmill walking, and bench stepping) and arm stations (rowing, arm cranking and wheeling, and wall pulleys and/or light weights). This method produces improvement in both aerobic fitness and upper body strength.

Because strength development is specific in regard to how the muscle is trained, a more specific strength-training routine is necessary at this state of recovery. Therefore, a combination of calisthenic and weight-lifting exercises can be used. For example, Figure 8–9 outlines an upper body strength routine that can be used by uncomplicated patients beginning the second week of an outpatient phase II program. Most patients begin the weight-training program with 3-pound weights and progress to 5- to 7-pound weights before the 6- to 8-week SL-GXT. Depending on test results and patient needs, they may increase their weight up to 12 to 15 pounds before completing the phase II program. French curls would not be recommended for use with the surgical patient until the sternum is adequately healed.

Additional leg exercises are not included (except for ROM) because most patients are already getting leg strengthening with their aerobic activities. For the abdominal muscles, a modified bent-legged sit-up is used. In this modification, most patients will rest their arms across the chest and sit up through just the first one third of the range of motion. Patients should be taught not to hold their breath during any exercise and to take a full inspiration and expiration with each repetition. Most of the exercises recommended for home use (see pp. 325 to 335) are still recommended.

For uncomplicated patients after the 6- to 8-week SL-GXT, many of the general restrictions on lifting or pushing weight with the arms and shoulders are eliminated. This may include the addition of arm and shoulder ergometer activities, i.e., a combination arm-leg cycle ergometer (Airdyne, produced by Excelsior Fitness Corporation, Chicago, Illinois), rowing machine, and so on. The Airdyne ergometer (see Fig 8–5) allows a participant to train with a combination of arms and legs, legs only, and arms only. The arm-shoulder action is a push-pull movement that develops the muscles that will be used in many commonly performed work and recreation types of activities.

Research is needed to determine safe limits for weight training using moderate-to-heavy weights (resistance). It seems probable that many patients without complications can train with heavier weights. Possibly, weight training without the hand-gripping component will allow patients to do more safely.

PATIENT EDUCATION, ADDITIONAL FORMS, AND PROGRAM PROGRESS REPORT

As mentioned with the inpatient program, patient education should be a continued process and an integral part of all phases of cardiac rehabilitation. For the formal outpatient program, examples of a physician referral form and informed consent were described earlier and are shown in Appendix B, Figures B–6 and B–7. Other forms that may be helpful include a daily exercise record, data record of pertinent information, and an outpatient progress report (see Appendix B, Figures B–8 to B–10). The daily exercise record is used to keep accurate records of the patient's program. Pertinent information is kept on the various phases of the program, such as warm-up,

WARM-UP

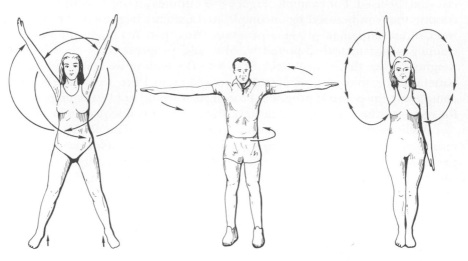

1. Full Body Stretch
    5–10 repetitions

2. Side Twist
    5 repetitions

3. Arm Circles
    5 repetitions–forward
    5 repetitions–backward

WEIGHT TRAINING

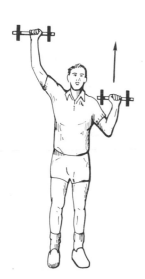
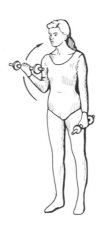
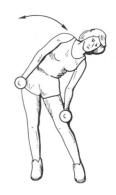

1. Shoulder Press
    2 sets of 8–12
    repetitions

2. Arm Curls
    2 sets of 8–12
    repetitions

3. Side Bends
    10–15 bends
    on each side

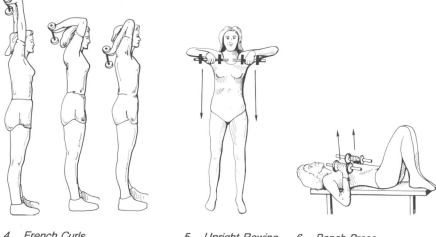

4. French Curls
    2 sets of 8–12 repetitions

5. Upright Rowing
    2 sets of 8–12
    repetitions

6. Bench Press
    2 sets of 8–12 repetitions

Figure 8–9. The upper body warm-up and weight training routine is introduced as early as 2 weeks after hospital discharge. This routine is used in the outpatient cardiac rehabilitation program, Mount Sinai Medical Center, Milwaukee, WI.

weight training, treadmill and/or cycle ergometer activity, and cool-down. In addition, ECG strips are taken each day (rest, peak exercise, and recovery) and are mounted separately.

The data record form summarizes important medical, physiological, and psychological information on each patient. Much of the information on this form should be self-explanatory. Line three lists risk factors and any special diet the patient may be on. Patient education (listed under V) includes initial assessment, introduction, risk factor education, and follow-up sessions. The body composition data are based on the sum of three skinfold fat measures (refer to the section on body composition measurement in Chapter 6).

Upon completion or termination of the outpatient program, patients are given a summary of their results (progress, potential problems, precautions, and so on) in the outpatient program. They are also given recommendations for a home program as well as a phase III community-based program. The outpatient progress report is mailed to the patient's referring physician.

COMMUNITY-BASED CARDIAC REHABILITATION PROGRAM—PHASE III

As mentioned earlier, the phase III program can be prescribed in an organized and supervised community-based setting or in an unsupervised home or community program. The discussion in this section will be directed toward the organized and supervised program, but many of the guidelines and suggestions can be applied to the unsupervised program.

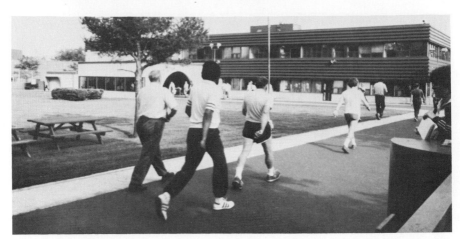

Figure 8–10. The outdoor walk-run track of the Toronto Rehabilitation Centre. The Nurse/exerise leader station at the right. The Centre's indoor facilities are shown in the background. (Courtesy of the Toronto Rehabilitation Centre, Toronto, Ontario, Canada. From J. Cardiac Rehab. 2:453–456, 1982.)

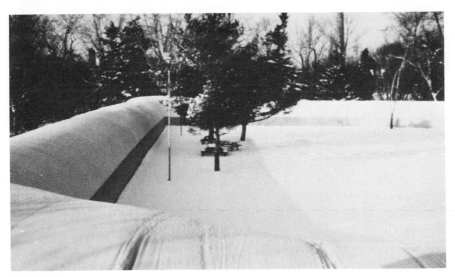

Figure 8–11. The outdoor walk-run track of the Toronto Rehabilitation Centre has a plastic bubble cover for the winter months. (Courtesy of the Toronto Rehabilitation Centre, Toronto, Ontario, Canada. From J. Cardiac Rehab. 2:453–456, 1982.)

A supervised phase III program is generally conducted at a YMCA, Jewish Community Center, community or private rehabilitation-prevention center, or university campus. Figures 8–10 to 8–12 show examples of indoor and combination indoor-outdoor facilities used for phase III cardiac rehabilitation programs. Both the Toronto Rehabilitation Centre and the Reh-Fit program do service some phase II patients. Although described under phase II programs, Figures 8–7 and 8–8 show facilities used for both

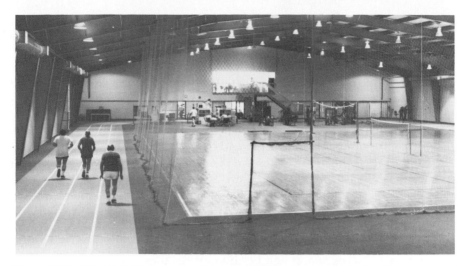

Figure 8–12. The Reh-Fit Program. A community-based program for healthy adults and cardiac patients. GXT and sports medicine rehabilitation equipment and facilities and program observation deck are located at the far end of the track. (Courtesy of the Reh-Fit Program, Winnepeg, Manitoba, Canada. From J. Cardiac Rehab. 2:453–456, 1982.)

phase II and phase III programs. Further descriptions of these programs are published elsewhere.[91]

A patient is admitted to the phase III program after receiving a physical examination and a SL-GXT and completing a medical history questionnaire. A physician referral form should also be required. Information related to medical status and the risk of further development of CAD is usually obtained during the physical examination, SL-GXT, and other tests. This information should be documented on the physician referral form. A current SL-GXT is important and should not be more than 3 months old. Phase III programs usually accept the same type of patient as described for the phase II program. Phase III patients have had more time to recover from their MI or surgical procedure and are generally more stable medically and stronger physically. The same contraindications to exercise and guidelines for modifying the training program described for the phase II program are also recommended for the phase III program. As a result of studies showing that the distance traveled to and from an exercise facility correlates well with program adherence,[103] patients should be recommended to attend the programs that are most convenient to their office or home.

The phase III facility is generally not attached or necessarily close to a hospital; thus a portable defibrillator with ECG recorder and monitoring scope, sphygmomanometer, and emergency drugs, equipment, and supplies should be on site for all training sessions.[46–48]

Table 8–4 shows the guidelines for exercise prescription used in the community-based phase III programs. At this phase of training, the exercise prescription is similar for both MI and CABG patients. In addition, the exercise prescription becomes more similar to that recommended for the healthy adult. The intensity of training is based on the patient's medical and physical status and on the results of the entry SL-GXT. The initial intensity prescribed is usually 70 per cent of the HRmax reserve. As a patient progresses in the program (1 to 6 months), the intensity can be adjusted upward and in some participants may reach 85 per cent of maximum. Some programs do not allow a significant upper limit target and training HR change until the patient has completed another SL-GXT. This SL-GXT is administered as a progress check between 3 and 6 months after entry into the phase III program. When patients enter the program 6 to 12 months after the MI or surgery and have already been quite active, they can progress at a faster rate. If such a patient is asymptomatic and has a high functional capacity, he or she could progress to a higher intensity HR after just a couple of orientation sessions. Usually a functional capacity of 8 to 10 METs is sufficient to be placed into a jogging regimen. Once patients are placed into a jogging type of program, it will be difficult for them to stay at the 70 per cent intensity level. If the patient has not been observed previously in a supervised program, however, waiting approximately a week to 1 month before increasing the intensity is recommended. As in the case of other phases of the program, the level of intensity is individualized, and the patient progresses only if it is considered safe and the patient so desires.

The duration of training is between 30 and 60 minutes and depends on available time and intensity of training. Table 8–12 shows a 16-step walk, walk-jog program for patients in a phase III program. The duration of training shown does not reflect the time needed for a warm-up or cool-down (see Table 8–3). The guidelines for progression in Table 8–12 are the same as those described for the outpatients, i.e., a patient should be considered stable for at least 1 to 2 weeks before advancing to a higher step. Initially, the patient is placed at the step that corresponds to his or her functional capacity and proven experience in another phase of the program. If there is any question regarding the proper step, take the conservative approach and place the patient in a lower step.

It should be noted that the starter programs and 20-week walking or walking-jogging programs listed in Chapter 7 may also be appropriate for use with cardiac patients. See Table 6–3 for assignment to the proper fitness category.

Patients with low functional capacities or those limited as a result of impaired coronary and ventricular function are not likely to progress to a jogging program. Although these patients cannot tolerate higher intensity work, they generally adapt well to activity of lower intensity and longer duration.[104,105] In this situation, the patient progresses by duration of training and in increments of 5 minutes. This situation should not be confused with the patient who has a low ejection fraction ($<$ 45 per cent) but has a moderate-to-normal functional capacity (8+ METs). These patients have a limited ventricular function but can often tolerate jog, walk-jog programs.[105] The suggested progression shown in Table 8–12 and subse-

TABLE 8–12. SIXTEEN-STEP WALK, WALK-JOG PROGRAM FOR CARDIAC
PATIENTS IN PHASE III (COMMUNITY BASED-HOME) EXERCISE PROGRAM

FUNCTIONAL CAPACITY (METs)	STEP	SPEED (mph)	DURATION (min)	METs	METs (avg/workout)	ENERGY COST (Kcal/min)
5 METs	1	2.5	30–60	2.5	2.5	3.0
	2	3.0	30–60	3.0	3.0	3.7
	3	3.25	30–60	3.25	3.25	4.0
5–8 METs	4	3.5	30–60	3.5	3.5	4.2
	5	3.75	30–60	4.0	4.0	4.9
	6	4.0	30–60	4.6	4.6	5.5
8 METs or greater	7	3.75 (2 min)[a]	30–45	4.0	4.6	4.9
		5.0 (30 sec)		6.9		8.3
	8	3.75 (2 min)[a]	30–45	4.0	5.0	4.9
		5.0 (1 min)		6.9		8.3
	9	3.75 (2 min)[a]	30–45	4.0	5.5	4.9
		5.0 (2 min)		6.9		8.3
	10	3.75 (1 min)[a]	30–45	4.0	6.0	4.9
		5.0 (2 min)		6.9		8.3
	11	3.75 (1 min)[a]	30–45	4.0	6.3	4.9
		5.0 (4 min)		6.9		8.3
	12	3.75 (1 min)[a]	30–45	4.0	6.5	4.9
		5.0 (6 min)		6.9		8.3
	13	3.75 (1 min)[a]	30–45	4.0	6.6	4.9
		5.0 (8 min)		6.9		8.3
	14	3.75 (1 min)[a]	30–45	4.0	6.6	4.9
		5.0 (10 min)		6.9		8.3
	15	3.75 (1 min)[a]	30–45	4.0	7.9	4.9
		5.5 (10 min)		8.3		10.1
	16	3.75 (1 min)[a]	30–45	4.0	8.0	4.9
		5.5 (12 min)		8.3		10.1

[a]Two lines denote interval training; for example, in step seven the patient will alternate 2 min of walking at 3.75 mph with 30 sec of jogging at 5.0 mph.

(Reprinted with permission from Pollock, M.L., Foster, C., and Ward, A.: Exercise prescription for rehabilitation of the cardiac patient. In Pollock, M.L., and Schmidt, D.H., editors: Heart Disease and Rehabilitation. New York, John Wiley and Sons, 1975, pp. 413–445.)

quent remarks are only guidelines; patient stability and perception of effort should override any predetermined plan.

The duration of training shown in steps 1 to 6 is longer than that of steps 7 to 16 because steps 1 to 6 are of lower intensity. The attempt is to fit the program to the patient's daily schedule or time frame and to increase the kilocaloric level (total work) of the program toward a 300-Kcal level.

Community-based programs usually require patients to attend class 3 days per week. Minimum acceptable attendance is usually 75 per cent. It is strongly recommended that the patients train 3 to 5 days per week. As previously mentioned in Chapter 3, 300 Kcal expenditure per training session and 1,000 Kcal per week seem to be important thresholds for developing and maintaining fitness. Concerning the latter, Sidney, Shephard, and Harrison[106] showed that older participants who trained at approximately 200 to 250 Kcal for a minimum of 4 days per week showed adequate improvement in cardiorespiratory function. The important point is that if the patient is training at a lower intensity, either or both the duration and frequency of training should be increased. Because of busy schedules, it is often difficult for patients to complete any more than a 30-minute aerobic program per session; thus, an increase in frequency (4 to 6 days per week) may be preferable. To maintain the necessary frequency of training, a home program is often needed. In this regard, a home program should follow the same guidelines as those described for the phase II outpatient program.

Table 8–4 shows that a wider variety of activities are available for the patient in a phase III program. The activity will still depend on medical status, functional capacity, needs and desires, time, and available facilities. Games and various endurance sport activities may not be recommended at this time. For example, unless a patient has successfully participated in a walk-jog, jog regimen for several weeks to 3 months, sport activities that include a jog-run component in it would not be recommended. In addition, activities such as golf and tennis may require the patient to have special preparation (strength and flexibility training) before starting. Once a patient has participated satisfactorily in the phase III program and can easily attain the MET requirement to take part in a specific activity (see Table 7–6), other activities can be encouraged. Highly competitive games and situations are not recommended. In certain situations, before a patient resumes normal work or leisure activities, he or she can perform the required or desired activity while being monitored by telemetry or Holter. In addition, it may be important to evaluate blood pressure. This type of monitoring may be useful in assessing the heart rhythm, blood pressure, and HR responses under conditions that simulate those of the unsupervised setting. Although this technique of evaluating patient activity has some limitations, the results tend to eliminate certain apprehensions and thus help the patient toward a full recovery.

Monitoring of the patient during the phase III program is accomplished through systematic checks of HR, blood pressure, and rhythm. Heart rate and rhythm strips are determined before, approximately halfway through, at the end of the training session, and before the patient leaves the exercise area (approximately 10 to 15 minutes). The rhythm monitoring may be accomplished with a defibrillator or quickly applied electrodes that are attached to a recorder. Blood pressure is checked before the training session and before the patient leaves the exercise area. If patients are symptomatic or have a questionable blood pressure response to exercise, then more frequent readings (during exercise and recovery) should be taken. Heart rate is usually checked by the patient using the palpation technique. In general, no routine continuous monitoring of patients with telemetry is usually done at this stage of training.

If local patients prefer to train at home rather than as part of a supervised program, they are encouraged to have periodic evaluations of their training routines. These evaluations may occur once every 2 weeks to several months, depending on their medical status and stage of training. These sessions can be conducted in either the community-based or the phase II outpatient setting, and the patients are monitored by telemetry under simulated exercise conditions. These specially monitored sessions are encouraged when the patient is making a major change in training intensity or duration.

As mentioned earlier, strength training and flexibility exercises should be an integral part of a well-rounded program. For patients with normal left ventricular function and average to above-average MET capacities, more strenuous exercise can be recommended. Other patients who are medically stable may also be encouraged to perform more strenuous activity, but they should initiate these activities under supervision. All patients should continue to avoid heavy static holds and other activities that include a moderate but steady static component, such as water skiing.

SURVEY OF EXPERTS

In the survey of experts in the field, 17 phase III programs were examined.[38] Of the 17 programs, 8 accepted patients at 8 weeks and 5 at 12 weeks after MI or surgery. The others accepted patients earlier, and these programs coincided with ongoing outpatient programs. All but one program required an SL-GXT before entry into the program. The one program required a GXT to 90 per cent of age-predicted HR max.

The frequency of training for the community-based programs was 3 days per week ($\pm$ 0.7). Several programs used a combination of supervised (community-based) and unsupervised (home) training sessions. Two of 17 programs had patients train 3 days per week in a supervised program for the first 3 months, then 2 days supervised and 1 day unsupervised for the next 3 months, and finally 1 day supervised and 2 days unsupervised for the next 3 months. The idea was to have the patients gradually become independent, so that they would not always have to rely on a supervised program. About 50 per cent of the programs encouraged their patients to walk at home on days they did not have to report to the formal program.

Duration of training (aerobic phase) averaged 31.3 minutes ($\pm$ 7.2) per exercise session. Although the duration of training ranged from 20 to 60 minutes, few programs increased the duration of aerobic work beyond 40 minutes (6 of 17). Two of 17 programs had durations of 20 to 25 minutes for aerobic training.

Intensity of training for phase III programs centered mainly on the following two methods: 60 to 85 per cent of HR max and 60 to 85 per cent of HR max reserve. Heart rate monitoring was accomplished by telemetry or hard wire hook-ups, using either quick hook-up electrodes from an ECG or paddles from a defibrillator, and by palpating the pulse. In 5 of 17 programs, patients were routinely monitored by telemetry or hard wire at least once a week for the first 2 to 4 weeks of training. Another three programs monitored workouts by telemetry on a few patients when deemed necessary. Most programs required the patients to check their HRs when they entered the exercise area, at the middle and end of their aerobic workouts, and before leaving the exercise area. Initially, blood pressure was determined before and after each training session in 13 of 17 programs. Less attention was paid to blood pressure monitoring and the number of times that HR was counted as the patients progressed in the program.

The community-based programs used a single mode of aerobic training (12 of 17), a single mode plus recreational game activities (4 of 17), or circuit training (1 of 17). Walking, walking-jogging, jogging, and stationary cycling were the activities most used.

Seven of 17 programs required a physician, and 8 of 17 required a nurse to be present at all training sessions. Three other programs always had a physician present in the building or adjacent area, and four programs had a physician present at least once a week. The physician generally used this time to review cases, to modify exercise prescriptions, and to speak with patients.

SUMMARY

This chapter has described in detail the manner in which exercise is prescribed to cardiac patients in an inpatient (phase I), outpatient (phase II), and community-based (phase III) program setting. The risks and medical problems associated with cardiac rehabilitation programs were discussed. The risks of fatal or nonfatal coronary events were shown to be low and significantly reduced in more recent years. Guidelines for staffing, medical safety, and monitoring patients were discussed. Although medical problems exist, it was shown that initiating programs early after MI or CABG surgery is safe and beneficial to the patient.

Inpatient programs for patients without complications usually begin 3 days after MI or 1 to 2 days after open heart surgery. Programs are conducted at a low intensity and emphasize ROM exercise, ambulation, and stair climbing. Outpatient programs are recommended for at least 8 to 12 weeks after hospital discharge, followed by 3 to 6 months in a community-based program.

The standards for exercise prescription were outlined, and the common features of training programs for normal healthy adults and cardiac patients were discussed. Because of the physical limitations of the cardiac patient, progression of exercise is slower, intensity is lower, frequency is greater, and duration is longer than in healthy individuals. In the early stages of rehabilitation, the patient cannot tolerate long bouts of exercise; thus, the prescription includes shorter periods of exercise conducted approximately two or three times per day. As for noncardiac patients (Chapter 7), 300 Kcal per exercise session or 1,000 Kcal per week of energy expenditure, is suggested as a minimal threshold for development and maintenance of cardiorespiratory fitness and weight control.

The need for a well-rounded training program for patients was discussed. It was recommended that strength training be included early in the recovery process (phase II) so that patients may be better prepared to carry out work and leisure activities. In addition, the importance and need for ROM exercise in surgical patients as early as 1 to 2 days after surgery was stressed.

Monitoring of exercise sessions was accomplished in a variety of ways. Early ambulation was usually monitored by direct wire or telemetry systems for HR and ECG rhythm. Although there were diverse opinions regarding how long and to what extent sophisticated monitoring should take place, most experts believed that 6 to 8 weeks of continuous or periodic monitoring was ideal. Longer periods of monitoring were recommended for patients at high risk and with dangerous rhythm disturbances. Guidelines for blood pressure monitoring and the use of the rating of perceived exertion scale for exercise prescription were discussed. During phases II and III, rhythm strips were often obtained periodically by a defibrillator or electrode hook-up, and blood pressure was frequently determined before and after exercise.

The results of a survey of experts in the field of cardiac rehabilitation revealed the diversity of methods by which exercise is currently prescribed as well as the lack of organized cardiac rehabilitation programs for which the experts felt a need. The experts surveyed differ in many aspects of the exercise prescription, particularly in the recommendation for exercise intensity. Depending on the phase of the various programs, for instance, there were 8 to 11 different methods of prescribing exercise intensity, and training intensities prescribed during phases II and III varied from 10 to 25 beats/min. To gain insight into the determination of exercise prescriptions, most directors administered a SL-GXT 6 to 12 weeks after surgery or MI. The predischarge GXT appeared to be developing as a standard procedure for both diagnosis and exercise prescription. In general, exercise prescription for the cardiac patient should start early but progress slowly, include rhythmical activity of low intensity, emphasize greater frequency and longer duration, be individualized, and help the patient become independent and return to a normal life.

REFERENCES

1. Lewis, T.: Disease of the Heart. New York, MacMillan, 1933, pp. 41–49.
2. Levine, S. A., and Lown, B.: The chair treatment of acute coronary thrombosis. Trans. Assoc. Am. Physicians 64:316–327, 1951.
3. Cain, H. D., Frasher, W. G., and Stivelman, R.: Graded activity program for safe return to self-care after myocardial infarction. J.A.M.A. 177:111–115, 1961.
4. Hellerstein, H. K., and Ford, A. B.: Rehabilitation of the cardiac patient. J.A.M.A. 164: 225–231, 1957.
5. Wenger, N. K.: The use of exercise in the rehabilitation of patients after myocardial infarction. J. S. C. Med. Assoc. 65:(Suppl. 1–12) 66–68, 1969.
6. Naughton, J., Bruhn, J. G., and Lategola, M. T.: Effects of physical training on physiologic and behaviorial characteristics of cardiac patients. Arch. Phys. Med. Rehabil. 49: 131–137, 1968.

7. Zohman, L. R.: Early ambulation of post–myocardial infarction patients: Montefiore Hospital. In Naughton, J. P., Hellerstein, H. K., and Mohler, L. C., editors: Exercise Testing and Exercise Training in Coronary Heart Disease. New York, Academic Press, 1973, pp. 329–336.

8. Karvonen, M. J., and Barry, A. J., editors: Physical Activity and the Heart. Springfield, IL, Charles C Thomas, Publisher, 1967.

9. Fox, S. M., Naughton, J. P., and Haskell, W. L.: Physical activity and the prevention of coronary heart disease. Ann. Clin. Res. 3:404–432, 1971.

10. Naughton, J. P., Hellerstein, H. K., and Mohler, L. C., editors: Exercise Testing and Exercise Training in Coronary Heart Disease. New York, Academic Press, 1973.

11. Amsterdam, E. A., Wilmore, J. H., and DeMaria, A. N., editors: Exercise in Cardiovascular Health and Disease. New York, Yorke Medical Books, 1977.

12. Wenger, N. K., and Hellerstein, H. K., editors: Rehabilitation of the Coronary Patient. New York, John Wiley and Sons, 1978.

13. Leon, A. S., and Blackburn, H.: Exercise rehabilitation of the coronary heart disease patient. Geriatrics 32:66–76, 1977.

14. Pollock, M. L., and Schmidt, D. H., editors: Heart Disease and Rehabilitation. New York, John Wiley and Sons, 1979.

15. Kellerman, J. J., editor: Comprehensive Cardiac Rehabilitation. Basel, S. Karger, 1982.

16. Kallio, V., Hamalainen, H., Hakkila, J., and Luurila, O. J.: Reduction in sudden deaths by a multifactorial intervention programme after acute myocardial infarction. Lancet 2 (8152):1091–1094, 1979.

17. Hjermann, I., Velve Dyre, K., and Holme, I.: Effect of diet and smoking intervention on the incidence of a randomized trial in healthy men. Lancet 2(8259):1303–1310, 1981.

18. Taylor, H. L., Henschel, A., Brozek, J., and Keys, A.: Effects of bed rest on cardiovascular function and work performance. J. Appl. Physiol. 2:223–239, 1949.

19. Saltin, B., Blomqvist, G., Mitchell, J., Johnson, R. L., Wildenthal, K., and Chapman, C. B.: Response to exercise after bed rest and after training. Circulation 37 and 38 (Supp. 7): 1–78, 1968.

20. Convertino, V., Hung, J., Goldwater, D., and DeBusk, R. F.: Cardiovascular responses to exercise in middle-aged men after 10 days of bed rest. Circulation 65:134–140, 1982.

21. Cassem, N. H., and Hackett, T. P.: Psychological rehabilitation of myocardial infarction patients in the acute phase. Heart Lung 2:382–388, 1973.

22. Morgan, W. P., and Pollock, M. L.: Physical activity and cardiovascular health: psychological aspects. In, Landry, F., and Orban, W. A. R., editors: Physical Activity and Human Well-being. Miami, Symposium Specialists, 1978, pp. 163–181.

23. Block, A., Maeder, J. P., Hassily, F. C., Felix, J., and Blackburn, H.: Early mobilization after myocardial infarction. A controlled study. Am. J. Cardiol. 34:152–157, 1974.

24. Haskell, W. L.: Cardiovascular complications during training of cardiac patients. Circulation 57:920–924, 1974.

25. Shephard, R. J.: Do risks of exercise justify costly caution? Phys. Sportsmed. 5:58–65, 1977.

26. Gibbons, L. W., Cooper, K. H., Meyer, B. M., and Ellison, R. C.: The acute cardiac risk of strenuous exercise. J.A.M.A. 244:1799–1801, 1980.

27. Hossack, K. F., and Hartwig, R.: Cardiac arrest associated with supervised cardiac rehabilitation. J. Cardiac Rehabil. 2:402–408, 1982.

28. American Heart Association: Exercise Testing and Training of Individuals with Heart Disease or at High Risk for its Development: A Handbook for Physicians. Dallas, American Heart Association, 1975.

29. American College of Sports Medicine: Guidelines for Graded Exercise Testing and Exercise Prescription, 2nd ed. Philadelphia, Lea and Febiger, 1980.

30. Granath, A., Sodermark, T., Winge, T., Volpe, U., and Zetterquist, S.: Early work load tests for evaluation of long-term prognosis of acute myocardial infarction. Br. Heart J. 39:758–763, 1977.

31. Theroux, P., Waters, D. D., Halphen, C., Debaisieux, J. D., and Mizgala, H. F.: Prognostic value of exercise testing soon after myocardial infarction. N. Engl. J. Med. 301: 341–345, 1979.

32. Dillahunt, P. H., and Miller, A. B.: Early treadmill testing after myocardial infarction. Chest 76:150–155, 1979.

33. Davidson, D. M., and DeBusk, R. F.: Prognostic value of a single exercise test 3 weeks after uncomplicated myocardial infarction. Circulation 61:236–242, 1980.

34. Starling, M. R., Crawford, M. H., Kennedy, G. T., and O'Rourke, R. A.: Exercise testing early after myocardial infarction: predictive value for subsequent unstable angina and death. Am. J. Cardiol. 46:909–914, 1980.
35. Koppes, G. M., Kruyer, W., Beckmann, C. H., and Jones, F. G.: Response to exercise early after uncomplicated acute myocardial infarction in patients receiving no medication: long-term follow-up. Am. J. Cardiol. 46:764–769, 1980.
36. McNeer, J. F., Margolis, J. R., Lee, K. L., Kisslo, J. A., Peter, R. H., Kong, Y., Behar, V. S., Wallace, A. G., McCants, C. B., and Rosati, R. A.: The role of the exercise test in the evaluation of patients for ischemic heart disease. Circulation 57:64–70, 1978.
37. Epstein, S. E.: Implications of probability analysis on the strategy used for noninvasive detection of coronary artery disease. Am. J. Cardiol. 46:491–499, 1982.
38. Pollock, M. L., Foster, C., and Ward, A.: Exercise prescription for rehabilitation of the cardiac patient. In Pollock, M. L., and Schmidt, D. H., editors: Heart Disease and Rehabilitation. New York, John Wiley and Sons, 1979, pp. 413–445.
39. Dion Faraher, W., Grevenow, P., Pollock, M. L., Squires, R. W., Foster, C., Johnson, W. D., and Schmidt, D. H.: Medical problems and physiologic responses during supervised inpatient cardiac rehabilitation: the patient after coronary bypass grafting. Heart Lung 11:248–255, 1982.
40. Savin, W. M., Haskell, W. L., Houston-Miller, N., and DeBusk, R. F.: Improvement in aerobic capacity soon after myocardial infarction. J. Cardiac Rehabil. 1:337–342, 1981.
41. American Heart Association/Wisconsin Affiliate: Recommendations for Insurance Coverage of Supervised Cardiac Exercise Rehabilitation Programs. Milwaukee, American Heart Association/Wisconsin Affiliate, 1980.
42. American Heart Association: Standards and guidelines for cardiopulmonary resuscitation (CPR) and emergency cardiac care (ECC). J.A.M.A. 244:453–509, 1980.
43. North Carolina Cardiac Rehabilitation Association: North Carolina Cardiac Rehabilitation Plan. Raleigh, North Carolina Division of Vocational Rehabilitation Services, 1983.
44. Fox, S. M.: Heart disease and rehabilitation: scope of the problem. In Pollock, M. L., and Schmidt, D. H., editors: Heart Disease and Rehabilitation. New York, John Wiley and Sons, 1979, pp. 3–14.
45. Brammel, H. L., Robertson, D. R., Darnell, R., McDaniel, J. W., and Niccoli, S. A.: Cardiac Rehabilitation Handbook for Vocational Rehabilitation Counselors. Denver, Webb-Waring Lung Institute, 1979.
46. Fardy, P. S., Bennett, J. L., Reitz, N. L., and Williams, M. D., editors: Cardiac Rehabilitation Implications for the Nurse and other Health Professionals. St. Louis, C. V. Mosby, 1980.
47. Wilson, P. K., Fardy, P. S., and Froelicher, V. F.: Cardiac Rehabilitation, Adult Fitness, and Exercise Testing. Philadelphia, Lea and Febiger, 1981.
48. Fry, G., and Berra, K.: YMCArdiac Therapy. Chicago, National Council of the YMCA, 1981.
49. Kavanagh, T., Shephard, R. J., Doney, H., and Pandit, V.: Intensive exercise in coronary rehabilitation. Med. Sci. Sports 5:34–39, 1973.
50. Wenger, N. K.: The physiological basis for early ambulation after myocardial infarction. In Wenger, N.K., editor: Exercise and the Heart. Philadelphia, F. A. Davis, 1978, pp. 107–116.
51. DeBusk, R. F., Houston, N., Haskell, W., Fry, G., and Parker, M.: Exercise training soon after myocardial infarction. Am. J. Cardiol. 44:1223–1229, 1979.
52. DeVries, H. A.: Physiological effects of an exercise training regimen upon men aged 52 to 88. J. Gerontol. 24:325–336, 1970.
53. Pollock, M. L., Dawson, G. A., Miller, H. S., Jr., Ward, A., Cooper, D., Headly, W., Linnerud, A. C., and Nomeir, M. M.: Physiologic responses of men 49 to 65 years of age to endurance training. J. Am. Geriatr. Soc. 24:97–104, 1976.
54. American College of Sports Medicine: Position statement on the recommended quantity and quality of exercise for developing and maintaining fitness in healthy adults. Med. Sci. Sports 10:vii–x, 1978.
55. Pollock, M. L., Foster, C., Knapp, D., and Schmidt, D. H.: Cardiac rehabilitation program at Mount Sinai Medical Center, Milwaukee. J. Cardiac Rehabil. 2:458–463, 1982.
56. Foster, C., Pollock, M. L., Anholm, J., Squires, R., Ward, A., Rod, J., Saichek, R., and Schmidt, D. H.: Randomized exercise and relaxation trials with myocardial revascularization surgery patients. J. Cardiac Rehabil. (in press).

57. Wenger, N. K.: Rehabilitation of the patient with acute myocardial infarction: early ambulation and patient education. *In* Pollock, M. L., and Schmidt, D. H., editors: Heart Disease and Rehabilitation. New York, John Wiley and Sons, 1979, pp. 446–462.
58. Åstrand, P. O., and Rodahl, K.: Textbook of Work Physiology, 2nd ed. New York, McGraw-Hill, 1977.
59. American Heart Association Professional Catalog for Physicians, Nurses, and Allied Health Professionals. Dallas, American Heart Association, 1982.
60. Billie, D. A., editor: Practical Approaches to Patient Teaching. Boston, Little, Brown, and Company, 1981.
61. Health/Patient Education Catalog. Bowie, MD, R. J. Brady Co., 1982.
62. Patient Education Materials 1982 Catalog. Atlanta, Pritchell and Hull Associates, 1982.
63. Hansen, M., Laughlin, J., Pollock, M. L., and Schmidt, D. H.: Heart Care—After Heart Attack. Redmond, WA, Medic Publishing Co., 1984.
64. Hansen, M., Laughlin, J., Pollock, M. L., and Schmidt, D. H.: Heart Care—After Heart Surgery. Redmond, WA, Medic Publishing Co., 1984.
65. Silvidi, G. E., Squires, R. W., Pollock, M. L., and Foster, C.: Hemodynamic responses and medical problems associated with early exercise and ambulation in coronary artery bypass graft surgery patients. J. Cardiac Rehabil. *2:*355–362, 1982.
66. Willius, F. A., and Keys, J. E.: Cardiac Classics. St. Louis, C. V. Mosby, 1941.
67. Hurst, W. J.: The Heart, 5th ed. New York, McGraw-Hill, 1982.
68. Champeau, L.: Grading of angina pectoris. Circulation *54:*522–523, 1976.
69. Borg, G., Holmgren, A., and Lindblad, I.: Quantitative evaluation of chest pain. Acta. Med. Scand. *644:*(Suppl.)43–45, 1981.
70. Richter, E. A., Ruderman, N. B., and Schneider, S. H.: Diabetes and Exercise. Am. J. Med. *70:*201–209, 1981.
71. Costill, D. L., Miller, J. M., and Fink, W. J.: Energy metabolism in diabetic distance-runners. Phys. Sportsmed. *8:*64–71, 1980.
72. Cantu, R. C.: A Practical, Positive Way to Control Diabetes, Diabetes and Exercise. New York, E. P. Dutton, 1982.
73. Superko, H. R.: The effects of cardiac rehabilitation in permanently paced patients with third degree heart block. J. Cardiac Rehabil. *3:*561–568, 1983.
74. Skinner, J. S., and Standness, P. E.: Exercise and intermittent claudication. II. Effect of physical training. Circulation *36:*23–29, 1967.
75. Hall, J. A., and Barnard, R. J.: The effects of an intensive 26-day program of diet and exercise on patients with peripheral vascular disease. J. Cardiac Rehabil. *2:*569–574, 1982.
76. Moser, K. M., Archibald, C., Hansen, P., Ellis, B., and Whelan, D.: Better Living and Breathing. A Manual for Patients. St. Louis, C. V. Mosby, 1980.
77. Wilson, P. K., Bell, C. W., and Norton, A. C.: Rehabilitation of the Heart and Lungs. Fullerton, CA, Beckman Instruments, 1980.
78. Unger, K. M., Moser, K. M., and Hansen, P.: Selection of an exercise program for patients with chronic obstructive pulmonary disease. Heart Lung *9:*68–76, 1980.
79. Rod, J. L., Squires, R. W., Pollock, M. L., Foster, C., and Schmidt, D. H.: Symptom-limited graded exercise testing soon after myocardial revascularization surgery. J. Cardiac Rehabil. *2:*199–205, 1982.
80. Epstein, S. E., Robinson, B. E., Kahler, R. L., and Braunwald, E.: Effects of beta-adrenergic blockade on the cardiac response to maximal and submaximal exercise in man. J. Clin. Invest. *44:*1745–1753, 1965.
81. Tesch, P. A., and Kaiser, P.: Effects of beta-adrenergic blockage on O_2 uptake during submaximal and maximal exercise. J. Appl. Physiol. *54:*901–905, 1983.
82. Pollock, M., Foster, C., Rod, J., Stoiber, J., Hare, J., and Schmidt, D.: Effect of propranolol dosage on the response to submaximal and maximal exercise. Am. J. Cardiol. (abstract)*49:*1000, 1982.
83. Powles, A. C. P., Sutton, J. R., Wicks, J. R., Oldridge, N. B., and Jones, N. L.: Reduced heart rate response to exercise in ischemic heart disease: the fallacy of the target heart rate in exercise testing. Med. Sci. Sports *11:*227–233, 1979.
84. Haskell, W. L., and DeBusk, R.: Cardiovascular responses to repeated treadmill exercise testing soon after myocardial infarction. Circulation *60:*1247–1251, 1979.
85. Squires, R. W., Rod, J. L., Pollock, M. L., and Foster, C.: Effect of propranolol on perceived exertion soon after myocardial revascularization surgery. Med. Sci. Sports Exer. *14:*276–280, 1982.

86. Pollock, M. L., and Foster, C.: Exercise prescription for participants on propranolol. J. Am. Coll. Cardiol. (abstract) 2:624, 1983.
87. Hellerstein, H. K., and Friedman, F. H.: Sexual activity and the post-coronary patient. Arch. Intern. Med. 125:987–999, 1970.
88. Skinner, J. S.: Sexual relations, and the cardiac patient. In Pollock, M. L., and Schmidt, D. H., editors: Heart Disease and Rehabilitation. New York, John Wiley and Sons, 1979, pp. 587–599.
89. Uno, M.: The so-called coition death. Jpn. J. Leg. Med. 17:333–340, 1963.
90. Scheuer, J., Greenberg, M. A., and Zohman, L. R.: Exercise training in patients with coronary artery disease. Mod. Concepts Cardiovasc. Dis. 47:85–90, 1978.
91. Froelicher, V. F., and Pollock, M. L., editors: Cardiac rehabilitation programs: state of the art 1983. J. Cardiac Rehabil. 2:429–514, 1982.
92. Pollock, M. L., Foster, C., Rod, J. L., and Wible, G.: Comparison of methods for determining exercise training intensity for cardiac patients and healthy adults. In Kellerman, J. J., editor: Comprehensive Cardiac Rehabilitation. Basel, S. Karger, 1982, pp. 129–133.
93. Gutmann, M. C., Squires, R. W., Pollock, M. L., Foster, C., and Anholm, J.: Perceived exertion-heart rate relationship during exercise testing and training in cardiac patients. J. Cardiac Rehabil. 1:52–59, 1981.
94. Magder, S., Linnarsson, D., and Gullstrand, L.: The effect of swimming of patients with ischemic heart disease. Circulation 63:979–986, 1981.
95. Thompson, D. L., Boone, T. W., and Miller, H. S.: Comparison of treadmill exercise and tethered swimming to determine validity of exercise prescription. J. Cardiac Rehabil. 2:363–370, 1982.
96. Holmer, I., Stein, E. M., Saltin, B., Ekblom, B., and Åstrand, P. O.: Hemodynamic and respiratory responses compared in swimming and running. J. Appl. Physiol. 37:49–54, 1974.
97. Fletcher, G. F., Cantwell, J. D., and Watt, E. W.: Oxygen consumption and hemodynamic response of exercises used in training of patients with recent myocardial infarction. Circulation 60:140–144, 1979.
98. Lind, A. R., and McNicol, G. W.: Muscular factors which determine the cardiovascular responses to sustained and rhythmic exercise. Can. Med. Assoc. J. 96:706–713, 1967.
99. Bezucha, G. R., Lenser, M. C., Hanson, P. G., and Nagle, F. J.: Comparison of hemodynamic responses to static and dynamic exercise. J. Appl. Physiol. 53:1589–1593, 1982.
100. Blomqvist, C. G., Lewis, S. F., Taylor, W. F., and Graham, R. M.: Similarity of the hemodynamic responses to static and dynamic exercise of small muscle groups. Circ. Res. (Suppl. II) 48:87–92, 1981.
101. Markiewicz, W., Houston, N., and DeBusk, R.: A comparison of static and dynamic exercise soon after myocardial infarction. Israel J. Med. Sci. 15:894–897, 1979.
102. DeBusk, R. F., Valdez, R., Houston, N., and Haskell, W.: Cardiovascular responses to dynamic and static effort soon after myocardial infarction. Application to occupational work assessment. Circulation 58:368–375, 1978.
103. Oldridge, N. B., Wicks, J. R., Hanley, C., Sutton, J. R., and Jones, N. L.: Non-compliance in an exercise rehabilitation program for men who have suffered a myocardial infarction. Can. Med. Assoc. J. 118:361–364, 1978.
104. Lee, A. P., Ice, R., Blessey, R., and Sanmarco, M. E.: Long-term effects of physical training on coronary patients with impaired ventricular function. Circulation 60:1519–1526, 1979.
105. Cohn, E. H., Sanders, R. S., and Wallace, A. G.: Exercise responses before and after physical conditioning in patients with severely depressed left ventricular function. Am. J. Cardiol. 49:296–300, 1982.
106. Sidney, K. H., Shephard, R. J., and Harrison, H.: Endurance training and body composition of the elderly. Am. J. Clin. Nutr. 30:326–333, 1977.

Chapter 9

SPECIAL CONSIDERATIONS IN PRESCRIBING EXERCISE

INTRODUCTION

Once the commitment has been made to begin an exercise program, attention must be given to a number of factors that can directly influence the program's success or failure. What type of clothing should be worn when exercising, and how important is proper footwear? What steps can be followed to minimize the possibility of serious orthopedic injury? Is warm-up necessary, and what is the proper way in which to cool down after a bout of vigorous exercise? How does altitude or extreme variations in temperature and humidity influence the daily workout? Does one's age or sex become factors in modifying the exercise program or limit the degree of improvement that might be expected to result from the exercise program? Can the exercise prescription be followed when traveling or when forced inside during inclement weather? How does one stay motivated to continue his or her exercise program from day to day or year to year? These and many other questions of a similar nature will be discussed in this chapter.

CLOTHING, SHOES, AND SPECIAL EQUIPMENT

The selection of improper or inappropriate clothing, shoes, or related equipment can create many problems for participants just beginning an exercise program. Overdressing or underdressing, wearing the wrong size or type of shoe, or using the wrong piece of equipment can lead to serious problems of heat or cold stress, disability, injury, overstress, or unnecessary expense.

CLOTHING

The choice of clothing will be totally dependent on the specific activity selected and the environmental conditions under which the activity will be performed. With swimming, the conditions are relatively stable throughout the year and, as a result, special considerations are not required when selecting a swimming suit. For hiking, walking, jogging, running, bicycling, or any other sporting activity that is performed outdoors, the attire should be comfortable, reasonably loose, and of the proper weight to insure protection from the sun, heat, cold, and wind. As a general rule, it is better to underdress than overdress, since the exercise itself will have a considerable warming effect on the body. Women should avoid restrictive support garments or clothing that would impede movement or blood flow. Bras may or may not be worn, depending on the size of the breasts. It is generally felt that a bra is beneficial for women with large breasts. Although men should wear supporters when participating in vigorous or contact sports, supporters are not essential during an activity such as jogging and may lead to skin irritations during long periods of activity.

Although there is a great deal of individual variation, the following suggestions should prove helpful. When a person is exercising at temperatures between 60 and 80°F, a light T-shirt or blouse and shorts would be adequate; between 40 and 60°F, a sweat shirt is advisable; and below 40°F, sweat pants and/or thermal underwear may be required. Gloves and stocking caps are also desirable when the temperature drops below 40°F. Kaufman[1] has recently summarized his work on short-term and long-term exposure to cold relative to clothing needs. At temperatures above 80°F, men may wish to exercise without a shirt and women may elect to wear a halter top. These recommendations are made on the assumption that there are moderate levels of humidity and wind. With higher humidities, the extremely high and low temperatures are considerably more stressful. Direct radiation from the sun is also an important consideration at the higher temperatures, and hats can be worn to reduce the radiant load.

Under no circumstances should one exercise while wearing rubberized or plastic clothing. This is common practice among individuals who are trying to use exercise as a means of losing weight. Athletes such as jockeys and wrestlers frequently use this technique to get down to their prescribed weight limit. The increased sweat loss does not result in a permanent loss of body weight, and this practice can be very dangerous.[2] The rubberized or plastic clothing does not allow the body sweat to evaporate. Since sweating is the principal manner in which the body regulates its temperature during exercise, lack of sweating or reduced evaporation of sweat can lead to a dramatic increase in body temperature, excessive dehydration and salt loss, and possible heat stroke or heat exhaustion.

Shoes and Socks

The type of shoe selected and the proper fit of the shoe are important considerations for any activity program. For most activities, a well-fitting tennis, basketball, or general gym shoe of good quality is perfectly adequate. For jogging or running activities, however, a special and carefully fitted shoe

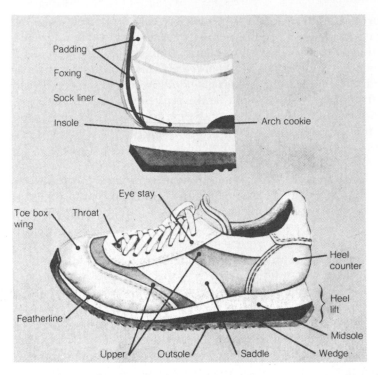

Figure 9–1. The anatomy of a running shoe. (Reprinted with permission from Bates, W.T.: Selecting a running shoe. Phys. Sports Med. *10:*15–155, 1982.)

designed specifically for these activities is highly recommended, since the foot strikes the ground, supporting the majority of the body weight, many times during a single workout. This places considerable stress on the foot and its associated structures. Thus, a shoe that gives good support and protection and has good shock-absorbing qualities is highly desirable. Most of the better running shoes have a strong, highly supportive heel counter, a heel wedge and midsole, a good arch support, a comfortable innersole, a relatively pliable outer sole, and a comfortable toe box.[3] The heel counter, which provides support and stabilization of the heel, should be firm and should fit snugly, and should come at least 4 inches forward from the rear point of the heel.[3] The heel wedge and midsole combine to form the heel lift, which helps to reduce pressure on the Achilles tendon and serves as the primary shock absorber. The outer sole should be durable and tough to prevent rapid wear but must be pliable. The toe box is often overlooked but is extremely important for total foot comfort. Black toenails result from blood blisters that form under the toenail and are caused by a toe box that has insufficient clearance between the toes and the underside of the toe box. The sockliner and the insole provide additional protection from shock and from blister formation and should feel comfortable with no seams to cause irritation. Prices will vary between $30 and $100 or more for a good pair of shoes. Several running magazines publish annual ratings of the various running shoes on the market. These publications should be consulted when selecting a running shoe for the first time or when changing from one shoe to another. Despite the ratings, however, the most important factor is proper shoe fit and comfort. Some brands come in different widths, and this is important for the individual with an extremely narrow or wide foot.

Socks are also important items for the beginning exerciser. Wool or cotton socks are appropriate, provided they fit properly after washing. Tube socks have become quite popular, for they fit a variety of sizes, do not shrink appreciably, and tend to stay fixed to the foot. This last point is important, since creeping socks tend to bunch up and cause painful blisters.

SPECIAL EQUIPMENT

An activity such as swimming or jogging requires no special equipment other than that described previously. If, however, the exercise prescription specifies games like tennis or racketball, or an indoor exercise device such as a stationary cycle, proper knowledge of the equipment under consideration is important. It would be impossible to discuss here all possible items of equipment likely to be used in an exercise program designed to promote cardiorespiratory fitness. However, there are certain guidelines that can be applied in the purchase of most specialized exercise equipment, including the following.

- **Deal with reputable businesses that will stand behind their products.**
- **Consult experts in the field or various consumer reports if there is any question about a company or its product. Most YMCAs, colleges, or universities have experts in this area who would be willing to provide valuable information.**
- **Avoid devices that claim to do all of the work. Active participation is essential to obtain the desired benefits of exercise.**
- **Do not be misled into thinking that the more expensive the item, the better job it does. Many items of equipment are greatly overpriced.**
- **Do not buy something that will not be used. Many expensive pieces of exercise equipment end up being stored in the garage, basement, or attic.**
- **Do not buy on impulse after receiving a high-powered sales pitch. Wait at least three days before making the final decision.**
- **Understand completely the purpose of the exercise device and its principle of operation.**

WARM-UP, COOL-DOWN, AND INJURY PREVENTION

WARM-UP PERIOD

It is particularly important to incorporate a brief, but basic, warm-up routine into the endurance training program. This was discussed in Chapter

7, and appropriate stretching exercises were illustrated. The stretching exercises develop and maintain flexibility as well as prepare the muscles, joints, and ligaments for the added stress of the cardiorespiratory endurance training session.[2] Barnard et al.[4] demonstrated serious electrocardiogram abnormalities when sudden exercise was undertaken without proper warm-up. Strength and muscular endurance exercises can be performed as a part of the initial warm-up period, but they should be preceded by the stretching exercises. If jogging or running, bicycling, hiking, or similar activities are the participant's main endurance activity, then strength and muscular endurance exercises should concentrate more on the upper body, because the lower body is the primary focus of these cardiorespiratory endurance programs. Proper warm-up may help alleviate many potential injuries such as muscle pulls, strains, sprains, and lower back discomfort, in addition to reducing the extent of muscle soreness.[2]

COOL-DOWN PERIOD

The cool-down period is equal to the warm-up period in importance. This is the period immediately after the cardiorespiratory endurance portion of each exercise session. The major purpose of the cool-down period is to keep the primary muscle groups, which were involved in the endurance exercise, continuously active. Since most cardiorespiratory endurance exercises involve the legs and are typically performed in an upright position, blood will pool in the lower half of the body if the individual does not perform light activity such as walking or slow jogging during the recovery period. This light activity allows the leg muscles to assist the return of the pooled blood to the heart. As the muscles in the legs contract, they create pressure against the veins, which in turn pushes the blood toward the heart, with the venous valves permitting blood to flow in only one direction—back to the heart. Without this light activity, blood will continue to pool in the lower body, and the participant may experience dizziness and can even pass out because of inadequate blood flow to the brain (vaso-vagal response).

Light activity during the cool-down period also helps to prevent extreme muscle soreness. This is particularly true if the cool-down period includes a few selected stretching exercises that concentrate on the legs and lower back. The length of the cool-down period need not exceed 5 to 10 minutes. After the workout, the participant should take a warm, *not hot,* shower, since hot showers after endurance exercise can create serious cardiovascular complications, i.e., peripheral dilation, increasing blood pooling in the periphery.

INJURY PREVENTION

The potential for serious injury exists in almost any exercise program if the proper precautions are not followed. As discussed earlier, sudden vigorous exercise has been shown to place a potentially lethal strain on the heart.[4] A proper warm-up period decreases the likelihood of this occurring. The participant must be aware of the various warning signs that may result from vigorous endurance exercise. Zohman, in her booklet *Beyond Diet . . . Exercise Your Way to Fitness and Heart Health,*[5] has listed a number of potential warning signs and symptoms that could occur either during or immediately after exercise. These may be grouped into the following two categories.

A. *Stop exercising.* See a physician before resuming if the following occur:

1. Abnormal heart activity, including arrhythmias, fluttering, jumping, or palpitations in the chest or throat; sudden burst of rapid heartbeats; or a sudden slowing of a rapid pulse rate.
2. Pain or pressure in the center of the chest, the arm, or the throat, during or immediately after exercise.
3. Dizziness, lightheadedness, sudden lack of coordination, confusion, cold sweating, glassy stare, pallor, cyanosis, or fainting.
4. Illness, particularly viral infections, can lead to myocarditis, that is, viral infection of the heart muscle. Avoid exercise during and immediately after an illness, particularly when fever is present.

B. *Attempt self-correction.*

1. Persistent rapid pulse rate throughout 5 to 10 minutes of recovery or longer. *Self correction technique:* Reduce the intensity of the activity (use a lower training heart rate) and progress to higher levels of activity at a slower rate. Consult a physician if the condition persists.
2. Nausea or vomiting after exercise. *Self-correction technique:* Reduce the intensity of the endurance exercise and prolong the cool-down period. Avoid eating for at least 2 hours before the exercise session.
3. Extreme breathlessness lasting more than 10 minutes after the cessation of exercise. *Self-correction technique:* Reduce the intensity of the endurance exercise. Consult a physician if the condition persists.
4. Prolonged fatigue up to 24 hours after exercise. *Self-correction technique:* Reduce the intensity of the endurance exercise and reduce the duration of the total workout session if this symptom persists. Consult a physician if these self-correcting techniques do not remedy the situation.

In addition to the preceding, there are a number of potential injuries or medical complications of an orthopedic nature that are usually minor but can also result in many participants dropping out of their exercise programs. Sharkey has listed a number of these in his book *Fitness and Work Capacity*[6] and has suggested a sound course of action to follow in an attempt to correct the situation. The list includes the following.

BLISTERS. These are a common problem, particularly when breaking in a pair of new shoes. Prevention begins with properly fitting shoes and socks that stay in place and do not creep or bunch up. When blisters occur, puncture the edge of the blister with a sterile needle, drain the fluid, apply a topical antiseptic, and cover with gauze or an adhesive bandage. Use precaution to avoid possible infection.

MUSCLE SORENESS.   Soreness usually accompanies the start of any exercise program or results from a sudden change in exercise habits, the exact cause of which is unknown. The degree of soreness can be reduced by starting at low levels of exercise and progressing slowly through the first few weeks and by thorough warm-up and cool-down periods that include stretching exercises. Massage and warm baths help to relieve the soreness when present.

MUSCLE CRAMPS.   These are involuntary muscle contractions that may be due to a salt and potassium imbalance in the muscle. Stretching and massaging the muscle usually bring immediate relief. Proper warm-up, replacement of electrolytes that were lost through sweating, and postexercise stretching should prevent most muscle cramps.

BONE BRUISES.   These are painful bruises, usually on the bottoms of the feet, caused by a single blow or repeated trauma to the bone. Ice and padding of the bruised area provide some relief, but proper footwear, including good midsoles, usually prevents the problem.

LOWER BACK PAIN.   Lower back pain is usually the result of poor flexibility, weak abdominal and back muscles, and poor posture. Stretching and muscle-strengthening exercises, along with a conscious effort to improve posture, remedy the problem in the majority of cases. See Chapter 7 for details on exercises for a healthy back.

KNEE PROBLEMS.   These can be caused or aggravated by the endurance conditioning program. This is a frequent area of complaint among joggers and runners. Wearing proper footwear and running on soft, even surfaces such as grass tend to reduce or eliminate the problem. Stay away from sharp turns or roads with high crowns. A physician or podiatrist should be consulted if the problem persists.

SHIN SPLINTS.   A shin splint is manifested as a sharp pain on the front aspect of the tibia. Shin splints are probably the result of a lowered arch, irritated membranes, tearing of muscle where it attaches to bone, hairline or stress fracture of the bone, or other factors. Although rest is the only sure cure, limited exercise is possible with the leg wrapped or taped, or an alternate form of exercise—e.g., cycling or swimming—may be chosen. Prevention of shin splints can be accomplished by proper footwear, running on soft surfaces such as grass, and strengthening the surrounding musculature.

ACHILLES TENDON INJURIES.   These injuries are a frequent source of trouble in distance runners. Improper footwear, including shoes without heel wedges, and high back shoes that rub against the Achilles tendon are considered to be the primary cause. Reduced activity or total rest combined with ice appears to be the only remedy, and surgical repair may be necessary. Prevention through selection of proper footwear and adequate warm-up is strongly advised. The warm-up should include a heel-stretching exercise, but caution must be exerted to prevent overstretching (see Chapter 7).

ANKLE PROBLEMS. These are a frequent problem for those who play sports that require a quick change in direction. A sprained ankle should be put on ice immediately to prevent major swelling and to facilitate recovery. Serious sprains should be examined by a physician. Prevention is best achieved by strengthening the surrounding musculature, by wearing high-topped gym or basketball shoes, and by preventive taping or ankle wraps.

If a jogger has an injury to the lower extremity and rest is required, he or she can use alternate activities such as cycling (stationary or free wheeling) or swimming. In this way, general fitness can be maintained while the jogging injury has a chance to heal. The reader is referred to several good textbooks on athletic injuries for a more comprehensive review of this area.[7-9]

ENVIRONMENTAL CONSIDERATIONS

In a temperature-controlled swimming pool or inside an air-conditioned or heated building, the environment remains stable from day to day and month to month, independent of changes in the outer environment. However, most individuals exercise outside these controlled conditions, and factors such as heat, cold, humidity, and quality of air become major considerations. In addition, whether exercising under controlled conditions or not, any marked change in altitude will also significantly influence one's ability to exercise.[10]

HEAT

The body's temperature is maintained consistently at approximately 98.6°F under normal conditions. When confronted with variations in outside temperature, the body makes rather remarkable adjustments to preserve its temperature. In extreme cold, the body shivers, which generates metabolic heat to maintain body temperature. In extreme heat, the body relies primarily on sweating to keep a constant temperature. Sweating is effective only as long as the sweat can evaporate, since it is the evaporation of the sweat that cools the body. Wind also aids in the evaporative process. In very humid weather, since the air is nearly saturated with water, evaporation becomes limited and thus the body has difficulty being cooled. The lethal combination of high temperature and high relative humidity has resulted in a number of deaths related to exercise, including football[11] and jogging.[12]

During exercise, the body temperature is maintained at a much higher level, from 100° to 104°F, which can be perfectly normal. The exercising body is more efficient at a higher body temperature. Exercise itself increases the heat production of the body, as evidenced by the fact that when an individual is cold, moving around and keeping active helps that person stay warm.

The ability of an individual to perform successfully in a hot environment depends on the magnitude of heat, the existing humidity, the air movement, the intensity and duration of the exercise, and the extent of his or her previous exposure to heat, i.e., acclimatization. The amount of direct radiation is also a critical factor, for direct exposure to the sun, as opposed to shade or cloud cover, is a major source of heat gain.

The higher the temperature, the greater the heat stress on the individual. With low humidity and acclimatization, the individual can tolerate air temperatures in excess of 90°F without too much trouble, since the individual can sweat at rates in excess of 2 liters per hour, and the dry air can evaporate most of the sweat.[2] As the humidity increases, the tolerable heat level reduces considerably. In a dry climate, the individual is not even aware he or she is sweating, since the sweat evaporates the moment it reaches the skin. Under conditions of moderate-to-high humidity, the individual is quite conscious of sweating, since very little is being absorbed by the already saturated air, and the sweat may roll off unceasingly. Another factor that is critical to determining the total thermal stress is air movement. The greater the air movement, the greater the cooling effect. Still air stagnates and becomes saturated with water, and evaporation is reduced.

The intensity and duration of the activity also contribute to the total heat stress.[13] Since the body produces heat as it exercises, the higher the intensity of the exercise and the longer the duration, the greater will be the resulting heat load and the subsequent stress to the body. It is possible to partially adapt or acclimatize to heat through repeated exposure, but total adaptation never occurs; i.e., heat will always be a major limitation to peak performance.[13]

One of the primary concerns when exercising in the heat is dehydration. With high sweat rates, the body loses a large volume of water. Since a major portion of this water loss comes from the blood volume, a serious situation exists unless rehydration is accomplished by consuming the appropriate fluids. Water and a diluted electrolyte solution appear to be the best fluids for quick rehydration. Fluids high in sugar content are not rapidly absorbed by the body.[14] Since a salt loss occurs with these high sweat rates, a liberal salting of food is recommended. Patients with hypertension and on salt-restricted diets or diuretics, or both, should consult their physicians.

Since people respond quite differently to heat, the adjustments to exercising in the heat should be made on an individual basis. In the summer, it is often important to exercise during the cooler parts of the day, preferably when the sun's radiation is minimal, i.e., early morning or early evening; to drink fluids abundantly before, during, and after the exercise session; and to avoid exercise altogether when the combination of temperature and humidity is such that severe heat stress resulting in heat exhaustion or heat stroke is unavoidable.[2,14] It is most likely that both the intensity and the duration of the activity will have to be reduced to maintain the same training heart rate. In 1975, the American College of Sports Medicine published a position statement on "Prevention of Heat Injuries During Distance Running." This is included in Appendix C.

Continued exposure to heat results in a gradual adaptation of the body to this stress, and the heat can be tolerated much more effectively. If a participant must play vigorous game activities or run races in the heat, then much of his or her training should be done under similar conditions. For example, many runners had a bad experience at the 1975 Boston Marathon when the temperature reached in excess of 90°F. They had not prepared themselves for the heat. One can become more than 90 per cent acclimatized in approximately 14 days. If one becomes sporadic in exercising in the heat and chooses to train during the cool part of the day, then part of the acclimatization is lost in just a few days.[13]

COLD

Exercise in the cold presents far fewer problems. The exercise itself provides considerable body heat, and additional clothing can always be worn. Since the hands, feet, and head are particularly sensitive to extreme cold, proper gloves, extra socks, and a stocking hat with a face mask are strongly advised. As with heat, the degree of humidity and air movement is important. The more humid the air and the greater the wind velocity, the greater the cold stress for the same absolute temperature. On the other hand, in a very dry, cold environment, care must be taken not to overdress, since sweating will occur once the individual warms up and the sweat-soaked clothing is subject to evaporation, which leads to rapid cooling and chills. If possible, easily unzipped layers of light clothing that can be ventilated (opened from the front) or even removed are often better than one or two heavy garments. Table 9–1 outlines the interaction between temperature and wind speed and should be used as a guide to plan winter exercise sessions. Kavanagh has prepared extensive guidelines for cardiac patients exercising outdoors in cold weather; these are included in Appendix C.

AIR POLLUTION

Air pollution has become a major consideration over the recent years because of its effect on the exercising subject.[15–18] Although this may not be a problem in many rural communities, it is a major problem in most large metropolitan areas. Carbon monoxide has a much greater affinity or attraction to hemoglobin than oxygen. Since almost all oxygen is transported through the blood by hemoglobin, high concentrations of carbon monoxide greatly reduce one's working capacity.[19] Other air pollutants, particularly ozone, have also been shown to have a significant negative effect on exercise

TABLE 9-1. WIND-CHILL-FACTOR CHART[a]

ESTIMATED WIND SPEED (mph)	ACTUAL THERMOMETER READING (°F)											
	50	40	30	20	10	0	-10	-20	-30	-40	-50	-60
	EQUIVALENT TEMPERATURE (°F)											
Calm	50	40	30	20	10	0	-10	-20	-30	-40	-50	-60
5	48	37	27	16	6	-5	-15	-26	-36	-47	-57	-68
10	40	28	16	4	-9	-24	-33	-46	-58	-70	-83	-95
15	36	22	9	-5	-18	-32	-45	-58	-72	-85	-99	-112
20	32	18	4	-10	-25	-39	-53	-67	-82	-96	-110	-124
25	30	16	0	-15	-29	-44	-59	-74	-88	-104	-118	-133
30	28	13	-2	-18	-33	-48	-63	-79	-94	-109	-125	-140
35	27	11	-4	-20	-35	-51	-67	-82	-98	-113	-129	-145
40	26	10	-6	-21	-37	-53	-69	-85	-100	-116	-132	-148

	Green	Yellow	Red
Wind speeds greater than 40 mph have little additional effect.	LITTLE DANGER (for properly clothed person). Maximum danger of false sense of security.	INCREASING DANGER Danger from freezing or exposed flesh.	GREAT DANGER

Trenchfoot and immersion foot may occur at any point on this chart.

[a] Adapted from *Runner's World 8:*28 (1973). Reproduced by permission of the publisher.

capacity. In certain areas of the United States, smog alerts have been instituted to warn individuals to stay indoors and to restrict physical activity levels on days when smog levels exceed a certain critical level. Exercising along heavily traveled roads can also expose the exerciser to fairly high, concentrated doses of pollutants, which are also potentially dangerous. Exercising in nonpolluted areas or restricting activity when pollution levels are high is strongly suggested. Raven has recently published an excellent summary of the national ambient air quality standards and recommended federal episode criteria for various pollutants (Table 9–2).[20]

ALTITUDE

The percentage of oxygen in the atmosphere at a 10,000-foot altitude is exactly the same as that at sea level. However, the atmospheric pressure is much less at the 10,000-foot altitude, and thus, pressure exerted by oxygen at that altitude is proportionally less than at sea level. As a result, it is more difficult to deliver oxygen to the working muscles of the body, and the absolute working capacity is reduced in direct proportion to the altitude.[10] This will have little, if any, effect on short bursts of activity such as sprinting, but it will greatly affect activities of an endurance nature. For

TABLE 9–2. NATIONAL AMBIENT AIR QUALITY STANDARDS AND RECOMMENDED FEDERAL EPISODE CRITERIA

POLLUTANT, UNITS/ AVERAGING TIME	SECONDARY	PRIMARY	ALERT*	WARNING*	EMERGENCY*	SIGNIFICANT HARM†
Sulfur dioxide $\mu g/m^3$ (ppm)						
1 year		80 (0.03)				
24 hours		365 (0.14)	800 (0.3)	1,600 (0.6)	2,100 (0.8)	2,620 (1.0)
3 hours	1,300 (0.5)					
Particulate matter $\mu g/m^3$ (COH)						
1 year	60	75				
24 hours	150	260	375 (3.0)	625 (5.0)	875 (7.0)	1,000 (8.0)
Product of sulfur dioxide and particulate matter $[\mu g/m^3]^2$ (ppm × COH)			6.5×10^4 (0.2)	2.61×10^5 (0.8)	3.93×10^5 (1.2)	4.90×10^5 (1.5)
Carbon monoxide mg/m^3 (ppm)						
8 hours	10 (9)	10 (9)	17 (15)	34 (30)	46 (40)	57.5 (50)
1 hour	40 (35)	40 (35)				144 (125)
Oxidents $\mu g/m^3$ (ppm)						
1 hour	160 (0.08)	160 (0.08)	200 (0.1)	800 (0.4)	1,200 (0.6)	1,400 (0.7)
Nitrogen dioxide $\mu g/m^3$ (ppm)						
1 year	100 (0.05)	100 (0.05)				
24 hours			282 (0.15)	565 (0.3)	750 (0.4)	938 (0.5)
1 hour			1,130 (0.6)	2,260 (1.2)	3,000 (1.6)	3,750 (2.0)
Hydrocarbons $\mu g/m^3$ (ppm) 3 hours (6 to 9 AM)	160 (0.24)	160 (0.24)				

*The federal episode criteria specify that meteorologic conditions are such that pollutant concentrations can be expected to remain at these levels for 12 or more hours or increase; or, in the case of oxidants, the situation is likely to reoccur within the next 24 hours unless control actions are taken.

†Priority I regions must have a contingency plan that shall, as a minimum, provide for taking any emission control actions necessary to prevent ambient pollutant concentration from reaching these levels at any location.

(Reprinted with permission from Raver, P.B.: Questions and Answers. J. Cardiac Rehabil. 2:411–414, 1982.)

the same heart rate, more work can be done at sea level than at high altitude. As a result, the intensity of the workout at high altitudes should be reduced to maintain approximately the same cardiovascular stress as experienced at sea level. The body starts to adapt to the stress of a particular altitude shortly after arriving at that altitude. After several weeks at that altitude, the body partially acclimatizes, but performance is still compromised.[2] Particular caution must be exerted by postcoronary and pulmonary patients.

AGE AND SEX CONSIDERATIONS

Do individuals adapt differently to exercise, depending upon their age and sex? Are we "over the hill" by the age of 30 years? Are women genetically inferior to men when it comes to exercise capacity? These questions have been asked for many years, and the answers are just now starting to surface.

First, endurance capacity does increase with age up to the middle to late twenties.[21,22] Strength, muscular endurance, and cardiovascular endurance follow similar patterns of development.[22] Women tend to reach their peak much earlier, that is, shortly after puberty.[21,23] Men tend to maintain their peak values until the age of thirty, after which there is a gradual decline throughout their lives.[21] Women start to decline shortly after attaining their peak and continue to do so gradually throughout the rest of their lives. The earlier peak and decline for women is thought to be a result of their lack of participation at an early age. Up to the point of puberty, there are essentially no differences between males and females for practically all aspects of physical performance, that is, speed, strength, power, agility, and muscular and cardiorespiratory endurance. Beyond puberty, men become considerably stronger in upper body strength, become faster, and have greater power and muscular and cardiorespiratory endurance.[23]

Two questions arise from the preceding observations. Are the sex differences seen after puberty genetically determined, or are they the result of different cultural and social conditions, i.e., the fact that women frequently discontinue participation in sports after puberty? Are the declines in physical ability noted with aging purely biological phenomena, or are they the result of an increasingly sedentary lifestyle? To answer the first question, studies that have compared highly trained female athletes with male athletes of similar training have found few physiological differences between the sexes, with the exception of upper body strength.[23] Therefore, it appears that the large differences seen between normal men and women beyond the age of puberty result from comparing moderately active males with relatively sedentary females. The implications are obvious. Women are not second-class citizens physically but can enjoy all the same benefits of exercise enjoyed by men!

With respect to the decline in performance with age,[24] recent studies have shown that individuals who have remained physically active, even to the point of international class competition for their age category, have not experienced the same rate of decline in physiological function.[25–27] There does appear to be a decrease, as would be expected, but the decrease is greatly accentuated by a decline in daily physical activity patterns. Since there are a large number of men and women who are vigorously active in their 50s, 60s, and 70s, and even older, including those who are competing in 26-mile, 385-yard marathon runs, it does appear that age is not a barrier to an active lifestyle.[28] For example, Kasch studied a group of middle-aged men ranging in age from 45 to 55 who trained for 10 years.[29] The men maintained their level of training (10 to 15 miles per week) during this period and showed no reduction in cardiorespiratory fitness. The older individual may need to start the exercise program at a much lower level and progress at a slower rate, but, given time, the benefits will be the same.[25]

SPECIFICITY OF TRAINING

Over the past few years, research has continued to confirm what many have suspected for years, i.e., training benefits are specific to the activity. Athletes who participate in both football and basketball are frequently shocked to find that all of the hard training that conditioned them for the sport of football did little to prepare them for a full court scrimmage on the first night of basketball practice. Playing basketball conditions players for a game of basketball but does little to prepare them for running a 5-mile race. Endurance training in a swimming pool has little or no carryover for long distance running. Changes that result from physical training are very specific to the actual muscles involved and to the pattern in which the muscles are used. This is an important concept to remember. Researchers are just now probing into why the training responses are so specific.[2,30]

EXERCISE PROGRAMS FOR TRAVELING AND AT HOME

Frequently, an individual just gets started on an exercise program when the program is interrupted by a vacation, business travel, or inclement weather. This problem has been of major concern to physicians, exercise physiologists, and program staff, since this interruption frequently signals the end of the program for that particular individual. By the time he or she returns or the weather improves, the urge to exercise has passed or considerable deconditioning has occurred.[2,30]

To combat such a situation, several approaches have been taken to develop indoor home and travel programs in order to maintain the continuity of the exercise program. Some good indoor activities are available. The stationary cycle is probably the best home exercise device. It can be set in front of the television or by an outside window to provide variety while exercising, thus eliminating potential boredom. Stationary cycles should have an adjustable knob to vary the resistance against which the individual pedals. The resistance should be set to provide an intensity of exercise equivalent to that used in the individual's jogging, running, or swimming program, i.e., should use the same training heart rate. Duration and frequency would also be the same as that prescribed for jogging, walking, or swimming. Because of the specificity of training, it will probably take a few workouts to get the legs sufficiently in shape for a full program.

Rope skipping and running in place are two additional exercises that can be performed indoors at home or when traveling on the road, although these would not be appropriate for some patient populations, e.g., post-coronary patients. Both exercises are excellent when performed correctly for the same duration and frequency and at the same intensity as stationary cycling. A word of caution is necessary, however. Extreme muscle soreness in the calf muscles is very common during the first few weeks of both rope-skipping and running-in-place programs. As with all other forms of exercise, the intensity is regulated on the basis of the training heart rate. In addition, calf-stretching exercises will help alleviate muscle soreness and cramping.

When traveling, it is also possible to substitute long, brisk walks or stair climbing for the activity normally pursued. It is also becoming widely acceptable for joggers and runners to take their workout gear with them on trips. Usually there are parks or lightly traveled roads within a short distance of most hotels or motels. Once the individual overcomes the embarrassment of riding the elevator and walking through the lobby in his or her running gear, the rest is easy!

MOTIVATION

The success or failure of any exercise program is directly related to the motivation of the individual participants. Those who are highly motivated will continue their exercise program indefinitely, even when faced with injury. Those who are poorly motivated will have great difficulty adhering to their exercise program. It has been estimated that only 60 to 85 per cent of those who start an exercise program will adhere to this program for 10 weeks or longer, whereas the remaining 15 to 40 per cent drop out.[31] Studies have attempted to identify those factors that might be responsible for adherence versus dropout. Some of these include the attitude of the participant's husband or wife toward involvement in the program, the participant's credit rating, the proximity of the participant to the testing and exercise facility, the intensity of training, being overweight, other commitments, and freedom from serious illness or injury.[32] Factors such as behavior pattern, health consciousness, attitude toward physical activity, level of physical fitness, and previous athletic experiences, apparently have little or no relationship to adherence rates.[31] Factors that have not been studied, but would appear to be important, include the degree of supervision and guidance provided in the exercise program and the optimization of the exercise prescription, i.e., mode, frequency, intensity, and duration.

Physical activity must be a lifetime pursuit, and therefore, proper motivation is critical to continued participation in the exercise program. One of the most important aspects of motivation is to have participants properly educated about why regular exercise should be an important component of their lifestyle. Films, books, booklets, lectures, seminars, workshops, and group discussions are all excellent methods to help them understand the importance of regular physical activity.

A second factor of equal importance is having participants engage in activities they enjoy or helping them to learn to enjoy activities that would be of greatest benefit to them. Unfortunately, too many people have been under the false impression that jogging and running are the only activities that have any long-term benefits and value. Many people simply do not enjoy jogging or running. To insist that all people must jog or run is creating a situation in which a high percentage of the participants will drop out of the exercise program after a relatively short period of time. Alternative activities that have a high aerobic or cardiorespiratory endurance component should be suggested and prescribed if they are more attractive to the participant. Brisk walking, hiking, swimming, bicycling, and vigorous sports such as handball, racquetball, and tennis would all be acceptable substitutes for jogging or running. Although individuals may not improve as rapidly with these alternative modes of exercise, the important factor is that they will improve, and they have an entire lifetime ahead of them in which to attain optimal levels of fitness.

It is argued by some, with good logic, that a sport should not be used to gain physical fitness, but rather to maintain fitness. In other words, as an example, rather than using tennis as an activity to get into shape, use an activity like jogging for several months to increase the basic level of fitness to a respectable level and then switch to tennis to maintain that optimal level. It is felt that the individual will be better able to enjoy participation in the sport if this approach is followed.

Other factors that have been shown to facilitate adherence include exercising at a regular time of day as a fixed part of a daily routine. Professionals who have conducted fitness programs for many years generally agree that the attrition rate is much lower for those who exercise in the early morning before going to work. First, there is the obvious advantage that there are few interruptions early in the morning—no phone calls, unscheduled meetings, early dinner, and so on. Second, when the weather is warm, this is an ideal time to exercise, since heat stress is minimized. However, it must be recognized that not everyone is a "morning person," and an early morning program would be largely unacceptable to some participants, particularly in winter months when it is dark and cold. Whatever the agreed-upon time, consistency is the critical factor.

Exercising with a partner or as a member of a formal group, as opposed to doing it alone, has been found to reduce the dropout rate. Companionship and knowing that others are waiting is a potent motivator to show up for group exercise sessions. A word of caution must be introduced at this point, however. Group participation frequently leads to competition, and this is usually not recommended. Almost everyone is intrigued by competition, but it is unwise for the novice who is just beginning his or her exercise program. The potential for orthopedic injury is there, as well as other medical risks.

Simple tests, self-administered on a regular basis, are also motivating, since progress can be seen from week to week. Monitoring the resting pulse rate before getting up in the morning, after a good night's sleep, should show a decrease of approximately 1 beat/min every two weeks for the first 15 to 20 weeks of training. After 10 weeks, it is not unusual to see a resting pulse rate of 70 beats/min drop to 65 beats/min. This change reflects improvement in cardiorespiratory efficiency, which is a positive reinforcement to the participant and acts to encourage the individual to continue the present program. Many simple tests are available, can be self-administered, and certainly help to maintain a high level of participant enthusiasm and motivation.

The ultimate in motivation has been noted by Glasser, who, in his book *Positive Addiction,*[33] has reported that joggers or runners who exercise 30 to 60 minutes per day for 4 days a week or more frequently become addicted to this routine. If illness, injury, travel, or some other interruption disrupts their exercise routine, these individuals actually go through withdrawal-like symptoms. Of course, this would be a highly desirable outcome, but unfortunately too many individuals do not have the patience, persistence, or psychological strength to get to this point of "positive addiction."

Most recently, attempts have been made to apply the concepts of behavioral modification to increase adherence to exercise programs. Since this is a new approach, it is too early to predict if it will be any more successful than traditional approaches. Behavior modification uses a system of rewards to promote changes in behavior. Many programs have provided rewards to their participants in the form of 100-Mile Club, 500-Mile Club, 1,000-Mile Club, and 10,000-Mile Club T-shirts. These programs have been shown to be very effective. It is somewhat ironic to watch mature men, who are wealthy enough to buy the entire company that makes the T-shirts, fight to get one of these relatively inexpensive rewards. If past experience provides any indication of the future, behavior modification techniques, applied more broadly, should have a significant impact on increasing adherence rates.

SUMMARY

Participation in any exercise program requires that attention be given to a number of factors, each of which directly influences how successful the individual participant will be in his or her exercise program. Ignoring such things as correct shoes, clothing, and special equipment; warm-up, cool-down, and injury prevention; and environmental factors such as heat, cold, humidity, air pollution, and altitude can lead the participant into an unpleasant if not hazardous situation that may have serious and sometimes tragic consequences. A knowledge of the specificity of training and how the sexes and individuals of varying ages differ in their response to an exercise program is also extremely important. Total education of the participant is important to prevent possible medical complications or injury and to promote a healthy, positive attitude toward the program. Exercise must become the reward and not the punishment.

REFERENCES

1. Kaufman, W. C.: Cold-weather clothing for comfort or heat conservation. Phys. Sportsmed. *10:* 71–75, 1982.
2. Wilmore, J. H.: Training for Sport and Activity: The Physiological Basis of the Conditioning Process. 2nd ed. Boston, Allyn and Bacon, 1982.
3. Bates, W. T.: Selecting a running shoe. Phys. Sportsmed. *10:* 154–155, 1982.
4. Barnard, R. J., Gardner, G. W., Diaco, N. V., MacAlpin, R. N., and Kattus, A. A.: Cardiovascular responses to sudden strenuous exercise—heart rate, blood pressure, and ECG. J. Appl. Physiol. *34:* 833–834, 1973.
5. Zohman, L. R.: Beyond Diet . . . Exercise Your Way to Fitness and Heart Health. Englewood Cliffs, NJ, Mazola Products, Best Foods, 1974.
6. Sharkey, B. J.: Fitness and Work Capacity. U.S. Department of Agriculture, Forest Service Equipment Development Center, Missoula, Montana, 1976.
7. Klafs, C. E., and Arnheim, D. D.: Modern Principles of Athletic Training. 4th ed. St. Louis, C. V. Mosby, 1977.
8. Kuprian, W., editor: Physical Therapy for Sports. Philadelphia, W. B. Saunders Co. 1982.
9. Fahey, T. D.: What To Do About Athletic Injuries. New York, Butterick Publishing, 1979.
10. Goddard, R. F., editor: The Effects of Altitude on Physical Performance. Chicago, The Athletic Institute, 1966.
11. Murphy, R., and W. Ashe.: Prevention of heat illness in football players. J.A.M.A. *194:* 650–654, 1965.
12. Sutton, J. R., and Bar-Or, O.: Thermal illness in fun running. Am. Heart J. *100:* 778–781, 1980.
13. Buskirk, E. R., and Bass, D. E.: Climate and exercise. *In* Johnson, W. R., editor: Science and Medicine in Exercise and Sports. New York, Harper and Brothers, 1960, pp. 311–338.
14. Costill, D. L.: A Scientific Approach to Distance Running. Los Altos, CA, Track and Field News, 1979.
15. Drinkwater, B. L., Raven, P. B., Horvath, S. M., Gliner, J. A., Ruhling, R. O., Bolduan, N. W., and Taguchi, S.: Air pollution, exercise, and heat stress. Arch. Environ. Health *28:* 177–181, 1974.
16. Gliner, J. A., Raven, P. B., Horvath, S. M., Drinkwater, B. L., and Sutton, J. C.: Man's physiologic response to long-term work during thermal and pollutant stress. J. Appl. Physiol. *39:* 628–632, 1975.
17. Horvath, S. M., Raven, P. B., Dahms, T. E., and Gray, D. J.: Maximal aerobic capacity at different levels of carboxyhemoglobin. J. Appl. Physiol. *38:* 300–303, 1975.
18. Raven, P. B., Drinkwater, B. L., Ruhling, R. O., Bolduan, N. W., Taguchi, S., Gliner, J. A., and Horvath, S. M.: Effect of carbon monoxide and peroxyacetyl nitrate on man's maximal aerobic capacity. J. Appl. Physiol. *36:* 288–293, 1974.
19. Raven, P. B., Drinkwater, B. L., Horvath, S. M., Gliner, J. A., Ruhling, R. O., Sutton, J. C., and Bolduan, N. W.: Age, smoking habits, heat stress, and their interactive effects with carbon monoxide and peroxyacetyl nitrate on man's aerobic power. Int. J. Biometeorol. *18:* 222–232, 1974.

20. Raven, P. B.: Questions and answers. J. Cardiac Rehabil. *2:* 411–414, 1982.
21. Åstrand, I.: Aerobic work capacity—its relation to age, sex, and other factors. Circ. Res. *20* and *21* (Suppl. I), *1:* 211–217, 1967.
22. Skinner, J. S.: Age and performance. *In* Limiting Factors of Physical Performance. Stuttgart: George Thieme, 1973, pp. 271–282.
23. Wilmore, J. H.: Inferiority of female athletes: myth or reality. J. Sports Med. *3:* 1–6, 1975.
24. Bottiger, L. E.: Regular decline in physical working capacity with age. Br. Med. J. *3:* 270–271, 1973.
25. Pollock, M. L., Dawson, G. A., Miller, Jr., H. S., Ward, A., Cooper, D., Headley, W., Linnerud, A. C., and Nomeir, M. M.: Physiologic responses of men 49 to 65 years of age to endurance training. J. Am. Geriatr. Soc. *24:* 97–104, 1976.
26. Wilmore, J. H., Miller, H. S., and Pollock, M. L.: Body composition and physiological characteristics of active endurance athletes in their eighth decade of life. Med. Sci. Sports *6:* 44–48, 1974.
27. Pollock, M. L., Foster, C., Rod, J., Hare, J., and Schmidt, D. H.: Ten year follow-up on aerobic capacity of champion Master's track athletes (abstract). Med. Sci. Sports Exer. *14:* 105, 1982.
28. Cureton, T. K.: A physical fitness case study of Joie Ray (improving physical fitness from age 60 to 70 years). J. Assoc. Phys. Mental Rehabil. *18:* 64–72, 1964.
29. Kasch, F. W.: The effects of exercise on the aging process. Phys. Sportsmed. *4:* 64–68, 1976.
30. Åstrand, P.-O., and Rodahl, K.: Textbook of Work Physiology. 2nd ed. New York, McGraw-Hill, 1977.
31. Pollock, M. L., Gettman, L. R., Milesis, C. A., Bah, M. D., Durstine, L., and Johnson, R. B.: Effects of frequency and duration of training on attrition and incidence of injury. Med. Sci. Sports *9:* 31–36 1977.
32. Morgan, W. P.: Involvement in vigorous physical activity with special reference to adherence. Proceedings, National College of Physical Education for Men, Orlando, FL, January 1977.
33. Glasser, W.: Positive Addiction. New York, Harper and Row, 1976.

Chapter 10

NUTRITION IN HEALTH AND DISEASE*

BASIC CONCEPTS IN NUTRITION

Simply defined, food includes all of the solid and liquid materials taken into the digestive tract that are utilized to maintain and build body tissues, regulate body processes, and supply body heat. Food can be categorized into six classes of nutrients, each with a unique chemical structure and a specific function within the body. The six categories include water, minerals, vitamins, proteins, fats, and carbohydrates. Each of these will be briefly discussed relative to their importance in general body function and in health and disease.

WATER

Seldom is water thought of as a food. Although it has no caloric value and does not provide any of the other nutrients, it is second in importance only to oxygen in maintaining life. Water constitutes between 55 and 70 per cent of the total body weight. However, although humans can survive for weeks or even months without food, they can go without water for only a few days. It has been estimated that one can lose up to 40 per cent of his or her body weight in fats, carbohydrates, and proteins and still survive, whereas a 20 per cent loss in body water will likely lead to death.

Water is necessary for digestion, absorption, circulation, and excretion. With respect to exercise, water plays two critical roles. First, it is important in maintaining the electrolyte balance in the body. Second, it is vital in controlling body temperature. This second function has been discussed in the previous chapter.

---

*Adapted in part from Wilmore, J. H.: Training for Sport and Activity: The Physiological Basis of the Conditioning Process. 2nd ed. Copyright © 1982 by Allyn and Bacon, Inc., Boston. Reprinted with permission.

Water intake is controlled largely by thirst sensations, which are received by a regulatory center in the hypothalamus. These sensations are activated by the osmotic pressure of the body fluids, i.e., as the osmotic pressure increases, thirst sensations are activated. It should be mentioned however, that the body's thirst mechanisms do not always keep up with its need for water. This has been referred to as "voluntary dehydration." This phenomenon is not well understood, but it does occur when working or exercising in hot climates. This voluntary dehydration will not usually have serious consequences over a period of a single day of exercise, but when the individual is faced with repeated exposures to exercise in the heat, this dehydration will be cumulative and can have serious, if not fatal, consequences. Evidently, such tremendous volumes of water are lost via sweating to maintain body temperature that the body finds it difficult to consume and absorb an equivalent volume of water over a 24-hour period. Thus, it is always important to drink more fluid than the thirst mechanisms dictate in an attempt to avoid voluntary dehydration. If too much water is ingested, the body can adapt readily by passing off the excess in the urine.

Water is normally ingested directly, in other fluids, or as a part of ingested food. The normal water intake of the average adult in a moderate climate will be approximately 2 liters per day. This will obviously increase in direct proportion to the fluid loss experienced by the individual through exercise and increased environmental temperature. With respect to foods, water constitutes 96 per cent of the total content of lettuce, 88 per cent of an orange, 87 per cent of milk, 74 per cent of eggs, 60 per cent of lean beef, and only 4 per cent of dry cereals and soda crackers. In addition to the water contained in the ingested food, water is also a by-product of the metabolism of stored food.

Ingested water is rapidly absorbed by the intestines, but it must first be emptied from the stomach. Considerable research has shown that the glucose content of the ingested solution largely dictates the speed of gastric emptying. Thus, to increase water absorption in the intestines, it is important to ingest either water or solutions that have a very low glucose content.

MINERALS

Minerals refer to the elements in their simple inorganic form. Although there are more than 20 mineral elements in the body, approximately 17 have been proved to be essential in the diet. Approximately 4 per cent of one's body weight is in the form of minerals, and most of this is in bone. Minerals such as calcium, phosphorus, and magnesium are needed in relatively large amounts and are referred to as macrominerals. Potassium, sulfur, sodium, and chlorine also fall into this category. Macrominerals, by definition, are minerals that are needed by the body in amounts of more than 100 mg per day. Microminerals, or trace elements, are those needed in amounts of less than 100 mg per day and include iron, zinc, selenium, manganese, copper, iodine, molybdenum, cobalt, fluorine, and chromium. Several of the more important macrominerals will be briefly discussed. In addition, Table 10–1 provides a list of the 17 essential minerals, their location in the body, their major function, the best food source, and the 1980 recommended dietary allowance for each.

Calcium is the most abundant mineral in the body, constituting 1.5 to 2.0 per cent of the total body weight and approximately 40 per cent of the total minerals present in the body. Of the total calcium in the body, 99 per cent is found in the bones and teeth. The major function of calcium is to build and maintain bones and teeth. It is essential for muscle contraction, blood clotting, control of cell membrane permeability, and nervous control of the heart. Milk and milk products are the best sources of calcium.

Phosphorus is closely linked to calcium and constitutes approximately 22 per cent of the total mineral content of the body. About 80 per cent of phosphorus is found in combination with calcium in the form of calcium phosphate, which provides strength and rigidity to the bones and teeth. It is also an essential part of metabolism, cell membrane structure, and the buffering system to maintain the blood at a constant pH. Meat, poultry, fish, eggs, and milk are the primary sources of phosphorus.

Iron is present in the body in relatively small amounts, i.e., 35 to 50 mg per kilogram of body weight. Iron plays an extremely critical role in the transportation of oxygen throughout the body. As was mentioned in earlier chapters, oxygen is carried in the blood primarily by its attachment to hemoglobin, an iron-containing protein. The iron combines with oxygen in the lungs and releases the oxygen at the level of the tissues. The myoglobin found in muscle, similar to hemoglobin, is also an iron-containing protein.

Iron deficiency is considered to be very prevalent throughout the world, with some estimates as high as 25 per cent of the world's population. The major problem associated with iron deficiency is iron deficiency anemia, in which there is a reduction in the oxygen-carrying capacity of the blood and a resulting feeling of general tiredness and lack of energy. The major dietary source of iron is liver. However, oysters, shellfish, lean meat, and other organ meats are good sources, as are leafy green vegetables and egg yolks.

Sodium, potassium, and chloride are classified as electrolytes and are found distributed throughout all body fluids and tissues, with sodium and chloride found predominantly extracellularly and potassium, intracellularly. These electrolytes function to maintain normal water balance and distribution, normal osmotic equilibrium, normal acid-base balance, and normal muscular irritability. The major sources of sodium chloride are normal table salt, seafood, milk, and meat. Potassium is found most readily in fruits, milk, meat, cereals, and vegetables.

VITAMINS

Vitamins are defined as a group of unrelated organic compounds. They

TABLE 10–1. MINERAL ELEMENTS IN THE BODY

MINERAL	PRIMARY LOCATION IN BODY	PRIMARY FUNCTION	FOOD SOURCES	1980 RECOMMENDED DIETARY ALLOWANCE
Calcium	Bone and teeth	Blood clotting, bone formation, transportation of fluids, muscle contraction	Milk and milk products, broccoli, sardines, clams, and oysters	1200 mg/day for ages 11–18 years and 800 mg/day for adults
Phosphorus	Bone and teeth	Bone formation, body's energy system, pH regulation	Cheese, egg yolk, milk, meat, fish, poultry, whole-grain cereals, legumes, and nuts	1200 mg/day for ages 11–18 years and 800 mg/day for adults
Magnesium	Bone and inside cells	Activation of enzymes	Whole-grain cereals, nuts, meat, milk, green vegetables and legumes	300–400 mg/day for teens and adults
Sodium	Bone and extracellular fluid	Regulation of body fluid osmolarity, pH, and body fluid volume	Table salt, seafood, milk and eggs, although abundant in most food except fruits	900–3,300 mg/day for teens and adults
Chloride	Extracellular fluid	Buffer and enzyme activation	Table salt, seafood, milk, meat and eggs	1,400–5,100 mg/day for teens and adults
Potassium	Intracellular fluid	Regulation of body fluid osmolarity, pH, and cell membrane transfer	Fruits, meat, milk, cereals, vegetables, and legumes	1,525–5,625 mg/day for teens and adults
Sulfur	Amino acids	Oxidation-reduction reactions	Protein foods, including meat, fish, poultry, eggs, milk, cheese, legumes, and nuts	None
Iron	Hemoglobin, liver, spleen, and bone	Oxygen transportation	Liver, meat, egg yolk, legumes, whole or enriched grains, dark green vegetables, shrimp, oysters	10–18 mg/day for teens and adults

Zinc	Most tissues, with higher amounts in liver, muscle, and bone	Constituent of essential enzymes and insulin	Milk, liver, shellfish, herring, and wheat bran	15 mg/day for teens and adults
Copper	All tissues, with larger amounts in the liver, brain, heart, and kidney	Constituent of enzymes	Liver, shellfish, whole grains, cherries, legumes, kidney, poultry, oysters, chocolate, and nuts	2.0–3.0 mg/day for teens and adults
Iodine	Thyroid gland	Essential constituent of thyroxin	Iodized table salt, seafood, water, and vegetables	150 mcg/day for teens and adults
Manganese	Bone, pituitary, liver, pancreas, and gastro-intestinal tissue	Constituent of essential enzymes	Grains, nuts, legumes, fruit, and tea	2.5–5.0 mg/day for teens and adults
Fluoride	Bone	Reduces dental caries and may reduce bone loss	Drinking water, tea, coffee, soybeans, spinach, gelatin, onions, and lettuce	1.5–2.5 mg/day for teens and 1.5–4.0 mg/day for adults
Molybdenum	Enzymes	Constituent of essential enzymes	Legumes, cereal grains, dark green, leafy vegetables, and organs	0.15–0.5 mg/day for teens and adults
Cobalt	In all cells	Essential to normal function of all cells	Liver, kidney, oysters, clams, poultry, and milk	None
Selenium	The cell	Fat metabolism	Grains, onions, meats, milk, and vegetables	0.05–0.2 mg/day for teens and adults
Chromium	The cell	Glucose metabolism	Corn oil, clams, whole-grain cereals, meats, and drinking water	0.05–0.2 mg/day for teens and adults

are needed in relatively small quantities, but they are essential for specific metabolic reactions within the cell and for normal growth and maintenance of health. Vitamins function primarily as catalysts in chemical reactions within the body. They are essential for the release of energy, for tissue building, and for controlling the body's use of food. Vitamins can be classified into one of two major categories, i.e., they are soluble in either fat or water. Fat-soluble vitamins—A, D, E, and K—are stored by the body in lipids. Because they are stored, there is the possibility that they could be consumed or taken in doses that would lead to vitamin toxicity. Vitamin C and the B complex vitamins are water-soluble and when taken in excess will be excreted, mainly in the urine. The major vitamins of interest in health and their functions will be briefly discussed in the following paragraphs. Refer to Table 10–2 for a more complete listing of each vitamin, its sources and functions, and the 1980 recommended dietary allowance.

Vitamin A, or retinol, was the first fat-soluble vitamin to be discovered (1913). Natural vitamin A is usually found esterified with a fatty acid. It is essential for night vision, as an integral part of the visual purple of the retina. Vitamin A is also essential for maintaining normal epithelial structure and is thus vital in the prevention of infection. It is important, as well, for normal bone development and tooth formation. The major dietary sources of vitamin A are liver, kidney, butter, egg yolk, whole milk, and dark green, leafy, and yellow vegetables. Approximately 90 per cent of the stored vitamin A is found in the liver, and toxicity results in bone fragility and stunted growth, loss of appetite, coarsening and loss of hair, scaly skin eruptions, enlargements of the liver and spleen, irritability, double vision, and skin rashes.

Vitamin D was discovered in 1930. It is absorbed with fats from the intestine in its ingested state, but it can also be absorbed from the skin directly into the blood. It is stored in the liver, skin, brain, and bones and is essential for normal growth and development and for normal bone and tooth formation. Rickets results from vitamin D deficiency, and toxicity leads to excessive calcification of bone, kidney stones, headache, nausea, and diarrhea.

Discovered in 1922, vitamin E consists of four different tocopherols: alpha, beta, gamma, and delta. Alpha tocopherol is biologically more active than the other three, and delta tocopherol is the most potent antioxidant. Vitamin E functions in metabolism and helps to enhance the activity of vitamins A and C. Vitamin E deficiency in humans is rare, and no toxic effects have been identified. Many claims have been made for vitamin E with respect to rheumatic fever, muscular dystrophy, coronary artery disease, sterility, menstrual disorders, and spontaneous abortion, among others, but the claims for cures or benefits for any of these areas lack supporting scientific evidence.

The B complex vitamins were at one time considered to be a single vitamin that was important in the prevention of the disease beriberi. At the

TABLE 10-2. VITAMINS AND THEIR FUNCTIONS, SOURCES, AND ASSOCIATED DEFICIENCY STATES

VITAMIN	PRIMARY FUNCTION	SOURCES	1980 RECOMMENDED DIETARY ALLOWANCE (units/day)
Fat-Soluble Vitamins			
A	Adaptation to dim light, resistance to infection, prevents eye and skin disorders, bone and tooth development	Liver, kidney, milk, butter, egg yolk, yellow vegetables, apricots, cantaloupe, and peaches	800 and 1,000 mcg for females and males, respectively—teens and adults
D	Facilitates absorption of calcium, bone, and tooth development	Sunlight, fish, eggs, fortified dairy products and liver	10 mcg for 11–18 years of age; 5–7.5 mcg for adults
E	Prevents oxidation of essential vitamins and fatty acids and protects red blood cells from hemolysis	Wheat germ, vegetable oils, green vegetables, milk fat, egg yolk, and nuts	8–10 mg for teens and adults
K	Blood clotting	Liver, soybean oil, vegetable oil, green vegetables, tomatoes, cauliflower, and wheat bran	70–140 mcg for teens and adults
Water-Soluble Vitamins			
B_1 (Thiamine)	Energy metabolism, growth, appetite, and digestion	Pork, liver, organs, meats, legumes, whole-grain and enriched cereals and breads, wheat germ and potatoes	1.0–1.5 mg for teens and adults
B_2 (Riboflavin)	Growth, health of eyes, and energy metabolism	Milk and dairy foods, organ meats, green vegetables, eggs, fish, and enriched cereals and breads	1.2–1.7 mg for teens and adults
Niacin	Energy metabolism and fatty acid synthesis	Fish, liver, meat, poultry, grains, eggs, peanuts, milk, and legumes	13–19 mg for teens and adults
B_6 (Pyridoxine)	Protein metabolism and growth	Pork, glandular meats, cereal bran and germ, milk, egg yolk, oatmeal, and legumes	1.8–2.2 mg for teens and adults
Pantothenic acid	Hemoglobin formation and carbohydrate, protein, and fat metabolism	Whole-grain cereals, organ meats, and eggs	4–7 mg for teens and adults
Biotin	Carbohydrate, fat, and protein metabolism	Liver, peanuts, yeast, milk, meat, egg yolk, cereal, nuts, legumes, bananas, grapefruit, tomatoes, watermelon, and strawberries	100–200 mcg for teens and adults
Folic acid (Folacin)	Growth, fat metabolism, and maturation of red blood cells	Green vegetables, organ meats, lean beef, wheat, eggs, fish, dry beans, lentils, asparagus, broccoli, and yeast	400 mcg for teens and adults
B_{12} (Cobalamin)	Red blood cell production, nervous system metabolism, and fat metabolism	Liver, kidney, milk and dairy foods, and meat	3.0 mcg for teens and adults
C (Ascorbic acid	Growth, tissue repair, and tooth and bone formation	Citrus fruits, tomatoes, strawberries, potatoes, melons, peppers, and pineapple	50–60 mg for teens and adults

present time, however, more than a dozen B complex vitamins that have very specific functions within the body have been identified. B complex vitamins play an essential role in the metabolism of all living cells, serving as cofactors in the various enzyme systems involved in the oxidation of food and the production of energy. The B complex vitamins have such a close interrelationship that a deficiency in one may impair the utilization of the others. Dry yeast is the single best source of the B complex vitamins.

Vitamin C, or ascorbic acid, was isolated in 1928 and is both the prevention and the cure for scurvy. Vitamin C functions as either a coenzyme or a cofactor in metabolism, is required for the production and maintenance of collagen, and has been postulated to assist in wound healing, to combat fever and infection, and to prevent or cure the common cold. Vitamin C deficiency is characterized by general weakness, poor appetite, anemia, swollen and inflamed gums and loosened teeth, shortness of breath, swollen joints, and neurotic disturbances.

PROTEINS

Proteins are nitrogen-containing compounds formed by amino acids, and they constitute the major structural component of the cell, antibodies, enzymes, and many hormones. Protein is necessary for growth, as well as for the repair and maintenance of body tissues; for the production of hemoglobin (iron and protein); for the manufacture of enzymes, hormones, mucus, milk, and sperm; for the maintenance of normal osmotic balance; and for protection from disease through antibodies. Proteins are also potential sources of energy, but they are generally spared when fat and carbohydrate arc available in ample supply. More than 20 amino acids have been identified, and, of these, 9 are considered to be essential as a part of the daily food intake. Although many of the amino acids can be synthesized by the body, these 9 indispensable ones cannot be synthesized by the body either at all or at a rate sufficient to meet the body needs; thus, they become a necessary part of the diet. If any one of these 9 is absent from the diet, protein cannot be synthesized or body tissue maintained. Protein sources in the diet that contain all of the essential amino acids in the proper ratio and in sufficient quantity are referred to as complete proteins. Meat, fish, and poultry are the three primary complete proteins. The proteins in vegetables and grains are referred to as incomplete proteins, since they do not supply all of the essential amino acids in appropriate amounts. This concept is important for individuals on vegetarian diets. This will be discussed in much greater detail in the next section of this chapter.

Approximately 5 to 15 per cent of the total calories consumed per day in the United States are in the form of protein. This is considered by many to be two to three times the actual amount of protein necessary for proper body function. The daily recommended allowance, published in 1980 by the

National Research Council, are 45 and 56 g per day for the teenage and adult male, respectively, and 44 to 46 g per day for the teenage and adult female. Since the allowance is dependent on the individual's body weight, an allowance of 0.8 g per kilogram of body weight is considered appropriate for the adult. These recommendations are substantially lower than the 1968 recommendations.

FATS

Fats, or lipids, are composed of about 98 per cent triglycerides, with the remainder including traces of mono- and diglycerides, free fatty acids, phospholipids, and sterols. Triglycerides are composed of three molecules of fatty acids and one molecule of glycerol. Although fat has generally been thought of in negative terms—i.e., a person is too fat, or the blood fats are elevated, placing the person at risk for coronary artery disease—fat provides many useful functions in the body. It is an essential component of cell walls and nerve fibers; it is a primary energy source, providing up to 70 per cent of the total energy when the body is in the resting state; it supplies support and cushion for vital organs; it is involved in the absorption and transport of the fat-soluble vitamins; and it provides a subcutaneous insulating layer for the preservation of body heat.

There are two types of fatty acids, saturated and unsaturated. The difference between the two is in the bonding between carbon and hydrogen atoms. Unsaturated fats contain one (monounsaturated) or more (polyunsaturated) double bonds between carbon atoms in a chain of carbon atoms. Each double bond in the chain takes the place of two hydrogen atoms. When the carbon chain is saturated with hydrogen atoms, i.e., two hydrogen atoms for each carbon atom, this is referred to as a saturated fatty acid. In practical terms, a saturated fat is in the form of a solid, i.e., animal fat, and an unsaturated fat is in the form of a liquid, i.e., fish and vegetable oil. Saturated fats are derived primarily from animal sources, and unsaturated fats come from plant sources.

Fat supplies approximately 40 to 45 per cent of the total caloric intake of the American population, and this represents a substantial increase over the percentage of fat consumed in the early 1900s. In addition, fat from animal sources has increased markedly, and that from vegetable sources has decreased. Most nutritionists recommend at least 25 per cent of the caloric intake in the form of fat, but this should not exceed 30 to 35 per cent. Although many agree that the reductions in fat intake should come from saturated fats, there is currently a great deal of controversy on specific recommendations for the intake of saturated fats, particularly in reference to egg and dairy products. Pritikin[1] has proposed reducing total fat content of the diet to less than 10 per cent of the total calories ingested.

CARBOHYDRATES

Carbohydrates are composed of sugars and starches and are classified as monosaccharides, disaccharides, oligosaccharides, or polysaccharides. Monosaccharides are the simple sugars (glucose and fructose are the primary simple sugars) that cannot be hydrolyzed to a simpler form. Disaccharides can be hydrolyzed to two molecules of the same or different monosaccharide (sucrose, lactose, and maltose). Oligosaccharides can be hydrolyzed to yield 3 to 10 monosaccharide units, and polysaccharides can provide more than 10 monosaccharide units. The major polysaccharides are starch, dextrin, cellulose, and glycogen, which are composed completely of glucose units. Glucose serves many functions in the body. First, it is a major source of energy, particularly during high-intensity exercise. Glucose also exerts an influence on both protein and fat metabolism, sparing the use of protein as an energy source and controlling the utilization of fat. Glucose is the sole source of energy for the brain and is necessary for the functional integrity of nerve tissue.

In the early 1900s, carbohydrates constituted over 55 per cent of the total caloric intake. In the 1970s, this figure dropped to approximately 45 per cent. In the early 1900s, starches constituted 68 per cent of the total carbohydrate intake, but this has dropped to below 50 per cent. Sugar intake, conversely, increased from 32 per cent to over 50 per cent during the same time period. The major sources of carbohydrates are grains, fruits, vegetables, milk, and concentrated sweets. Refined sugar, syrup, and cornstarch are examples of pure carbohydrates, and many of the concentrated sweets such as candy, honey, jellies, molasses, and soft drinks contain few, if any, other nutrients. These foods have been said to contain empty calories, for they contribute no nutrients but just calories to the diet.

THE ATHLETE'S DIET

Since athletes are placing considerable demands on their bodies every day they train and compete, it is important that the body be as finely tuned as possible. This, by necessity, must include optimal nutrition. Too often, the athlete spends considerable time and effort in perfecting his or her skills and in attaining top physical condition, only to ignore proper nutrition and sleep. It is not uncommon to trace the deterioration of an athlete's performance to poor nutrition. What, then, is the best diet for an athlete? Will the dietary demands vary with the sport?

Although considerable research is currently being conducted and additional study is needed, the available evidence suggests that the dietary requirements of the athlete are no different from those of the nonathlete, with the exception of the total number of calories consumed. Thus, the optimum diet for athletes, as for nonathletes, must contain adequate quantities of water, calories, proteins, fats, carbohydrates, minerals, and vitamins in the proper proportions, independent of the sport or the event within a sport. In other words, a well-balanced diet appears to be all that is necessary.

What is a well-balanced diet? In the early 1940s, the Food and Nutrition Board of the National Research Council of the National Academy of Sciences was formed to define the nutrient requirements of the American population. At the conclusion of their deliberations, they published a report that became known as the "Recommended Dietary Allowances," called RDAs. The allowances were designed to provide a guideline for planning and evaluating food intake. In 1980, the National Research Council published its most recent of a number of revisions. The allowances for minerals and vitamins have been listed in Tables 10–1 and 10–2, and the protein allowance was discussed in the preceding section. With respect to energy intake, males 11 to 50 years of age should consume between 2,700 and 2,900 Kcal, and females should take in between 2,000 and 2,200 Kcal. These figures are calculated on the basis of the average height and weight of the population, for individuals doing light work. Obviously, athletes in intensive training would have considerably higher energy intake demands.

One of the problems associated with the RDAs was the inability of the average individual to understand the specific allowance value and its units of measure and to translate this information into meaningful terms. This led to a grouping of foods and the simplified "Basic Seven Food Plan." In 1956, this was simplified even further into the "Four Food Group Plan," which was published in the United States Department of Agriculture's publication *The Essentials of an Adequate Diet.* The "Four Food Group Plan" consists of the following four groups: milk and milk products, meat and high-protein foods, fruits and vegetables, and cereal and grain foods. Table 10–3 outlines the basics of the "Four Food Group Plan," including the number of servings per day and the major contributions of each food group. These suggestions are based on the minimal requirements and will have to be increased by either larger servings or more servings for individuals who are active and expend a considerable amount of additional energy each day. This basic dietary plan is recommended as a foundation, since it will assure the athlete of a well-balanced diet with no deficiencies, provided the energy intake is matching the energy expenditure. With respect to the balance between the basic food groups, protein should constitute 10 to 20 per cent of the total caloric intake, fats 30 to 35 per cent, and carbohydrates 50 to 55 per cent. For athletes who are training to exhaustion on successive days, the carbohydrate fraction could be as high as 70 per cent. More recently, a diet of less than 30 per cent fat has been advocated by preventive medicine experts.

VEGETARIAN DIETS

More people appear to be reducing their intake of meat and increasing their intake of vegetables. In some cases, people have made the complete transition to vegetarianism. Vegetarian diets are chosen for a number of health, ecological, and economical reasons. Vegetarians eat almost any food

TABLE 10–3. THE BASIC FOUR FOOD GROUP PLAN

FOOD GROUP	DAILY AMOUNTS FOR ADULTS	NUTRITIONAL CONTRIBUTION
Milk and milk products	Two or more servings per day as either a milk beverage or a milk product such as cheese and ice cream; serving would be one cup or its equivalent	Protein Calcium Riboflavin Vitamin D
Meat and high-protein products	Two or more servings of meat, fish, poultry, eggs, or vegetables such as dried beans, lentils, peas, and nuts; serving of meat, fish, or poultry would be 3.5 ounces of lean and boneless meat	Protein Thiamine Iron Niacin Riboflavin
Fruit and vegetables	Four or more servings per day of ½ cup or more	Vitamin A Vitamin C Folic acid
Cereal and grain	Four or more servings per day with one serving equal to one slice of bread, ½ to ¾ cup of cooked cereal, macaroni, and spaghetti.	Protein Thiamine Riboflavin Niacin Iron

from plant sources. However, there are several types of vegetarians. Vegans are strict vegetarians and eat only food from plant sources. Lactovegetarians eat plant foods and dairy products. Ovovegetarians eat plant foods and eggs, and lacto-ovovegetarians eat plant foods, dairy products, and eggs. Fruitarians eat fruits, nuts, olive oil, and honey.

Can an athlete survive on a vegetarian diet? The answer is a qualified yes. If the athlete is a strict vegan, he or she must be very careful in the selection of the plant foods he or she eats, to provide a good balance of the essential amino acids and adequate sources of vitamin A, riboflavin, B_{12}, vitamin D, calcium, iron, and sufficient calories. More than one professional athlete has noted significant deterioration in athletic performance after switching over to a strict vegetarian diet. The problem was later traced to an unwise selection of plant foods. Inclusion of milk and eggs is highly recommended, since they will lessen the likelihood of nutritional deficiencies. Anyone contemplating a switch from a normal to a vegetarian diet would be well advised to read authoritative reference material on the subject.

DIETARY SUPPLEMENTS

The food industry makes a considerable amount of money each year with dietary supplements. Is there a need for vitamin and mineral or protein supplementation? For the individual who is eating a well-balanced diet with the appropriate number of calories and who is moderately to highly active, dietary supplementation appears to be totally unnecessary. Supplements may be necessary for the individual or the athlete who is on a restricted caloric diet, in which the total energy intake is insufficient to provide the essential requirements. However, for the athlete in training whose total caloric intake is in excess of 3,000 Kcal and is as high as 10,000 Kcal, evidence would indicate that there is nothing to be gained by supplementation of any of the dietary constituents. The requirements for the various nutrients increase in direct proportion to the rise in energy expenditure, and the nutrient intake increases correspondingly.

PRECONTEST MEAL

For years, the athlete has been given the traditional steak dinner several hours before competition. Possibly, this practice originated from the early belief that the muscle consumed itself as fuel for muscular activity and that steak provided the necessary protein to counteract this loss. It is now recognized that this is probably the worst possible meal that the athlete could eat before competition. Steak contains a high percentage of fat, which takes many hours to be fully digested. The digestive process competes for the available blood with the muscles that are used in the contest. Because of this, the precontest meal, no matter what its content, should be given no later than 3 hours before the contest. Another factor to consider is the emotional climate at the time of this meal. The athlete is frequently extremely nervous, and even the choicest steak is not enjoyed. The steak would be psychologically more satisfying to the athlete either the night before or the night after the contest.

In his book *Food for Sport*, Smith[2] lists five goals that should be considered in planning the precontest diet. These are as follows:

1. Energy intake should be adequate to ward off any feeling of hunger or weakness during the entire period of the competition. Although precontest food intakes make only a minor contribution to the immediate energy expenditure, they are essential for the support of an adequate level of blood sugar and for avoiding the sensations of hunger and weakness.
2. The diet plan should insure that the stomach and upper bowel are empty at the time of competition.
3. Food and fluid intakes before and during prolonged competition should guarantee an optimal state of hydration.
4. The precompetition diet should offer foods that will minimize upset in the gastrointestinal tract.
5. The diet should include food that the athlete is familiar with and is convinced will "make him win."

It is also important that the athlete not eat anything with a high sugar content 2 hours or less before competition. Some athletes will ingest 2 or 3 candy bars with a very high sugar content 30 minutes to 1 hour before competition. With such a heavy sugar load, the body reacts by substantially increasing the insulin levels in the blood. In fact, the body overreacts and produces more insulin than is needed. This results in a very sharp decrease in the blood sugar level, and the athlete may become hypoglycemic. This condition will definitely reduce the performance potential of the athlete. It has recently been found that glucose feedings 30 to 45 minutes before endurance exercise increase the rate of carbohydrate oxidation and impede the mobilization of free fatty acids, thereby reducing the exercise time to exhaustion by 19 per cent.

Many athletes are starting to use a liquid pregame meal, since it is palatable, digests relatively easily, and is less likely to result in nervous indigestion, nausea, vomiting, and abdominal cramps. Those who have experimented with liquid precontest meals have found them to be highly satisfactory. At the present time, this would appear to be the best available choice as a pregame meal.

SUMMARY

The present chapter has reviewed the six classes of nutrients—i.e., water, minerals, vitamins, proteins, fats, and carbohydrates—discussing the importance of each relative to general nutrition, health, and disease. It was concluded that the optimum diet must contain adequate quantities of water, calories, proteins, fats, carbohydrates, minerals, and vitamins in the proper proportions. A well-balanced diet, as exemplified by the "Four Food Group Plan," appears to be the foundation for all individuals, athletes and nonathletes alike, provided the total caloric intake is sufficient. Vegetarian diets supply adequate nutrition provided plant food sources are carefully selected, thus insuring a good balance of the essential amino acids and adequate sources of vitamin A, riboflavin, vitamin B_{12}, vitamin D, calcium, iron, and sufficient calories.

REFERENCES

1. Pritikin, N., Kern, J., and Kaye, S. M.: Diet and exercise as a total therapeutic regimen for the rehabilitation of patients with severe peripheral vascular disease. Arch. Phys. Med. Rehabil. 56:558, 1975.
2. Smith, N. J.: Food for Sport. Palo Alto, CA, Bull Publishing Co., 1976.

Additional Readings

1. American Association for Health, Physical Education and Recreation: Nutrition for Athletes. A Handbook for Coaches. Washingtond, D.C., 1971.
2. Briggs, G. M., and Calloway, D. H., editors: Bogert's Nutrition and Physical Fitness. 10th ed. Philadelphia, W. B. Saunders Co., 1979.
3. Costill, D. L.: A Scientific Approach to Distance Running. Los Altos, CA, Tafnews Press, 1979.
4. Darden, E.: Nutrition and Athletic Performance. San Marino, CA, Athletic Press, 1976.

5. Farquhar, J. W.: The American Way of Life Need Not Be Hazardous to Your Health. New York, W. W. Norton and Co., 1978.
6. Katch, F. I., and McArdle, W. D.: Nutrition, Weight Control, and Exercise. Boston, Houghton Mifflin Co., 1977.
7. Krause, M. V., and Hunscher, M. A.: Food, Nutrition and Diet Therapy. 5th ed. Philadelphia, W. B. Saunders Co., 1972.
8. Nutrition and athletic performance. Dairy Council Digest. *46:*7–10, 1975.
9. Nutrition and human performance. Dairy Council Digest. *51:*13–17, 1980.
10. Stare, F. J., and McWilliams, M.: Living Nutrition. New York, John Wiley and Sons, 1973.
11. Williams, M. H.: Nutritional Aspects of Human Physical and Athletic Performance. Springfield, IL, Charles C Thomas, 1976.
12. Williams, M. H.: Nutrition for Fitness and Sport. Dubuque, IA: Wm. C. Brown Company Publishers, 1983.
13. Young, D. R.: Physical Performance Fitness and Diet. Springfield, IL, Charles C Thomas, 1977.
14. Zohman, L. R.: Beyond Diet . . . Exercise Your Way to Heart Health. Englewood Cliffs, NJ, Best Foods, 1974.

Appendix A

MEDICAL SCREENING
AND EXERCISE

MEDICAL
HISTORY
QUESTIONNAIRE

**Institute for Aerobics Research
11811 Preston Road
Dallas, Texas 75230**

This is your medical history form for your visit to The Institute for Aerobics Research. All information will be kept confidential. The doctor or exercise physiologist you see at the Institute will use this information in his evaluation of your health. You will want to make it as accurate and complete as possible, yet free of meaningless details. Please fill out this form carefully and thoroughly. Then check it over to be sure you haven't left out anything.

Note: Please PRINT all responses so that your data will be compatible with computer storage and analysis.

Name _____ Exam Date _____ ,19 _____

Figure A–1. Medical history questionnaire. (Published with permission of the Institute for Aerobics Research, Dallas, Texas, and John Wiley and Sons, New York, New York.)

Patient Medical History Form

Institute for Aerobics Research
11811 Preston Road
Dallas, Texas 75230

DO NOT WRITE IN THIS SPACE; FOR OFFICE USE ONLY.

PATIENT NUMBER	VISIT	CARD	FORM	CLINIC
		0 1	M 0	2 B

All information is private and confidential. Please Print.

I. GENERAL INFORMATION

☐ Mr. NAME
☐ Ms.
☐ Miss   FIRST   MIDDLE   LAST
☐ Mrs.
☐ Dr.

ADDRESS

NUMBER AND STREET

0 2

CITY   STATE   ZIP CODE

COUNTRY (IF OUTSIDE U.S.A.)

HOME PHONE   SOCIAL SECURITY NUMBER   DATE OF BIRTH   TODAY'S DATE

(   )   -   -   -   MONTH DAY YEAR   MONTH DAY YEAR
AREA CODE

FAMILY PHYSICIAN

Dr.
        FIRST NAME, IF KNOWN   INITIAL LAST NAME

DOCTOR'S ADDRESS (if known)

NUMBER AND STREET   PHONE

0 4
CITY   STATE   ZIP CODE   (   )   -
                                                      AREA CODE

May we send a copy of your consult to your physician?   Yes ☐   No ☐

MARITAL STATUS
        Single ☐   Married ☐   Divorced ☐   Widowed ☐   Separated ☐

SEX
        Male ☐   Female ☐   PRESENT AGE ☐☐☐

EDUCATION (Check highest level attained)
        ☐ Grade School   ☐ High School   ☐ College Graduate
        ☐ Junior High School   ☐ Two-year College (or 4-year college;   ☐ Postgraduate School
                                     degree not completed)

OCCUPATION

FOR OFFICE USE ONLY
OCCUP CODE ☐

EMPLOYER (use abbreviations if necessary)

0 5

EMPLOYER'S ADDRESS

NUMBER AND STREET

BUSINESS PHONE

0 6
CITY   STATE ZIP CODE   (   )   -
                                                     AREA CODE

What is/are your purpose(s) in coming to the Institute?

        ☐ To participate in a research study.

        ☐ To determine my current level of physical fitness and to receive recommendations for an exercise program.

        ☐ Other (please explain):

0 7

PLEASE PRINT

Figure A–1. *Continued.*

When dates are required, please use numbers to represent the months as follows:

January 01	May 05	September 09
February 02	June 06	October 10
March 03	July 07	November 11
April 04	August 08	December 12

For addresses, please use the official Post Office two-letter abbreviations listed below.

Abbreviations for States (and Territories)

AL	Alabama		NE	Nebraska
AK	Alaska		NV	Nevada
AZ	Arizona		NH	New Hampshire
AR	Arkansas		NJ	New Jersey
CA	California		NM	New Mexico
CZ	Canal Zone (Panama)		NY	New York
CO	Colorado		NC	North Carolina
CT	Connecticut		ND	North Dakota
DE	Delaware		OH	Ohio
FL	Florida		OK	Oklahoma
GA	Georgia		OR	Oregon
GU	Guam		PA	Pennsylvania
HI	Hawaii		PR	Puerto Rico
ID	Idaho		RI	Rhode Island
IL	Illinois		SC	South Carolina
IN	Indiana		SD	South Dakota
IA	Iowa		TN	Tennessee
KS	Kansas		TX	Texas
KY	Kentucky		UT	Utah
LA	Louisiana		VT	Vermont
ME	Maine		VA	Virginia
MD	Maryland		VI	Virgin Islands
MA	Massachusetts		WA	Washington (state)
MI	Michigan		DC	Washington, D. C.
MN	Minnesota		WV	West Virginia
MS	Mississippi		WI	Wisconsin
MO	Missouri		WY	Wyoming
MT	Montana			

Figure A–1. *Continued.*

Medical History

DO NOT WRITE IN THIS SPACE; FOR OFFICE USE ONLY.

PATIENT NUMBER	VISIT	CARD	FORM	CLINIC
		1 0	M 0 2	B

PRESENT HISTORY 2

Check the box in front of those questions to which your answer is yes. Leave others blank.

10
- ☐ Has a doctor ever said that your blood pressure was too high or too low?
- ☐ Do you ever have pain in your heart or chest?
- ☐ Are you often bothered by a thumping of the heart?
- ☐ Does your heart often race like mad?
- ☐ Do you ever notice extra heart beats or skipped beats?
- ☐ Are your ankles often badly swollen?
- ☐ Do cold hands or feet trouble you even in hot weather?
- ☐ Has a doctor ever said that you had or have heart trouble, an abnormal electrocardiogram (ECG or EKG), heart attack, or coronary?
- ☐ Do you suffer from frequent cramps in your legs?
- ☐ Do you often have difficulty breathing?
- ☐ Do you get out of breath long before anyone else?
- ☐ Do you sometimes get out of breath when sitting still or sleeping?
- ☐ Has a doctor ever told you your cholesterol level was high?

Comments:

Do you now have or have you recently had:

14
- ☐ A chronic, recurrent or morning cough?
- ☐ Any episode of coughing up blood?
- ☐ Increased anxiety or depression?
- ☐ Problems with recurrent fatigue, trouble sleeping or increased irritability?
- ☐ Migraine or recurrent headaches?
- ☐ Swollen or painful knees or ankles?
- ☐ Swollen, stiff or painful joints?
- ☐ Pain in your legs after walking short distances?
- ☐ Back pain?
- ☐ Kidney problems such as passing stones, burning, increased frequency, decreased force of stream of difficulty in starting or stopping your stream?
- ☐ Prostate trouble (men only)?
- ☐ Any stomach or intestinal problems such as recurrent heartburn, ulcers, constipation or diarrhea?
- ☐ Any significant vision or hearing problem?
- ☐ Any recent change in a wart or mole?
- ☐ Glaucoma or increased pressure in the eyes?
- ☐ Exposure to loud noises for long periods?

Comments:

WOMEN ONLY answer the following:

16
- ☐ Do you have any menstrual period problems?
- ☐ Do you have problems with recurrent itching or discharge?
- ☐ Did you have any significant childbirth problems?
- ☐ Do you have any breast discharges or lumps?
- ☐ Do you sometimes lose urine when you cough, sneeze or laugh?

Please give number of: Pregnancies ⌞—⌟ Living children ⌞—⌟ First day of last menstrual period MONTH DAY YEAR

Date of last pelvic exam and/or Paps smear: month ⌞—⌟ year 19 ⌞—⌟ Results: Normal ☐ Abnormal ☐

Comments:

PLEASE PRINT

Figure A–1. *Continued.*

Medical History

DO NOT WRITE IN THIS SPACE: FOR OFFICE USE ONLY.
PATIENT NUMBER   VISIT   CARD   FORM   CLINIC

2 5 | M | 0 | 2 | B | 3

MEN and WOMEN answer the following:

List any prescribed medications you are now taking:

| 25 |

List any self-prescribed medications or dietary supplements you are now taking:

| 26 |

Date of last complete physical examination: ____ 19 ____ never ☐ can't remember ☐ Normal ☐ Abnormal ☐
| 27 | month   year

Date of last chest x-ray: ____ 19 ____ never ☐ can't remember ☐ Normal ☐ Abnormal ☐
                          month   year

Date of last electrocardiogram: ____ 19 ____ never ☐ can't remember ☐ Normal ☐ Abnormal ☐
                                month   year

Date of last dental check-up: ____ 19 ____ never ☐ can't remember ☐ Normal ☐ Abnormal ☐
                              month   year

List any other medical or diagnostic test you have had in the past two years:

| 28 |

| 29 |

List hospitalizations including dates of and reasons for hospitalization:

| 30 |

| 31 |

| 32 |

List any drug allergies:

| 33 |

PAST HISTORY

Have you ever had:

| 34 |

☐ Heart Attack, how many years ago? ____
☐ Rheumatic Fever
☐ Heart murmur
☐ Diseases of the arteries
☐ Varicose veins
☐ Arthritis of legs or arms
☐ Diabetes or abnormal blood sugar test
☐ Phlebitis
☐ Dizziness or fainting spells
☐ Epilepsy or fits
☐ Strokes
☐ Diphtheria
☐ Scarlet fever
☐ Infectious mononucleosis
☐ Anemia

☐ Thyroid problems
☐ Pneumonia
☐ Bronchitis
☐ Asthma
☐ Abnormal chest x-ray
☐ Other lung diseases
☐ Injuries to back, arms, legs or joints
☐ Broken bones
☐ Jaundice or gallbladder problems
☐ Polio
☐ Urinary tract infections, kidney stones, or prostate problems.
☐ Any nervous or emotional problems

Comments:

| 35 |

PLEASE PRINT

Figure A–1. *Continued.*

Medical History

DO NOT WRITE IN THIS SPACE; FOR OFFICE USE ONLY.

PATIENT NUMBER	VISIT	CARD	FORM	CLINIC
		4 0	M 0 2	B

FAMILY MEDICAL HISTORY

40 FATHER: Alive ☐ Current age |___| General health now: excellent ☐ good ☐ fair ☐ poor ☐ don't know ☐
Deceased ☐ Age at death |___| Cause of death or reason for poor health now: |_____|

MOTHER: Alive ☐ Current age |___| General health now: excellent ☐ good ☐ fair ☐ poor ☐ don't know ☐
Deceased ☐ Age at death |___| Cause of death or reason for poor health now: |_____|

41 SIBLINGS: No. of brothers |___| No. of sisters |___| Age range |___|—|___| Health Problems: |_____|

FAMILIAL DISEASES: Have any of your blood relatives had any of the following?
Include grandparents, aunts, and uncles, but exclude cousins, relatives by marriage, and half relatives.

42
☐ Heart attacks under age 50
☐ Strokes under age 50
☐ High blood pressure
☐ Elevated cholesterol
☐ Diabetes
☐ Asthma or hay fever

☐ Congenital heart disease
☐ Heart operations
☐ Glaucoma
☐ Obesity (20 or more lbs. overweight)
☐ Leukemia or cancer under age 60

Comments: |_____|

43 OTHER HEART DISEASES RISK FACTORS

SMOKING

44
Have you ever smoked cigarettes, cigars or a pipe? yes ☐ no ☐
If no, skip to Diet section.
Do you smoke presently? yes ☐ no ☐
If you did or do smoke cigarettes, how many per day? |___| Age you started: |___|
If you did or do smoke cigars, how many per day? |___| Age you started: |___|
If you did or do smoke a pipe, how many pipefuls per day? |___| Age you started: |___|
If you have quit smoking, when was it? |___| 19 |___|
MONTH YEAR

DIET

45
What do you consider a good weight for yourself? |_____| pounds

What is the most you have ever weighed? (including when pregnant) |_____| lbs. At what age? |___| yrs.

Weight: Now |___| lbs. One year ago |___| lbs. At age 21 |___| lbs.

Number of meals you usually eat per day. ☐

Average number of eggs you usually eat per week: |__| (Do not count those in cooking and baking, cakes, casseroles, etc.)

Number of times per week you usually eat:

Beef |__| Fish |__| Desserts |__|
Pork |__| Fowl |__| French fried foods |__|

Number of servings (cups, glasses or containers) per week you usually consume of:

Homogenized (whole) milk |__| Buttermilk |__|
Skim (non-fat) milk |__| Tea (iced or hot) |__|
Two percent (2% fat) milk |__| Coffee |__|

Do you ever drink alcoholic beverages? yes ☐ no ☐

If yes, what is your approximate intake of these beverages?

	None	Occasional	Often	If often, how many drinks per week?
Beer	☐	☐	☐	☐
Wine	☐	☐	☐	☐
Hard Liquor	☐	☐	☐	☐

At any time in the past were you a heavy drinker (consumption of 6 oz. of hard liquor per day or more)? yes ☐ no ☐

46 Comments: |_____|

PLEASE PRINT

Figure A–1. *Continued.*

Medical History

DO NOT WRITE IN THIS SPACE; FOR OFFICE USE ONLY.
PATIENT NUMBER | VISIT | CARD | FORM | CLINIC | 5

5 0 | M | 0 | 2 | B

EXERCISE

50 Are you currently involved in a regular exercise program? yes ☐ no ☐

Do you regularly walk or run one or more miles continuously? yes ☐ no ☐ don't know ☐

If yes, average no. of miles you cover per workout or day: ☐·☐ miles

What is your average time per mile? ☐:☐ minutes: seconds don't know ☐

Do you practice weight lifting or home calisthenics? yes ☐ no ☐

Are you now involved in the Aerobics program? yes ☐ no ☐

If yes, your average Aerobics points per week: ☐

Have you taken in the past 6 months: ☐ 12 minute test ☐ 1.5 mile ☐ neither

If yes, your miles in 12 minutes: ☐·☐ or your time for 1.5 miles: ☐:☐ minutes : seconds

Do you frequently participate in competitive sports? yes ☐ no ☐

If yes, which one or ones?

☐ Golf ☐ Bowling ☐ Tennis ☐ Handball ☐ Soccer

☐ Basketball ☐ Volleyball ☐ Football ☐ Baseball ☐ Track

☐ Other

Average number of times per month ☐

51 In which of the following high school or college athletics did you participate?

☐ None ☐ Football ☐ Basketball ☐ Baseball ☐ Soccer

☐ Track ☐ Swimming ☐ Tennis ☐ Wrestling ☐ Golf

☐ Other

In which of the following high school or college athletics did you earn a varsity letter?

☐ None ☐ Football ☐ Basketball ☐ Baseball ☐ Soccer

☐ Track ☐ Swimming ☐ Tennis ☐ Wrestling ☐ Golf

☐ Other

52 What activity or activities would you prefer in a regular exercise program for yourself?

☐ Walking and/or running ☐ Bicycling (outdoors) ☐ Swimming

☐ Stationary running ☐ Stationary cycling ☐ Tennis

☐ Jumping rope ☐ Handball, basketball or squash

☐ Other

53 Comments:

Explain any other significant medical problems that you consider important for us to know:

5 5

5 6

5 7

5 8

5 9

6 0

6 1

PLEASE PRINT

MOUNT SINAI MEDICAL CENTER
Milwaukee, Wisconsin
NONINVASIVE LABORATORY
CARDIAC WORK EVALUATION LAB

I understand that this exercise test is being done to: **1.** determine the functional capacity of my heart and circulation and **2.** detect the possible presence of heart disease. *I hereby consent to voluntarily engage in an exercise test to determine the state of my heart and circulation.*

The tests which I will undergo will be performed on a treadmill, bicycle, or other methods designed to gradually increase the demands on the heart. This increase in effort will continue until symptoms such as chest discomfort or pain, excessive shortness of breath or fatigue would indicate that I should stop.

During the performance of the test, a physician and trained observer will keep under surveillance my pulse, electrocardiogram, and clinical appearance. Other tests may also be measured during or after the exercise.

There exists the possibility of certain changes occuring during the exercise tests. They include abnormal blood pressure, rapid or very slow heart beat, and very rare instances of heart attack. Every effort will be made to minimize them by the constant surveillance during testing. Emergency equipment and trained personnel are available to deal with unusual situations which may arise.

The information which is obtained will be treated as privileged and confidential and will not be released or revealed to any person other than my physician without my expressed written consent. The information obtained, however, may be used for a statistical or scientific purpose with my right of privacy retained.

I have read the foregoing, and I understand it; any questions which may have occurred to me have been answered to my satisfaction.

Signed: _____
PATIENT

_____
WITNESS

_____
PHYSICIAN SUPERVISING THE TEST

_____
DATE

Figure A–2. An example of an informed consent for graded exercise testing used mainly for diagnostic purposes. (Courtesy of Cardiac Work Evaluation Lab, Mount Sinai Medical Center, Milwaukee, WI.)

Human Performance Laboratory
Mount Sinai Medical Center
950 N. 12th Street
Milwaukee, Wisconsin 53233

CONSENT TO GRADED EXERCISE TESTING

PATIENT NAME _____

Date _____ Time _____

    I authorize Drs. _____ and such assistants or designees as may be selected by them to perform a symptom-limited graded exercise test to determine maximal oxygen uptake and cardiovascular function. During the test heart rate and electrocardiogram will be intermittently monitored. This test will facilitate evaluation of cardiopulmonary function and assist the physician or exercise physiologist in prescribing or evaluating exercise programs. It is my understanding that I will be questioned and examined by a physician prior to taking the test and will be given a resting electrocardiogram to exclude contraindications to such testing.

    Exercise testing will be performed on a treadmill, cycle ergometer or other device that allows workload to gradually increase until fatigue, breathlessness or when other signs or symptoms dictate cessation of the test. Blood pressure and electrocardiogram will be monitored by a physician, nurse, or exercise physiologist. In the latter cases, a physician will be readily available in case of emergency.

    There exists the possibility that certain abnormal changes may occur during the progress of the test. These changes could include abnormal heart beats, abnormal blood pressure response, and in rare instances heart attack. Professional care in selection and supervision of individuals provides appropriate precaution against such problems.

    The benefits of such testing are the scientific assessment of working capacity and the clinical appraisal of health hazards which will facilitate prescription of an exercise/rehabilitative program.

    I have read the foregoing information and understand it. Questions concerning this procedure have been answered to my satisfaction. I have also been informed that the information derived from this test is confidential and will not be disclosed to anyone other than my physician or others that are involved in my care or exercise prescription without my permission. However, I am in agreement that information from this test not identifiable to me can be used for research purposes.

Patient/Participant Signature _____

Witness Signature _____

Test Supervisor _____

Figure A-3. An example of an informed consent for graded exercise testing used for the purpose of entering an exercise program. (Courtesy of Human Performance Laboratory, Mount Sinai Medical Center, Milwaukee, WI.)

TABLE A-1. PHYSICAL FITNESS AND HEALTH STANDARDS FOR MEN 20 TO 29 YEARS OF AGE*

	PERCENTILE RANKINGS	RESTING (SITTING) Heart Rate (beats/min)	Blood Pressure SYSTOLIC (mm Hg)	Blood Pressure DIASTOLIC (mm Hg)	MAXIMUM Oxygen Uptake† (ml/kg·min⁻¹)	MAXIMUM Heart Rate (beats/min)	CHOLESTEROL (mg %)	TRIGLYCERIDES (mg %)	GLUCOSE (mg %)	BODY FAT (%)
High	99	40	94	60	60.0	214	120	27	75	7.2
High	95	46	102	64	51.5	209	142	48	83	9.6
High	90	50	110	70	47.5	205	154	55	88	11.6
Above Average	85	52	110	70	46.5	202	160	62	90	12.9
Above Average	80	54	112	72	45.0	200	165	66	93	13.9
Above Average	75	56	116	75	43.8	200	172	71	95	15.3
Average	70	58	118	78	43.8	199	178	76	96	16.2
Average	65	59	120	78	42.5	198	185	82	98	17.1
Average	60	60	120	80	41.8	197	190	87	100	18.0
Average	55	62	120	80	41.0	196	195	93	100	19.1
Average	50	63	121	80	39.1	194	199	100	102	20.1
Average	45	65	124	80	38.2	193	202	106	102	20.5
Below Average	40	66	128	80	37.0	192	203	110	103	21.2
Below Average	35	68	130	82	36.3	191	207	123	104	22.3
Below Average	30	70	130	84	35.6	190	211	137	105	23.4
Below Average	25	71	132	85	35.5	188	218	148	105	25.4
Low	20	72	136	88	33.5	186	222	170	106	27.4
Low	15	76	140	90	32.5	183	229	180	109	28.6
Low	10	80	140	90	31.5	180	240	200	110	30.5
Low	5	88	150	100	29.0	179	251	234	113	32.8
Low	1	99	158	110	22.8	170	269	296	118	38.0
							300	762	123	49.0
	Population size	358	367	367	371	371	273	271	271	248
	Average	64	124	80	40.0	192	200	133	101	21.6
	Standard deviation	12.5	13.4	9.6	6.4	12.2	39.1	107.8	14.5	9.1

*Data from the Cooper Clinic Coronary Risk Factor Profile Charts, which are from data collected on patients being evaluated at the Cooper Clinic and standards being established at the Institute for Aerobics Research, Dallas, Texas, 1978. Reprinted with permission from Pollock, M.L., Wilmore, J.H., and Fox, S.M.: Health and Fitness Through Physical Activity. New York, copyright © John Wiley and Sons, 1978.
†Maximum oxygen uptake was estimated from treadmill time.

TABLE A–2. PHYSICAL FITNESS AND HEALTH STANDARDS FOR MEN 30 TO 39 YEARS OF AGE*

PERCENTILE RANKINGS		RESTING (SITTING)			MAXIMUM		CHOLESTEROL (mg %)	TRIGLYCERIDES (mg %)	GLUCOSE (mg %)	BODY FAT (%)
		Heart Rate (beats/min)	Blood Pressure SYSTOLIC (mm Hg)	DIASTOLIC (mm Hg)	Oxygen Uptake† (ml/kg·min⁻¹)	Heart Rate (beats/min)				
99	High	40	96	50	54.4	210	135	35	75	7.1
95	Above Average	46	102	58	49.5	204	158	50	85	11.1
90		50	108	70	46.5	200	169	60	89	13.4
85		52	110	70	45.0	200	175	67	91	14.8
80		55	110	74	43.7	198	182	75	94	16.2
75		56	114	76	42.5	196	188	80	95	17.2
70		58	116	78	41.3	194	193	87	96	18.2
65		59	118	80	41.0	192	197	93	99	19.2
60	Average	60	120	80	39.0	191	203	100	100	20.1
55		62	120	80	39.0	190	208	105	100	21.1
50	Average	63	120	80	37.0	189	215	113	102	22.0
45		64	122	80	37.0	188	220	120	104	22.8
40		65	124	81	35.7	186	224	129	105	23.6
35		67	126	84	35.7	184	230	140	105	24.4
30	Below Average	68	130	85	34.6	183	235	150	107	25.5
25		70	130	88	33.5	181	240	169	110	26.4
20		72	132	90	32.9	180	250	187	110	28.0
15		74	138	90	31.5	177	256	207	114	29.8
10	Low	77	140	92	30.2	174	271	241	115	32.2
5		82	146	100	27.1	168	289	324	120	36.0
1		95	168	110	22.7	150	340	756	133	45.9
Population size		1538	1615	1615	1632	1632	1387	1377	1376	1223
Average		63	123	81	37.5	188	217	143	103	22.4
Standard deviation		11.0	13.6	9.6	—	11.7	41.2	114.0	18.2	7.9

*Data from the Cooper Clinic Coronary Risk Factor Profile Charts, which are from data collected on patients being evaluated at the Cooper Clinic and standards being established at the Institute for Aerobics Research, Dallas, Texas, 1978. Reprinted with permission from Pollock, M.L., Wilmore, J.H., and Fox, S.M.: Health and Fitness Through Physical Activity. New York, copyright © John Wiley and Sons, 1978.

† Maximum oxygen uptake was estimated from treadmill time.

TABLE A–3. PHYSICAL FITNESS AND HEALTH STANDARDS FOR MEN 40 TO 49 YEARS OF AGE*

| PERCENTILE RANKINGS | | RESTING (SITTING) | | | MAXIMUM | | CHOLESTEROL (mg %) | TRIGLYCERIDES (mg %) | GLUCOSE (mg %) | BODY FAT (%) |
| | | Heart Rate (beats/min) | Blood Pressure | | Oxygen Uptake† (ml/kg·min⁻¹) | Heart Rate (beats/min) | | | | |
			SYSTOLIC (mm Hg)	DIASTOLIC (mm Hg)						
99	High	42	96	60	52.5	205	145	37	80	9.2
95		47	104	70	48.0	200	165	53	87	13.0
90	Above Average	50	110	70	45.0	196	175	63	90	14.9
85		52	110	74	43.7	193	186	72	93	16.6
80		54	111	76	42.5	191	193	78	95	17.7
75		56	115	78	41.0	190	199	85	97	18.8
70	Average	58	118	80	40.0	188	204	91	99	19.7
65		58	120	80	39.0	186	209	98	100	20.7
60		60	120	80	37.0	185	214	105	101	21.5
55		61	120	80	36.3	183	220	112	103	22.2
50		62	121	80	35.7	182	225	121	105	23.0
45		64	124	82	35.3	180	230	130	105	23.8
40	Average	65	126	84	34.3	180	235	139	107	24.6
35		67	130	85	33.6	178	240	150	109	25.4
30		69	130	88	32.9	176	245	162	110	26.3
25	Below Average	71	131	90	31.5	174	250	180	111	27.4
20		72	138	90	31.1	171	257	200	114	28.5
15		75	140	92	30.2	168	265	227	115	30.0
10	Low	78	142	98	27.6	164	275	269	120	32.2
5		84	150	100	24.1	158	295	363	125	36.1
1		99	166	110	19.6	139	338	590	160	44.4
Population size		1826	1880	1880	1898	1898	1681	1665	1662	1537
Average		64	124	83	36.0	181	226	151	106	23.4
Standard deviation		11.5	14.5	10.0	—	13.3	39.7	110.5	21.0	7.1

*Data from the Cooper Clinic Coronary Risk Factor Profile Charts, which are from data collected on patients being evaluated at the Cooper Clinic and standards being established at the Institute for Aerobics Research, Dallas, Texas, 1978. Reprinted with permission from Pollock, M.L., Wilmore, J.H., and Fox, S.M.: Health and Fitness Through Physical Activity. New York, copyright © John Wiley and Sons, 1978.

† Maximum oxygen uptake was estimated from treadmill time.

TABLE A–4. PHYSICAL FITNESS AND HEALTH STANDARDS FOR MEN 50 TO 59 YEARS OF AGE*

PERCENTILE RANKINGS		RESTING (SITTING) Heart Rate (beats/min)	Blood Pressure SYSTOLIC (mm Hg)	Blood Pressure DIASTOLIC (mm Hg)	MAXIMUM Oxygen Uptake[†] (ml/kg·min⁻¹)	MAXIMUM Heart Rate (beats/min)	CHOLESTEROL (mg %)	TRIGLYCERIDES (mg %)	GLUCOSE (mg %)	BODY FAT (%)
99	High	42	98	60	51.6	200	149	44	80	9.0
95	High	47	108	70	45.4	192	173	55	88	13.1
90	Above Average	50	110	72	43.7	188	185	67	92	15.8
85	Above Average	52	114	75	41.0	186	193	75	95	17.4
80	Above Average	55	116	78	39.0	183	201	83	96	18.4
75	Above Average	56	119	80	37.0	180	205	89	99	19.6
70	Above Average	58	120	80	36.0	180	211	95	100	20.4
65	Average	60	120	80	35.7	178	215	100	101	21.4
60	Average	60	122	80	34.6	176	220	107	103	22.1
55	Average	62	125	80	33.5	175	225	116	105	22.9
50	Average	63	128	82	32.9	173	230	124	105	23.8
45	Average	64	130	84	32.2	172	235	133	108	24.6
40	Average	65	130	86	31.5	170	240	142	110	25.4
35	Below Average	66	132	88	30.8	168	245	153	110	26.1
30	Below Average	68	138	90	30.2	166	250	165	113	27.0
25	Below Average	70	140	90	29.2	163	255	185	115	28.0
20	Below Average	72	140	90	29.0	160	264	200	116	29.1
15	Below Average	75	144	95	26.2	157	274	230	120	30.9
10	Low	77	150	100	24.5	150	285	270	124	32.8
5	Low	82	160	102	21.0	140	300	370	135	35.9
1	Low	95	180	114	16.5	118	344	690	180	44.8
Population size		1046	1073	1075	1087	1087	942	936	935	847
Average		63	129	34	33.6	171	233	157	108	24.1
Standard deviation		11.0	17.2	10.4	—	15.9	40.5	120.9	21.2	7.0

*Data from the Cooper Clinic Coronary Risk Factor Profile Charts, which are from data collected on patients being evaluated at the Cooper Clinic and standards being established at the Institute for Aerobics Research, Dallas, Texas, 1978. Reprinted with permission from Pollock, M.L., Wilmore, J.H., and Fox, S.M.: Health and Fitness Through Physical Activity. New York, copyright © John Wiley and Sons, 1978.

†Maximum oxygen uptake estimated from treadmill time.

TABLE A–5. PHYSICAL FITNESS AND HEALTH STANDARDS FOR MEN 60+ YEARS OF AGE*

PERCENTILE RANKINGS		RESTING (SITTING)			MAXIMUM		CHOLESTEROL (mg %)	TRIGLYCERIDES (mg %)	GLUCOSE (mg %)	BODY FAT (%)
		Heart Rate (beats/min)	Blood Pressure		Oxygen Uptake† (ml/kg·min⁻¹)	Heart Rate (beats/min)				
			SYSTOLIC (mm Hg)	DIASTOLIC (mm Hg)						
99	High	38	98	60	49.5	195	152	43	83	10.5
95	Above Average	48	108	68	44.5	186	173	55	89	12.3
90		52	112	70	41.0	184	180	66	92	14.1
85		54	118	72	36.6	180	190	73	94	16.2
80		55	120	76	35.7	175	196	76	96	17.2
75	Above Average	56	120	78	35.0	172	201	82	100	18.0
70		58	124	80	33.6	170	205	89	102	18.9
65		58	128	80	32.2	170	210	95	104	19.9
60	Average	60	130	80	31.0	165	214	100	105	20.8
55		60	130	80	30.2	163	217	106	106	21.5
50	Average	62	131	81	29.0	162	225	115	108	22.3
45		64	135	84	29.0	160	228	122	110	23.3
40		65	140	84	26.2	159	234	129	110	24.4
35		67	140	86	25.9	156	240	142	112	25.4
30	Below Average	68	140	88	24.5	152	250	150	115	26.9
25		70	145	90	22.7	148	256	160	118	28.0
20	Below Average	72	150	90	21.8	145	264	170	120	28.9
15	Low	75	152	94	20.1	140	268	195	124	30.1
10		77	160	98	17.5	131	280	233	129	32.5
5		81	168	100	15.7	121	291	291	140	35.6
1		94	184	118	14.0	104	345	552	170	42.4
Population size		267	275	275	279	249	243	241	241	211
Average		63	135	83	30.0	159	228	139	110	23.1
Standard deviation		10.4	18.3	11.0	—	19.5	39.1	99.4	23.4	7.2

*Data from the Cooper Clinic Coronary Risk Factor Profile Charts, which are from data collected on patients being evaluated at the Cooper Clinic and standards being established at the Institute for Aerobics Research, Dallas, Texas, 1978. Reprinted with permission from Pollock, M.L., Wilmore, J.H., and Fox, S.M.: Health and Fitness Through Physical Activity. New York, copyright © John Wiley and Sons, 1978.
† Maximum oxygen uptake was estimated from treadmill time.

TABLE A–6. PHYSICAL FITNESS AND HEALTH STANDARDS FOR FEMALES 20 TO 29 YEARS OF AGE*

PERCENTILE RANKINGS		RESTING (SITTING) Heart Rate (beats/min)	Blood Pressure SYSTOLIC (mm Hg)	Blood Pressure DIASTOLIC (mm Hg)	MAXIMUM Oxygen Uptake† (ml/kg·min⁻¹)	MAXIMUM Heart Rate (beats/min)	CHOLESTEROL (mg %)	TRIGLYCERIDES (mg %)	GLUCOSE (mg %)	BODY FAT (%)
99	High	48	90	56	45.0	213	135	30	56	7.8
95	High	52	97	60	41.0	208	144	43	75	9.6
90	Above Average	55	100	63	38.0	203	150	45	81	11.6
85	Above Average	58	100	65	37.0	199	160	47	85	14.5
80	Above Average	59	101	68	35.7	198	165	50	86	15.1
75	Above Average	60	105	70	34.3	196	170	52	87	16.1
70	Above Average	60	106	70	33.6	194	170	58	90	18.3
65	Average	62	110	70	32.9	192	174	60	92	20.2
60	Average	63	110	72	31.5	190	182	65	94	23.2
55	Average	64	110	74	30.9	190	185	72	94	24.1
50	Average	65	112	75	30.2	188	190	76	95	24.9
45	Average	68	115	75	30.0	187	195	81	97	25.6
40	Below Average	70	118	78	29.6	186	196	88	99	26.2
35	Below Average	70	118	78	29.2	184	200	107	99	27.3
30	Below Average	72	120	80	29.0	182	210	109	100	28.2
25	Below Average	74	120	80	27.6	181	215	120	100	30.3
20	Below Average	75	120	80	25.3	180	219	126	101	33.3
15	Low	80	122	80	24.0	174	224	138	103	36.4
10	Low	84	130	82	21.8	172	251	158	105	38.5
5	Low	86	140	88	20.4	168	265	235	115	45.5
1	Low	100	141	90	19.2	160	380	635	200	51.4
Population size		115	118	118	119	119	68	68	67	61
Average		67	114	74	31.1	188	195	102	96	25.0
Standard deviation		11.2	12.0	7.8	—	11.8	41.8	89.7	20.9	11.5

*Data from the Cooper Clinic Coronary Risk Factor Profile Charts, which are from data collected on patients being evaluated at the Cooper Clinic and standards being established at the Institute for Aerobics Research, Dallas, Texas, 1978. Reprinted with permission from Pollock, M.L., Wilmore, J.H., and Fox, S.M.: Health and Fitness Through Physical Activity. New York, copyright © John Wiley and Sons, 1978.

†Maximum oxygen uptake estimated from treadmill time.

TABLE A–7. PHYSICAL FITNESS AND HEALTH STANDARDS FOR FEMALES 30 TO 39 YEARS OF AGE*

PERCENTILE RANKINGS		RESTING (SITTING)			MAXIMUM		CHOLESTEROL (mg %)	TRIGLYCERIDES (mg %)	GLUCOSE (mg %)	BODY FAT (%)
		Heart Rate (beats/min)	Blood Pressure SYSTOLIC (mm Hg)	Blood Pressure DIASTOLIC (mm Hg)	Oxygen Uptake† (ml/kg·min⁻¹)	Heart Rate (beats/min)				
99	High	48	90	60	43.7	210	124	25	60	5.1
95	High	52	98	60	40.0	200	141	37	79	10.1
90	High	55	100	65	37.0	196	158	44	83	13.1
85	Above Average	57	100	70	35.7	194	165	48	85	14.8
80	Above Average	58	104	70	35.0	192	168	51	88	16.7
75	Above Average	60	106	70	33.6	190	172	55	90	18.3
70	Average	62	110	70	32.9	189	176	59	91	19.3
65	Average	62	110	71	31.5	187	184	62	92	20.5
60	Average	65	110	74	31.5	185	188	68	95	21.5
55	Average	66	110	75	30.2	185	191	73	95	22.5
50	Average	68	114	76	30.2	184	195	77	95	23.6
45	Average	68	116	80	29.3	183	200	80	97	24.6
40	Average	70	118	80	29.0	182	204	85	99	25.5
35	Below Average	72	120	80	27.6	180	206	88	100	26.3
30	Below Average	74	120	80	26.2	180	211	93	100	27.6
25	Below Average	75	120	80	25.7	178	218	100	101	29.0
20	Below Average	76	122	82	24.5	176	224	108	103	31.3
15	Below Average	80	125	85	23.1	174	231	120	105	34.6
10	Low	82	130	90	21.7	170	240	132	107	38.1
5	Low	85	140	90	21.0	164	255	157	111	42.9
1	Low	108	160	110	17.0	148	300	428	116	50.2
Population size		280	301	301	309	309	220	220	220	192
Average		68	115	77	30.3	183	197	89	95	24.8
Standard deviation		11.5	13.3	9.9	—	14.8	36.0	68.0	14.8	11.0

* Data from the Cooper Clinic Coronary Risk Factor Profile Charts, which are from data collected on patients being evaluated at the Cooper Clinic and standards being established at the Institute for Aerobics Research, Dallas, Texas. 1978. Reprinted with permission from Pollock, M.L., Wilmore, J.H., and Fox, S.M.: Health and Fitness Through Physical Activity. New York, copyright © John Wiley and Sons, 1978.

† Maximum oxygen uptake estimated from treadmill time.

TABLE A–8. PHYSICAL FITNESS AND HEALTH STANDARDS FOR FEMALES 40 TO 49 YEARS OF AGE*

PERCENTILE RANKINGS		RESTING (SITTING)			MAXIMUM		CHOLESTEROL (mg %)	TRIGLYCERIDES (mg %)	GLUCOSE (mg %)	BODY FAT (%)
		Heart Rate (beats/min)	Blood Pressure SYSTOLIC (mm Hg)	DIASTOLIC (mm Hg)	Oxygen Uptake† (ml/kg·min⁻¹)	Heart Rate (beats/min)				
99	High	43	90	58	43.7	208	130	35	75	7.3
95		52	100	60	37.0	196	158	45	82	12.0
90	Above Average	55	100	65	35.0	192	171	49	86	15.8
85		58	102	70	32.9	189	178	56	88	17.9
80		60	105	70	31.5	186	184	58	90	19.6
75	Average	60	110	70	30.9	185	190	63	91	21.0
70		62	110	70	30.2	183	195	67	92	21.9
65		63	110	74	30.2	180	198	73	94	22.7
60		64	112	75	29.0	180	201	77	95	23.9
55		65	114	78	29.0	178	205	82	95	24.9
50	Average	66	118	80	26.7	177	210	86	96	25.9
45		68	120	80	26.2	175	213	91	98	26.7
40		70	120	80	25.3	173	217	98	100	27.6
35		72	120	80	24.5	172	223	105	100	28.2
30		72	120	80	24.5	170	228	110	100	29.1
25	Below Average	74	124	80	22.9	169	235	118	104	30.2
20		76	130	82	22.7	165	241	130	105	31.4
15		80	132	85	21.0	162	252	148	107	33.7
10	Low Average	80	138	90	21.0	158	264	162	111	37.4
5		87	150	94	19.2	148	283	223	117	43.1
1	Low	100	164	100	15.7	133	319	450	153	49.7
Population size		260	282	232	286	286	218	216	215	183
Average		68	118	78	28.0	175	214	106	98	26.1
Standard deviation		10.7	15.7	10.2	—	14.8	39.4	89.9	16.6	8.6

*Data from the Cooper Clinic Coronary Risk Factor Profile Charts, which are from data collected on patients being evaluated at the Cooper Clinic and standards being established at the Institute for Aerobics Research, Dallas, Texas, 1978. Reprinted with permission from Pollock, M.L., Wilmore, J.H., and Fox, S.M.: Health and Fitness Through Physical Activity. New York, copyright © John Wiley and Sons, 1978.

†Maximum oxygen uptake estimated from treadmill time.

TABLE A–9. PHYSICAL FITNESS AND HEALTH STANDARDS FOR FEMALES 50 TO 59 YEARS OF AGE*

PERCENTILE RANKINGS	RESTING (SITTING) Heart Rate (beats/min)	Blood Pressure SYSTOLIC (mm Hg)	DIASTOLIC (mm Hg)	MAXIMUM Oxygen Uptake[†] (ml/kg·min⁻¹)	Heart Rate (beats/min)	CHOLESTEROL (mg %)	TRIGLYCERIDES (mg %)	GLUCOSE (mg %)	BODY FAT (%)
99 (High)	45	90	58	42.5	202	158	39	78	10.8
95 (Above Average)	52	100	64	35.7	190	170	50	85	15.9
90 (Above Average)	55	108	69	32.9	185	180	60	89	18.2
85	58	110	70	31.5	182	192	68	91	21.0
80	60	110	70	30.2	180	198	70	93	22.7
75	60	115	74	30.2	179	202	77	95	23.9
70 (Average)	61	118	75	29.0	176	205	82	95	25.1
65	62	120	76	27.6	174	214	91	97	26.1
60	64	120	79	26.2	173	218	98	99	27.0
55	65	120	80	25.3	172	221	105	100	27.7
50 (Average)	67	122	80	24.5	170	225	110	100	28.4
45	68	128	80	24.5	168	230	115	102	29.6
40	69	130	82	23.6	167	234	118	105	30.4
35	70	130	84	22.7	164	236	125	105	31.4
30 (Below Average)	72	134	85	22.7	162	241	130	108	32.5
25	74	140	88	21.9	160	249	145	110	33.4
20	75	140	90	21.0	160	260	165	110	34.7
15	78	142	90	20.4	156	267	175	111	37.1
10 (Low)	83	148	92	19.2	152	275	218	115	39.7
5	89	160	100	17.6	144	295	242	120	44.4
1	105	172	110	14.4	128	320	395	135	52.2
Population size	162	167	167	169	169	137	136	137	127
Average	68	126	80	25.7	169	228	123	102	29.3
Standard deviation	11.7	16.8	10.6	—	14.5	27.3	67.1	15.1	9.5

*Data from the Cooper Clinic Coronary Risk Factor Profile Charts, which are from data collected on patients being evaluated at the Cooper Clinic and standards being established at the Institute for Aerobics Research, Dallas, Texas, 1978. Reprinted with permission from Pollock, M.L., Wilmore, J.H., and Fox, S.M.: Health and Fitness Through Physical Activity. New York, copyright © John Wiley and Sons, 1978.

[†]Maximum oxygen uptake estimated from treadmill time.

TABLE A–10. PHYSICAL FITNESS AND HEALTH STANDARDS FOR FEMALES 60+ YEARS OF AGE*

| PERCENTILE RANKINGS | | RESTING (SITTING) | | | MAXIMUM | | CHOLESTEROL (mg %) | TRIGLYCERIDES (mg %) | GLUCOSE (mg %) | BODY FAT (%) |
| | | Heart Rate (beats/min) | Blood Pressure | | Oxygen Uptake[†] (ml·kg·min⁻¹) | Heart Rate (beats/min) | | | | |
			SYSTOLIC (mm Hg)	DIASTOLIC (mm Hg)						
99	High	46	110	66	37.0	178	127	42	75	6.8
95		50	118	70	31.5	178	180	46	80	13.1
90	Above Average	52	120	70	30.2	176	185	62	88	17.7
85		56	120	71	30.2	170	188	72	90	19.3
80		57	120	75	26.9	165	210	80	91	22.2
75		59	122	75	25.3	162	220	87	94	24.0
70		60	125	76	25.3	160	223	90	97	25.1
65		60	125	78	24.5	158	235	93	98	26.6
60	Average	62	128	80	24.5	155	235	97	100	27.1
55		64	130	80	23.9	155	238	105	100	27.9
50		64	130	80	21.8	153	240	110	102	29.8
45		64	132	80	21.3	151	245	124	104	30.4
40		66	136	80	21.0	150	245	129	105	30.8
35		70	139	81	20.1	150	246	134	107	31.2
30	Below Average	72	140	84	20.1	145	262	140	110	31.7
25		72	140	86	19.2	142	265	164	110	32.5
20		74	142	88	18.3	140	269	183	110	34.7
15		75	150	90	17.5	128	275	210	110	35.2
10	Low	79	160	98	16.1	126	276	228	115	36.3
5		80	165	100	15.7	120	310	277	120	39.9
1		85	188	100	12.3	106	335	400	130	51.2
Population size		43	46	46	46	46	40	39	39	32
Average		65	135	81	22.9	151	237	131	102	28.3
Standard deviation		9.6	16.2	8.8	—	17.5	40.9	71.5	14.9	8.5

*Data from the Cooper Clinic Coronary Risk Factor Profile Charts, which are from data collected on patients being evaluated at the Cooper Clinic and standards being established at the Institute for Aerobics Research, Dallas, Texas, 1978. Reprinted with permission from Pollock, M.L., Wilmore, J.H., and Fox, S.M.: Health and Fitness Through Physical Activity. New York, copyright © John Wiley and Sons, 1978.

† Maximum oxygen uptake estimated from treadmill time.

24-HOUR HISTORY

NAME: _____ DATE: _____

TIME: _____

HOW MUCH SLEEP DID YOU GET LAST NIGHT? (Please circle one)
     1 2 3 4 5 6 7 8 9 10 (hours)

HOW MUCH SLEEP DO YOU NORMALLY GET? (Please circle one)
     1 2 3 4 5 6 7 8 9 10 (hours)

HOW LONG HAS IT BEEN SINCE YOUR LAST MEAL OR SNACK? (Please circle one)
     1 2 3 4 5 6 7 8 9 10 11 12 13 14 (hours)

LIST THE ITEMS EATEN BELOW:

_____

WHEN DID YOU LAST:

    Have a cup of coffee or tea _____

    Smoke a cigarette, cigar, or pipe _____

    Take drugs (including aspirin) _____

    Drink alcohol _____

    Give blood _____

    Have an illness _____

    Suffer from respiratory problems _____

WHAT SORT OF PHYSICAL EXERCISE DID YOU PERFORM YESTERDAY?

WHAT SORT OF PHYSICAL EXERCISE DID YOU PERFORM TODAY?

DESCRIBE YOUR GENERAL FEELINGS BY CHECKING ONE OF THE FOLLOWING:

_____ Excellent _____ Bad

_____ Very, Very Good _____ Very Bad

_____ Very Good _____ Very, Very Bad

_____ Neither Bad nor Good _____ Terrible

Figure A–4. This is an example of a 24-hour history form used to document and standardize testing conditions.

TABLE A-11. PERCENTILE RANKINGS FOR RECOVERY
HEART RATE AND PREDICTED MAXIMAL OXYGEN
CONSUMPTION FOR MALE AND FEMALE COLLEGE STUDENTS*

PERCENTILE RANKING	RECOVERY HR FEMALE	PREDICTED $\dot{V}O_2$ MAX (ml/kg min^{-1})	RECOVERY HR MALE	PREDICTED $\dot{V}O_2$ MAX (ml/kg min^{-1})
100	128	42.2	120	60.9
95	140	40.0	124	59.3
90	148	38.5	128	57.6
85	152	37.7	136	54.2
80	156	37.0	140	52.5
75	158	36.6	144	50.9
70	160	36.3	148	49.2
65	162	35.9	149	48.8
60	163	35.7	152	47.5
55	164	35.5	154	46.7
50	166	35.1	156	45.8
45	168	34.8	160	44.1
40	170	34.4	162	43.3
35	171	34.2	164	42.5
30	172	34.0	166	41.6
25	176	33.3	168	40.8
20	180	32.6	172	39.1
15	182	32.2	176	37.4
10	184	31.8	178	36.6
5	196	29.6	184	34.1

*See Chapter 6 for explanation of submaximal bench stepping test.

Reprinted with permission from Katch, F.I., and McArdle, W.D.: Nutrition, Weight Control, and Exercise. 2nd ed. Philadelphia, Lea and Febiger, 1983.

TABLE A-12. Y's WAY TO PHYSICAL FITNESS NORMS FOR MALES

Percentage Ranking	Rating	PWC Max Kgm	Maximum Oxygen Uptake LITERS/MIN	Maximum Oxygen Uptake ML/KG	METS	Trunk Flexion In.	Bench Press Repetitions	Sit ups 1 min Reps	3 Min Step Test Post Ex. HR 1 min BPM	Resting HR BPM
35 YEARS AND UNDER										
95	Excellent	2000	4.61	54	15.	21	35	45	81	51
85	Good	1800	3.89	49	14.	19	29	41	99	59
75	Above Av.	1700	3.49	46	13.	17	24	37	103	65
50	Average	1500	3.08	36	10.	15	20	33	120	72
30	Below Av.	1300	2.67	32	9.	12	15	28	123	78
15	Fair	1200	2.27	28	8.	9	11	23	127	84
5	Poor	1000	1.55	24	7.	7	7	18	136	92
36-45 YEARS OF AGE										
95	Excellent	1800	4.35	53	15.	22	30	42	84	54
85	Good	1600	3.65	45	13.	19	24	38	98	60
75	Above Av.	1500	3.26	39	11.	16	19	32	112	66
50	Average	1300	2.86	33	9.	14	17	27	120	72
30	Below Av.	1100	2.46	29	8.	12	14	21	125	78
15	Fair	1000	2.07	25	7.	10	10	18	129	84
5	Poor	900	1.37	23	6.	5	3	11	138	92
46 YEARS AND ABOVE										
95	Excellent	1700	3.64	43	12.	20	28	38	90	54
85	Good	1500	3.07	38	11.	17	22	33	102	59
75	Above Av.	1400	2.74	34	10.	15	19	26	111	64
50	Average	1200	2.41	30	9.	13	16	21	120	72
30	Below Av.	1000	2.08	27	8.	11	12	18	124	78
15	Fair	900	1.75	24	7.	8	8	15	130	84
5	Poor	800	1.18	20	6.	5	3	10	138	95

Reprinted with permission from Golding, L.A., Myers, C.R., and Sinning, W.E., editors: The Y's Way to Physical Fitness (revised). Chicago, The YMCA of the USA, 1982.

TABLE A–13. Y's WAY TO PHYSICAL FITNESS NORMS FOR FEMALES

Percentage Ranking	Rating	PWC Max Kgm	Maximum Oxygen Uptake LITERS/ MIN	ML/KG	METS	Trunk Flexion In.	Bench Press Repetitions	Sit ups 1 min Reps	3 Min Step Test Post Ex. HR 1 min BPM	Resting HR BPM
				35 YEARS AND UNDER						
95	Excellent	1700	3.32	55	15.	23	30	39	79	59
85	Good	1500	2.74	45	13.	21	24	34	94	63
75	Above Av.	1300	2.42	39	11.	20	20	30	109	68
50	Average	1100	2.09	34	10.	18	16	25	118	72
30	Below Av.	900	1.76	30	9.	15	13	20	122	80
15	Fair	700	1.44	26	7.	14	10	15	129	84
5	Poor	500	.86	20	6.	11	5	10	137	92
				36–45 YEARS OF AGE						
95	Excellent	1600	3.04	49	14.	23	29	39	79	59
85	Good	1400	2.55	43	12.	21	21	29	90	64
75	Above Av.	1200	2.27	37	10.	19	18	22	106	70
50	Average	1000	1.99	33	9.	17	15	18	118	75
30	Below Av.	800	1.71	29	8.	14	11	12	125	80
15	Fair	600	1.43	26	7.	12	7	9	134	88
5	Poor	400	.95	22	6.	10	4	4	145	92
				46 YEARS AND ABOVE						
95	Excellent	1500	2.80	46	13.	22	30	24	84	59
85	Good	1300	2.32	38	11.	19	22	20	97	63
75	Above Av.	1100	2.04	32	9.	18	18	17	108	67
50	Average	900	1.77	27	8.	15	14	14	118	73
30	Below Av.	700	1.50	24	7.	14	9	11	124	78
15	Fair	500	1.22	20	6.	11	5	7	130	84
5	Poor	300	.74	18	5.	9	2	2	145	92

Reprinted with permission from Golding, L.A., Myers, C.R., and Sinning, W.E., editors: The Y's Way to Physical Fitness (revised). Chicago, The YMCA of the USA, 1982.

UNIVERSITY HOSPITAL
University of California
Medical Center, San Diego

REPORT OF
TREADMILL EXERCISE TEST
(Page One)

Rev. Code **750**

SEND REPORT TO	Source	Date	
			Patient Identification
			Procedure No. 013 ☐

TMT NO.	AGE	SEX	WT (lbs)	HT (in)	CLINICAL REASONS FOR TEST

DIAGNOSIS OF ATYPICAL SENSATION OR PAIN POSSIBLY DUE TO ASCVD (Explain) ☐

☐ INPATIENT   DATE (Mo., Day, Yr.)   24 HR. TIME
☐ OUTPATIENT

PREVIOUS TEST   > 3 HRS. SINCE LAST MEAL   EVALUATION OF ANGINA
☐ No ☐ Yes, when: ☐ Yes   ☐ No   ☐ Typical   ☐ Variant   ☐ Unstable

MEDICATIONS
☐ Calcium Antagonist
☐ Digitalis   ☐ Nitrates
☐ Beta-Blocker   ☐ Quinidine/Pronestyl
☐ Anti-HBP   ☐ Other

DYSRHYTHMIA EVALUATION
☐ PVCs   ☐ SVT   ☐ HB   ☐ Sick Sinus   ☐ Other
OTHER HEART DISEASE   ☐ Valvular   ☐ Heart Muscle
☐ Mitral Prolapse   ☐ Congenital   ☐ Other
EVALUATION POST AMI ☐   TIME SINCE LAST INFARCT
Weeks   Months   Years

ACTIVITY STATUS
☐ Recent Bed Rest   ☐ Sedentary   ☐ Active   ☐ Athletic

SCREENING ASYMPTOMATIC INDIVIDUAL ☐   FUNCTIONAL CAPACITY EVALUATION ☐

PROBABILITY OF ASCVD BY HISTORY PRIOR TO TEST
☐ Unlikely   ☐ Possible   ☐ Probable   ☐ Very Probable

CORONARY BYPASS SURGERY   DATE OF SURGERY & TYPE
☐ Pre   ☐ Post

PHYSICAL EXAM (PRE) S_3 ☐ Yes ☐ No S_4 ☐ Yes ☐ No   MURMUR ☐ Yes ☐ No   OTHER ☐

STAGE	MPH/GRADE	METS	MIN/SEC IN STAGE	HR	BP	P.E.	DESCRIBE: CHEST PAIN/DYSRHYTHMIA/ ST SLOPE/AMOUNT J-JCT UP OR DOWN/LEAD(S)
				(AT END OF STAGE)			
SUPINE							
HV FOR 30 SEC	3.5cc O_2/kg·min = 1 MET						
STAND	If 2.0 mph, 2/3 the O_2 cost						
1A	2.0/0%	2					
1B	3.3/0%	4					
2	3.3/5%	6					
3	3.3/10%	8					
4	3.3/15%	10					
5	3.3/20%	13					
6	3.3/25%	15					

REASON FOR STOPPING
☐ Angina   ☐ Other chest pain
☐ Claudication   ☐ Other leg pain
☐ ECG changes   ☐ Dysrhythmia
☐ Maximal effort   ☐ Other

IMMED	MAX SBP (_____) x
2 MIN	MAX HR (_____) =
5 MIN	___ ___ . ___ x 10³
___ MIN	Estimated Maximal O_2 Cost = _____ METS

B248(3-83)6   WHITE - Medical Record   CANARY - Referring MD   PINK - Cardiology File   GOLD - Research File

Figure A–5. Data collection form and summary sheet for graded exercise testing. (Courtesy of Victor F. Froelicher, M.D., School of Medicine, University of California, San Diego.

UNIVERSITY HOSPITAL
University of California
Medical Center, San Diego

Rev. Code **750**

**REPORT OF
TREADMILL EXERCISE TEST**
(Page Two)

Source _____ Date _____

Patient Identification

Procedure No. 013 ☐

PHYSICAL EXAM (POST)	S_3 ☐ Yes ☐ No	S_4 ☐ Yes ☐ No		SIGNS/SYMPTOMS CHF		MURMUR ☐ Yes ☐ No	TYPE			
ECG RESPONSE	DYSRHYTHMIA	NO EXPLAIN		OCC PVC		FREQ PVC	VT	SVT		AF
	ST SEGMENTS	NL EXPLAIN		BORDERLINE	ABNL		ELEVATE		NORMALIZE	
	CONDUCTION	NL EXPLAIN		LBBB		RBBB		BLOCK		AXIS SHIFT

PATIENT RESPONSE	MAX HR ☐ NL ☐ HI ☐ LO		MAX SYSTOLIC BP ☐ NL ☐ HI ☐ LO ☐ Drop			FUNCTIONAL CAPACITY ☐ NL ☐ HI ☐ LO	
	ANGINA ☐ Yes ☐ No	ATYPICAL CHEST PAIN ☐ Yes ☐ No	CHF ☐ Yes ☐ No		OTHER COMPLICATIONS ☐ Yes ☐ No	MAXIMAL EFFORT ☐ Yes ☐ No	

RESTING ECG ☐ Normal ☐ Abnormal	DESCRIBE

INTERPRETATION

INTERPRETED BY _____ DATE _____

APPROVED BY _____ DATE _____

B248(3-83)6   WHITE - Medical Record   CANARY - Referring MD   PINK - Cardiology File   GOLD - Research File

Figure A–5. *Continued.*

Figure A–6. Recording form for anthropometric measures. (Adapted with permission from form developed by the Institute for Aerobic Research, Dallas, Texas.)

TABLE A–14. ESTIMATION OF TARGET WEIGHT FOR MALES*

% Fat	|———————————————————————— BODY WEIGHT (pounds) ————————————————————————|

% Fat	120	125	130	135	140	145	150	155	160	165	170	175	180	185	190	195	200	205	210	215	220	225	230	235	240
16	120	125	130	135	140	145	150	155	160	165	170	175	180	185	190	195	200	205	210	215	220	225	230	235	240
18	117	122	127	132	137	142	146	151	156	161	166	171	176	181	186	190	195	200	205	210	215	220	225	229	234
20	114	119	124	129	133	138	143	148	152	157	162	167	171	176	181	186	190	195	200	205	210	214	219	224	229
22	111	116	121	125	130	135	139	144	149	153	158	162	167	172	176	181	186	190	195	200	204	209	214	218	223
24	109	113	118	122	127	131	136	140	145	149	154	158	163	167	172	176	181	186	190	195	199	204	208	213	217
26	106	110	115	119	123	128	132	137	141	145	150	154	159	163	167	172	176	181	185	189	194	198	203	207	211
28	103	107	111	116	120	124	129	133	137	141	146	150	154	159	163	167	171	176	180	184	189	193	197	201	208
30	100	104	108	113	117	121	125	129	133	137	142	146	150	154	158	162	167	171	175	179	183	188	192	196	200
32	97	101	105	109	113	117	121	125	130	134	138	142	146	150	154	158	162	166	170	174	178	182	186	190	194
34	94	98	102	106	110	114	118	122	126	130	134	137	141	145	149	153	157	161	165	169	173	177	181	185	189
36	91	95	99	103	107	110	114	118	122	126	130	133	137	141	145	149	152	156	160	164	168	171	175	179	183
38	89	92	96	100	103	107	111	114	118	122	125	129	133	137	140	144	148	151	155	159	162	166	170	174	177
40	86	89	93	96	100	104	107	111	114	118	121	125	129	132	136	139	143	146	150	154	157	161	164	168	173

*Target weight is based on 16 per cent fat. To determine target weight, find present weight at the top of the table and then descend vertically to horizontal row corresponding to per cent of fat. See Chapter 6 (body composition) for equation to determine target weight. Reprinted with permission from Golding, L.A., Myers, C.R., and Sinning, W.E., editors: The Y's Way to Physical Fitness (revised). Chicago, The YMCA of the USA, 1982.

TABLE A–15. ESTIMATION OF TARGET WEIGHT FOR FEMALES*

% Fat	105	110	115	120	125	130	135	140	145	150	155	160	165	170	175	180	185	190	195
										WEIGHT (pounds)									
24	104	109	114	118	123	128	133	138	143	148	153	158	163	168	173	178	183	188	192
25	102	107	112	117	122	127	131	136	141	146	151	156	161	166	170	175	180	185	190
26	101	106	111	115	120	125	130	135	139	144	149	154	159	163	168	173	178	183	187
27	100	104	109	114	119	123	128	133	137	142	147	152	156	161	166	171	175	180	185
28	98	103	108	112	117	122	126	131	136	140	145	150	154	159	164	168	173	178	182
29	97	101	106	111	115	120	124	129	134	138	143	148	152	157	161	166	171	175	180
30	95	100	105	109	114	118	123	127	132	136	141	145	150	155	159	164	168	173	177
31	94	99	103	108	112	116	121	125	130	134	139	144	149	152	157	161	166	170	175
32	93	97	102	106	110	115	119	124	129	132	137	141	146	150	155	159	163	168	172
33	91	96	100	104	109	113	117	122	126	131	135	139	144	148	152	157	161	165	170
34	90	94	99	103	107	111	116	120	124	129	133	137	141	146	150	154	159	163	167
35	89	93	97	101	106	110	114	118	122	127	131	135	139	144	148	152	156	160	165
36	87	91	96	100	104	108	112	116	121	125	129	133	137	141	145	150	154	158	162
37	86	90	94	98	102	106	110	115	119	123	127	131	135	139	143	147	151	155	160
38	85	89	93	97	101	105	109	113	117	121	125	129	133	137	141	145	149	153	157
39	83	87	91	95	99	103	107	111	115	119	123	127	131	135	139	143	147	151	154
40	82	86	90	94	97	101	105	109	113	117	121	125	129	132	136	140	144	148	152

*Target weight is based on 23 per cent fat. To determine target weight, find present weight at the top of the table and then descend vertically to horizontal row corresponding to per cent of fat. See Chapter 6 (body composition) for equation to determine target weight. Reprinted with permission from Golding, L.A., Myers, C.R., and Sinning, W.E., editors: The Y's Way to Physical Fitness (revised). Chicago, The YMCA of the USA, 1982.

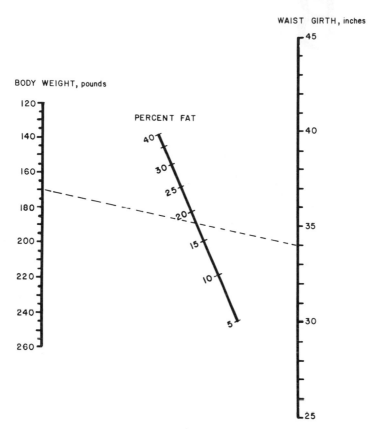

Figure A–7. Prediction of per cent body fat in men from waist circumference and body weight.[8,176] (Courtesy of Professor Brian Sharkey, University of Montana, Missoula, MT.)

Appendix B

ADDITIONAL INFORMATION AND FORMS USED IN CARDIAC REHABILITATION PROGRAMS

TABLE B-1. EMERGENCY CART—RECOMMENDED EQUIPMENT AND SUPPLIES FOR HOSPITAL-BASED PROGRAMS

Top
Life-Pak (monitor/defibrillator)
Saline pads
Electrode gel
Airway

Side
Cardiac board
Clipboard:
  Cart content list
  Resuscitation record
  Emergency protocol
Oxygen tank
Suction
Back-up drug box

First Drawer
(2) Medium airways
Laryngoscope with curved blade
(2) Extra laryngoscope batteries
(1) Extra laryngoscope bulb
Endotracheal tubes:
(1) #6
(1) #7
(1) #8
(1) #9
Macgill forceps and stylet
(1) 10 cc syringe without needle
(1) Hemostat with rubber ends
(1) Oxygen mask
(1) Oxygen cannula
(1) Oxygen extension tubing
(1) Suction connecting tubing
(1) Oxygen flowmeter (on tank)
(1) Suction connecting tubing
(2) Suction kits
(1) Yankaur suction tube
(1) Nasogastric tube
(1) Lubrafax small tube
(1) 60 cc Toomey syringe
(4) Arterial blood gas kits
(1) Flashlight

Second Drawer
Syringes with needles:
(4) TB
(2) 3 cc
(6) 10 cc
(2) 30 cc syringes without needle
Extra needles:
(2) 18 gauge
(2) 21 gauge
(2) Intracardiac needles

Second Drawer (continued)
(6) Jelco IV catheters—2"—18 gauge
(2) Intercath 8"—19 gauge
(2) Subclavian 12"–16 gauge
(2) IV catheter plugs
(2) Dual injection sites
Band-Aids
(4) Tourniquets
Alcohol wipes
Sepps
(1) 30 cc sterile water
(1) 30 cc sterile saline
Adhesive tape:
(2) 1"
(2) 2"
Spinal needles, 18 gauge
Scalpel

Third Drawer

NaHCO$_3$ (44.6 or 50 mEq/ 50 cc)	5 syringes
Epinephrine (1:10,000; 1 mg/ 10 cc prefilled syringe)	2 syringes
Epinephrine (1:1000; 1 mg/cc amp)	4 ampules
Atropine SO$_4$ (1 mg/cc; gr 1/60)	4 ampules
Isuprel (1 mg/5 cc amp)	2 ampules
Valium (10 mg/2 cc syringe)	2 syringes
Lidocaine (40 mg/cc; 1 gm/ 25 cc vial)	2 vials
Lidocaine (100 mg/5 cc syringe)	3 syringes
Pronestyl (100 mg/cc; 10 cc vial)	2 vials
Levophed (1 mg/1 ml; 4 ml amp)	2 ampules
Dopamine (200 mg/5 ml vial)	2 ampules
Calcium Cl (1 gm/10 cc amp)	2 ampules
Dextrose (50% 50 cc syringe)	1 syringe
Bretylium (500 mg/10 ml ampules)	2 ampules

Fourth Drawer

NaHCO$_3$ (44.5 or 50 mEq/ 50 cc)	5 syringes
Epinephrine (1:10,000; 1 mg/ 10 cc prefilled syringe)	3 syringes
(6) 4 × 4's	
(4) Sterile towels	

Fifth Drawer
(4) 250 cc D5W
(2) 250 cc NS
(2) 500 cc D5NS
(2) Regular IV administration set

(continued)

TABLE B-1. EMERGENCY CART—RECOMMENDED EQUIPMENT AND SUPPLIES FOR HOSPITAL-BASED PROGRAMS (Continued)

Fifth Drawer (continued)
- (3) Mini-drip
- (2) IV extension tubing
- CVP manometer (McGraw)
- Prep Tray:
- (2) Novacaine/xylocaine amps
- (2) 000 silk without needle
- (2) 000 silk on curved needle
- (1) Bottle iodine liquid
- Betadine ointment
- Disposable razor

Bottom of Cart
- Venous access/pneumothorax tray
- Ambu bag with mask and O_2 tubing
- Surgeon's gloves:
  - (2) Size 7½
  - (2) Size 8
  - (2) Size 8½
- Normal saline (sterile) 1000 cc
- Oxygen humidifier
- Chest tube (28 Fr./16")

List compiled and recommended by the American College of Sports Medicine, 1 Virginia Avenue, Indianapolis, IN. Published with permission.

TABLE B-2. EMERGENCY CART—RECOMMENDED EQUIPMENT AND SUPPLIES FOR COMMUNITY-BASED PROGRAMS

EQUIPMENT	SUPPLIES
1. Defibrillator—monitor with ECG electrodes—defibrillator paddles, or portable DC defibrillator and portable ECG monitor	1. Sodium bicarbonate IV
2. Airways—nasopharyngeal and oral (endotracheal desirable)	2. Catecholamine agents Epinephrine IV Isoproterenol IV Dobutamine IV
3. Face mask and Robert Shaw valve	3. Atropine sulfate
4. Oxygen	4. Antiarrhythmic agents Lidocaine IV Procainamide IV Propranolol IV/oral
5. Suction apparatus	5. Morphine sulfate
6. Syringes	6. Calcium chloride
7. Intravenous sets	7. Vasoactive agent Norepinephrine
8. Intravenous stand	8. Corticosteroids Methylprednisolone sodium succinate Dexamethasone phosphate
9. Adhesive tape	9. Digoxine IV/oral
10. Laryngoscope (desirable)	10. Lasix IV
	11. Dextrose 5% in water
	12. Nitroglycerin tablets
	13. Amyl nitrite pearls

Reprinted with permission from American College of Sports Medicine. Guidelines for Graded Exercise Testing and Exercise Prescription. 2nd ed. Philadelphia, Lea and Febiger, 1980.

```
┌─────────────────────────────────────────────────────────────────────────┐
│                                                                         │
│              EMERGENCY PHYSICIAN'S ORDERS FOR                           │
│          INPATIENT AND OUTPATIENT CARDIAC REHABILITATION               │
│                                                                         │
│  Emergency Protocol for Unstable Angina, Serious Arrhythmias or Cardiac Arrest: │
│          1) Stop exercise.                                              │
│          2) Start and maintain oxygen therapy by nasal cannula or mask. │
│                                                                         │
│  THEN IF:                                                               │
│                                                                         │
│          1) Angina                                                      │
│                                                                         │
│             A. Nitroglycerin gr 1/150 prn and monitor blood pressure.  │
│             B. Obtain 12 lead ECG STAT.                                 │
│          2) Symptomatic Bradycardia                                     │
│                                                                         │
│             A. Start intravenous 500 cc D5W and keep open.             │
│             B. Give atropine 0.5 to 1.0 mg IV bolus.                    │
│          3) Ventricular Dysrhythmias                                    │
│                                                                         │
│             Serious Ventricular Arrhythmias                             │
│                                                                         │
│             A. Start intravenous 500 cc D5W and keep open.             │
│             B. For uncontrolled and/or symptomatic PVC's, give lidocaine 100 mg │
│                IV STAT. May repeat with 50 mg every 5 minutes for a total dose of │
│                250 mg.                                                  │
│             C. Begin lidocaine drip with 1 gram in 250 cc D5W at 2 mg/minute (range │
│                1–4 mg/minute as needed).                                │
│             Ventricular Tachycardia–Ventricular Fibrillation           │
│                                                                         │
│             A. Defibrillate with 300–400 watt-seconds when life threatening. │
│          4) Cardiac Arrest                                              │
│                                                                         │
│             A. CPR.                                                     │
│             B. Sodium bicarbonate 1 amp IV following defibrillation.    │
│                                                                         │
│   NOTIFY M.D. IMMEDIATELY AFTER ABOVE ACTION HAS BEEN TAKEN            │
│                                                                         │
│                                                                         │
│   Signature of Physician: _____  │
│                                                                         │
│                                                                         │
│   Date: _____  │
│                                                                         │
└─────────────────────────────────────────────────────────────────────────┘
```

Figure B–1. Emergency physician's orders for cardiac rehabilitation. (Courtesy of Cardiac Rehabilitation Program, Cardiovascular Disease Section, Mount Sinai Medical Center, Milwaukee, WI.)

INPATIENT MEDICAL EVALUATION

Patient's Name: _____ Age: _____ Date: _____

Attending Physician: _____ Cardiologist: _____ Surgeon: _____

Specific Cardiac Diagnoses: _____

_____

_____ Surgery: Type_____ Date: _____

_____ MI: Type and Date: _____

_____

_____ CHF _____

_____ Other
         (describe): _____

_____

Pertinent Medical History: _____ Risk Factors: _____

_____   _____

_____   _____

_____   _____

Nuclear Studies, Cath Data, etc.: _____

_____

_____

_____

Medications and Dose: _____

_____

_____

Allergies: _____

Drug Reactions: _____

Physical Exam: _____

Weight: _____ Height: _____

Resting Heart Rate (range): _____

Resting Systolic Blood Pressure (range): _____

Resting Diastolic Blood Pressure (range): _____

Temperature: _____

Lab Results: Hct_____ Hgb_____ K+_____

Chest X-ray: _____

ECG (most recent): _____

CPK_____ MB_____% Others: _____

Complications post-op: _____

_____

_____

Additional Comments: _____

_____

Completed by: _____

Figure B–2. Inpatient medical evaluation. (Courtesy of the Cardiac Rehabilitation Program, Cardiovascular Disease Section, Mount Sinai Medical Center, Milwaukee, WI.)

INPATIENT EXERCISE RECORD—INPATIENT EXERCISE CENTER

Name _____

Age _____   Sex _____   Cardiologist _____   Surgeon _____

Address _____

street   city   state   zip   Date of Surgery/MI _____

Exercise

TM = Treadmill
BI = Bicycle
ST = Stairs
PT = Physical Therapy
OT = Other (specify)

ECG Changes

1 = ST-T Depression (≥ 1 mm)
2 = ST-T Elevation (≥ 1 mm)
3 = Unifocal PVC (indicate #/min)
4 = Multifocal PVC (indicate #/min)
5 = SVT
6 = V Tach
7 = Other (specify)

Signs and Symptoms

A = Chest pain and discomfort
B = Faintness, syncope, dizziness
C = Fatigue
D = Dyspnea
E = Hypertension
F = Hypotension
G = Pallor
H = Other (specify)

Body Composition

Axilla _____ mm
Triceps _____ mm
Suprailium _____ mm
% Fat _____
Ideal Wt _____ lb

Date	Weight (lb/kg)	Workload				Heart Rate			Blood Pressure				RPE	Comments/Signature (ECG changes, signs, symptoms, drugs, etc)
		Exer	mph, rpm	Resist	Duration	Rest	Exer	Rest	Imm Post-Ex	Post-Ex	5′	Post-Ex		

(Revised 2/1/81)

Figure B–3. Inpatient exercise record in an inpatient exercise center. (Courtesy of Cardiac Rehabilitation Program, Cardiovascular Disease Section, Mount Sinai Medical Center, Milwaukee, WI.)

Conversion Table for Upper Limit/Target Heart Rate

beats/10 sec		beats/min	beats/10 sec		beats/min	beats/10 sec		beats/min
9	=	54	15	=	90	21	=	126
10	=	60	16	=	96	22	=	132
11	=	66	17	=	102	23	=	138
12	=	72	18	=	108	24	=	144
13	=	78	19	=	114	25	=	150
14	=	84	20	=	120	26	=	156

Perceived Exertion Scale

6
7 Very, Very Light
8
9 Very Light
10
11 Fairly Light
12
13 Somewhat Hard
14
15 Hard
16
17 Very Hard
18
19 Very, Very Hard
20

MOUNT SINAI ✡ MEDICAL CENTER
Cardiac Rehabilitation
950 North 12th Street
Milwaukee, Wisconsin
(414) 289-8040

Revised 2/20/81

ACTIVITY LOG
FOR

MOUNT SINAI
MILWAUKEE

*"The journey of a thousand miles
starts with a single step"*

Upper Limit/Target HR _____

Date	Distance	Duration	Pre HR	Mid HR	End HR	Perceived Exertion	Comments

Figure B–4. Activity log. (Courtesy of the Cardiac Rehabilitation Program, Cardiovascular Disease Section, Mount Sinai Medical Center, Milwaukee, WI.)

INPATIENT PROGRESS REPORT

Dear Dr. _____ :

The following report is a summary of your patient, _____ 's, progress in the Inpatient Cardiac Rehabilitation Program, which he/she entered on

_____ .

Age:

Date of MI:

Date of Surgery:

Predischarge low-level Graded Exercise Test   Date:

      See enclosed report.

Exercise Data:

Started walking on treadmill for _____ minutes at _____ mph 0% grade on _____. Upon discharge was able to walk at _____ mph 0% grade for _____ minutes and climb _____ stairs.

ECG Changes and Problems: _____

_____

_____

_____

_____

_____

Recommendations: _____

_____

_____

_____

_____   _____

Program Director   Medical Director

_____

Inpatient Program Coordinator

Figure B–5. Inpatient progress report. (Courtesy of the Cardiac Rehabilitation Program, Cardiovascular Disease Section, Mount Sinai Medical Center, Milwaukee, WI.)

OUTPATIENT REFERRAL FORM

Patient's Name: _____ Date: _____

         Last   First   Middle

Address: _____ Age: _____ Phone: _____

_____ Cardiac Surgery (Type & Date): _____

_____ MI (Type & Date): _____

_____ CHF: _____

_____ Post MI/Surgery Complications: _____

_____

Medical Hx: _____

_____

_____

Angina: _____ Date of Onset: _____ Stable: _____ Unstable: _____

    Precipitated By: _____

    Therapy: _____

Hypertension: _____ Date of Onset: _____ Therapy: _____

Arrhythmias (Type): _____

    Date(s): _____ Therapy: _____

Cardiac Catheterization (most recent, post incident/surgery): Date: _____

    Cardiologist: _____ Location: _____

    Coronary Angiography (patency of grafts if post surgical): _____

_____

    Ventricular Function: _____ Ejection Fraction: _____

Nuclear Cardiology: _____

    Rest & Exercise Dynamics: _____ Date: _____

    Resting Ejection Fraction: _____ Resting Wall Motion: _____

    Exercise Ejection Fraction: _____ Exercise Wall Motion: _____

MI Scan: _____ Date: _____ Neg ☐   Pos ☐   Equiv ☐

    Positive Area: _____

Exercise Tolerance Test: Please enclose complete report and ECG.

    Yes ☐   No ☐   Date: _____

    If it is outdated (past 3 months), may this patient be tested: Yes ☐   No ☐

    If not, when? _____ Will you schedule the test?   Yes ☐   No ☐

    Shall we schedule and perform the test here at M.S.M.C.?   Yes ☐   No ☐

Risk Factors for Coronary Heart Disease: (please check those which apply to this patient)

☐ Smoking   ☐ Hypertension   ☐ Family History   ☐ Obesity

☐ Diabetes   ☐ Hyperlipidemia, Please Specify: ☐ Cholesterol   ☐ Triglycerides

Allergies: _____

Additional medical or orthopedic problems which may alter program participation (i.e.,

    insulin-dependent diabetes, claudication, COPD, asthma, prosthesis, psychiatric

    problems, etc.): _____

_____

_____

OUTPATIENT REFERRAL FORM (CONTINUED)

Present Medications (date and dosage):

_____   _____   _____

_____   _____   _____

_____   _____   _____

_____   _____   _____

Has patient been participating in an exercise program: □ Yes   □ No

    If yes, please describe: _____

I recommend the above-named patient to participate in Mount Sinai Medical Center's Outpatient Cardiac Rehabilitation Program.

_____   _____

Date   Signature of Referring Physician

Name of Physician: _____

Address: _____

_____   Phone: _____

_____   _____

Date   Signature of Medical Director

Figure B–6. Outpatient referral form. (Courtesy of the Cardiac Rehabilitation Program, Cardiovascular Disease Section, Mount Sinai Medical Center, Milwaukee, WI.)

INFORMED CONSENT FOR OUTPATIENT EXERCISE REHABILITATION

I voluntarily consent to participate in a medically supervised exercise rehabilitation program in conjunction with the Mount Sinai Medical Center Cardiac Rehabilitation Program which has been prescribed for me by my physician, Doctor _____. This program is part of my treatment to hasten improvement in my cardiovascular function.

Before I enter the exercise phase of the outpatient rehabilitation program, I will have had a clinical evaluation within the last three months which will include a medical history questionnaire, a physical examination, laboratory tests, a chest X-ray, a resting electrocardiogram, measurements of resting heart rate and blood pressure, and a graded exercise tolerance test. The purpose of this evaluation is to detect any condition which would indicate that I should not participate in a medically supervised exercise program and aid in exercise prescription.

The program will follow an exercise prescription prepared by the medical and program directors of the Cardiac Rehabilitation Program in conjunction with the personal physician and will be carefully monitored by the program coordinator and a coronary care nurse. The exercise rehabilitation program will consist of physical therapy, flexibility exercise, and endurance activity, e.g., walking, stationary cycling, stair-climbing, arm pedaling, and jogging as tolerated. The amount of exercise will be regulated on the basis of my functional capacity.

The exercise activities are designed to place a graduated increased work load on the cardiovascular system, thus improving its function. I understand that my heart rate and electrocardiogram will be monitored continuously by telemetry prior to, during, and at least 10 minutes post-exercise in order to detect abnormal responses to the exercise. In addition, my blood pressure will be measured before and following exercise. However, I realize that the response of the cardiovascular system to exercise cannot be predicted with complete accuracy and, consequently, there is a risk of certain changes occurring during or following the exercise. These changes include disorders of heart beats, abnormal blood pressure responses, and, in rare instances, heart attack or cardiac arrest. Proper care in selection and supervision of patients and proper exercise prescription and monitoring provide appropriate precautionary measures to reduce or eliminate such problems. Before starting the program, I will be instructed as to the signs and symptoms that will alert me to stop or slow down my activities. Also, I will be observed by trained personnel who will be alert to changes which would suggest that I modify my exercise. Furthermore, trained medical personnel, emergency equipment, and supplies for my safety will be present for all exercise sessions.

The benefits to me of an exercise program are the enhancement of my recovery from surgery or heart attack, improvement in cardiovascular function in order to perform daily activities, observation of daily activities for life-endangering signs and symptoms, and the scientific assessment of exercise rehabilitation as therapy for heart disease. The information which is obtained during the laboratory evaluations and exercise sessions of this program will be treated as privileged and confidential and will not be released to any unauthorized nonmedical person without my expressed written consent. The information obtained, however, may be used for a statistical or scientific purpose with my right of privacy retained. I also approve of periodic progress reports being sent to my physician of data relating to my laboratory evaluations and exercise sessions.

I have read and understand the preceding information. In addition, the program and its benefits and risks have been discussed with me by the medical or program director of the Cardiac Rehabilitation Program and any questions which have arisen or occurred to me have been answered to my satisfaction. If at any time during my program of rheabilitation I have any additional questions regarding the exercises or procedures in which I am involved, I may freely go to the medical or program directors or program coordinator with my questions. Further, I am guaranteed the right to withdraw from the program at any time.

Date of Signature: _____

Patient: _____

Witness: _____

Medical or Program Director: _____

Figure B–7. Informed consent. (Courtesy of the Cardiac Rehabilitation Program, Cardiovascular Disease Section, Mount Sinai Medical Center, Milwaukee, WI.)

OUTPATIENT EXERCISE RECORD

Name: _____

GXT _____

Date: _____

□ LL   □ SL

RHR: _____

MHR: _____

METS: _____

THR: _____

M.D. Comments: _____

Exercise Codes

TM = Treadmill
AE = Arm Ergometer
BI = Stationary Bicycle
AD = Air Dyne
RE = Rowing Ergometer
SR = Stretching
OT = Other, Specify: _____

Date	Wt (lb)	Resting HR	Resting B/P	Exer Code	Workload mph, rpm	Workload resist	Duration	Exercise HR	Exercise BP	RPE	Post HR	Post BP	Comments
							:						
							:						
							:						
							:						
							:						
							:						
							:						
							:						
							:						
							:						
							:						

Figure B–8. Outpatient exercise record. (Courtesy of the Cardiac Rehabilitation Program, Mount Sinai Medical Center, Milwaukee, WI.)

DATA RECORD—OUTPATIENT PROGRAM

Name _____ Age _____ Cardiologist _____ Surgeon _____

MI _____ Surgery _____ Phase II Entry Date _____

Smoking   Obesity   Hypertension   Cholesterol   Heredity   Diet: _____

Medical History: _____

Phase I: _____

I. Stress Test Data

Date					
☐ LL ☐ SL	☐ LL ☐ SL	☐ LL ☐ SL	☐ LL ☐ SL	☐ LL ☐ SL	
Double Product					
RHR					
MHR					
METS					
THR					
Results					
Time Mph-Grade					

III. Tests

Holter Monitor				
Echo				
Spirometry				
Psychological				

Allergies: _____

V. Patient Education

	Assess	Int.	R.F.	Ed. #1	Ed. #2
Date					

II. Nuclear Cardiology Data

Date				
R EF				
Wall Motion				
Exer EF				
Wall Motion				

MI Scan

Date _____ Pre Pos ☐ Neg ☐ Equiv ☐

Positive Area _____

Date _____ Post Pos ☐ Neg ☐ Equiv ☐

Positive Area _____

Cardiac Cath

Date _____: _____

Grafts _____

Date _____: _____

_____

Grafts _____

IV. Body Composition

Date				
Sum				
Fat %				
Weight/ Ht.				
Ideal Wt.				

Figure B–9. Data record in the outpatient program. (Courtesy of the Cardiac Rehabilitation Program, Mount Sinai Medical Center, Milwaukee, WI.)

OUTPATIENT PROGRESS REPORT

Date: _____

Dear Dr. _____:

The following report is a summary of your patient, _____'s, progress in the Outpatient Cardiac Rehabilitation Program, which he/she entered on

_____.

Age: _____ MI (Type & Date): _____

Surgery (Type & Date): _____

Other (please specify): _____

Graded Exercise Test (GXT)	Graded Exercise Test (GXT)
Date: _____	Date: _____
☐ Low Level GXT	☐ Low Level GXT
☐ Symptom-Limited GXT	☐ Symptom-Limited GXT
Standing Resting Heart Rate: _____	Standing Resting Heart Rate: _____
Maximum Heart Rate: _____	Maximum Heart Rate: _____
METs: _____	METs: _____
Results: _____	Results: _____
Double Product (at 5 METs): _____	Double Product (at 5 METs): _____
Nuclear Dynamics	Nuclear Dynamics
Date: _____	Date: _____
Resting E.F.: _____	Resting E.F.: _____
Resting Wall Motion: _____	Resting Wall Motion: _____
Exercise E.F.: _____	Exercise E.F.: _____
Exercise Wall Motion: _____	Exercise Wall Motion: _____

Exercise Data

Entrance Week #1 Dates: _____	Final Week # _____ Dates: _____
Body Weight (lb): _____	Body Weight (lb): _____
Percent Fat (%): * _____	Percent Fat (%)* _____
Target Heart Rate: † _____	Target Heart Rate: † _____

Week #1	Final Week
Activity: _____	Activity: _____
MET level: _____	MET level: _____
Duration: _____	Duration: _____
Workload: _____	Workload: _____

Figure B–10. Outpatient progress report. (Courtesy of the Cardiac Rehabilitation Program, Mount Sinai Medical Center, Milwaukee, WI.)

OUTPATIENT PROGRESS REPORT (CONTINUED)

Exercise Data (continued)

HR Achieved: _____   HR Achieved: _____

Perceived Exertion: _____   Perceived Exertion: _____

Total Calories/Session: _____   Total Calories/Session: _____

Stretching/Wt. Training: _____   Stretching/Wt. Training: _____

Attendance: _____

ECG Changes and Problems: _____

_____

_____

_____

_____

Summary: _____

_____

_____

_____

_____

Recommendations: _____

_____

_____

_____

_____

_____   _____
Program Director   Medical Director

_____
Coordinator, Outpatient Program

Figure B–10. Continued.

For Per Cent Fat: <19% recommended for males; <23% recommended for females.

†*Target Heart Rate:* Formula used in determining THR from Symptom-Limited GXT: (Max HR − Standing RHR) × Per Cent + Standing RHR. Percentage may change with progression in the program as patient tolerates (70→ 75→ 80).

PREVENTION OF HEAT INJURIES DURING DISTANCE RUNNING*

The Purpose of this Position Statement is:

(a) To alert local, national and international sponsors of distance running events of the health hazards of heat injury during distance running, and

(b) To inform said sponsors of injury preventive actions that may reduce the frequency of this type of injury.

The recommendations address only the manner in which distance running sports activities may be conducted to further reduce incidence of heat injury among normal athletes conditioned to participate in distance running. The Recommendations Are Advisory Only.

Recommendations concerning the ingested quantity and content of fluid are merely a partial preventive to heat injury. The physiology of each individual athlete varies; strict compliance with these recommendations and the current rules governing distance running may not reduce the incidence of heat injuries among those so inclined to such injury.

RESEARCH FINDINGS

Based on research findings and current rules governing distance running competition, it is the position of the American College of Sports Medicine that:

1) Distance races (> 16 km or 10 miles) should *not* be conducted when the wet bulb temperature—globe temperature (adapted from Minard, D. Prevention of heat casualties in Marine Corps recruits. *Milit. Med.* 126:261, 1961. WB–GT=0.7 [WBT] + 0.2 [GT] + 0.1 [DBT]) exceeds 28°C (82.4°F).[1,2]

2) During periods of the year when the daylight dry bulb temperature often exceeds 27°C (80°F), distance races should be conducted before 9:00 A.M. or after 4:00 P.M.[2,7–9]

3) It is the responsibility of the race sponsors to provide fluids which con-

*Position statement of the American College of Sports Medicine. Med. Sci. Sports 7: vii–viii, 1975. Reprinted with permission.

tain small amounts of sugar (less than 2.5 g glucose per 100 ml of water) and electrolytes (less than 10 mEq sodium and 5 mEq potassium per liter of solution).[5,6]

4) Runners should be encouraged to frequently ingest fluids during competition and to consume 400–500 ml (13–17 oz.) of fluid 10–15 minutes before competition.[5,6,9]

5) Rules prohibiting the administration of fluids during the first 10 kilometers (6.2 miles) of a marathon race should be amended to permit fluid ingestion at frequent intervals along the race course. In light of the high sweat rates and body temperatures during distance running in the heat, race sponsors should provide "water stations" at 3–4 kilometer (2–2.5 mile) intervals for all races of 16 kilometers (10 miles) or more.[4,8,9]

6) Runners should be instructed in how to recognize the early warning symptoms that precede heat injury. Recognition of symptoms, cessation of running, and proper treatment can prevent heat injury. Early warning symptoms include the following: piloerection on chest and upper arms, chilling, throbbing pressure in the head, unsteadiness, nausea, and dry skin.[2,9]

7) Race sponsors should make prior arrangements with medical personnel for the care of cases of heat injury. Responsible and informed personnel should supervise each "feeding station." Organizational personnel should reserve the right to stop runners who exhibit clear signs of heat stroke or heat exhaustion.

It is the position of the American College of Sports Medicine that policies established by local, national, and international sponsors of distance running events should adhere to these guidelines. Failure to adhere to these guidelines may jeopardize the health of competitors through heat injury.

The requirements of distance running place great demands on both circulation and body temperature regulation.[4,8,9] Numerous studies have reported rectal temperatures in excess of 40.6°C (105°F) after races of 6 to 26.2 miles (9.6 to 41.9 kilometers).[4,8,9] Attempting to counterbalance such overheating, runners incur large sweat losses of 0.8 to 1.1 liters/m²/hr.[4,8,9] The resulting body water deficit may total 6–10% of the athlete's body weight. Dehydration of these proportions severely limits subsequent sweating, places dangerous demands on circulation, reduces exercise capacity and exposes the runner to the health hazards associated with hyperthermia (heat stroke, heat exhaustion and muscle cramps).[2,3,9]

Under moderate thermal conditions, e.g., 65–70°F (18.5–21.3°C), no cloud cover, relative humidity 49–55%, the risk of overheating is still a serious threat to highly motivated distance runners. Nevertheless, distance races are frequently conducted under more severe conditions than these. The air temperature at the 1967 U.S. Pan American Marathon Trial, for example, was 92–95°F (33.6–35.3°C). Many highly conditioned athletes failed to finish the race and several of the competitors demonstrated overt symptoms of heat stroke (no sweating, shivering and lack of orientation).

The above consequences are compounded by the current popularity of distance running among middle-aged and aging men and women who may possess significantly less heat tolerance than their younger counterparts. In recent years, races of 10 to 26.2 miles (16 to 41.9 kilometers) have attracted several thousand runners. Since it is likely that distance running enthusiasts will continue to sponsor races under adverse heat conditions, specific steps should be taken to minimize the health threats which accompany such endurance events.

Fluid ingestion during prolonged running (two hours) has been shown to effectively reduce rectal temperature and minimize dehydration.[4] Although most competitors consume fluids during races that exceed 1–1.5 hours, current international distance running rules prohibit the administration of fluids until the runner has completed 10 miles (16 kilometers). Under such limitations, the competitor is certain to accumulate a large body water deficit (–3%) before any fluids would be ingested. To make the problem more complex, most runners are unable to judge the volume of fluids they consume during competition.[4] At the 1968 U.S. Olympic Marathon Trial, it was observed that there were body weight losses of 6.1 kg, with an average total fluid ingestion of only 0.14 to 0.35 liter.[4] It seems obvious that the rules and habits which prohibit fluid administration during distance running preclude any benefits which might be gained from this practice.

Runners who attempt to consume large volumes of sugar solution during competition complain of gastric discomfort (fullness) and an inability to consume fluids after the first few feedings.[4-6] Generally speaking, most runners drink solutions containing 5–20 grams of sugar per 100 milliliters of water. Although saline is rapidly emptied from the stomach (25 ml/min), the addition of even small amounts of sugar can drastically impair the rate of gastric emptying.[5] During exercise in heat, carbohydrate supplementation is of secondary importance and the sugar content of the oral feedings should be minimized.

REFERENCES

1. Adolph, E. F. *Physiology of Man in the Desert.* New York: Interscience, 1947.
2. Buskirk, E. R. and W. C. Grasley. Heat Injury and Conduct of Athletes. Ch. 16 in *Science and Medicine of Exercise and Sport,* 2nd Edition. W. R. Johnson and E. R. Buskirk, Editors, New York; Harper and Row, 1974.
3. Buskirk, E. R., P. F. Iampietro and D. E. Bass. Work performance after dehydration: effects of physical conditioning and heat acclimatization. *J. Appl. Physiol.* 12:189–194, 1958.
4. Costill, D. L., W. F. Kammer and A. Fisher. Fluid ingestion during distance running. *Arch. Environ. Health* 21:520–525, 1970.
5. Costill, D. L. and B. Saltin. Factors limiting gastric emptying during rest and exercise. *J. Appl. Physiol.* 37(5):679–683, 1974.
6. Fordtran, J. A. and B. Saltin. Gastric emptying and intestinal absorption during prolonged severe exercise. *J. Appl. Physiol.* 23:331–335, 1967.
7. Myhre, L. G. Shifts in blood volume during and following acute environmental and work stresses in man. (Doctoral Dissertation). Indiana University: Bloomington, Indiana, 1967.
8. Pugh, L. G. C., J. I. Corbett and R. H. Johnson. Rectal temperatures, weight losses and sweating rates in marathon running. *J. Appl. Physiol.* 23:347–353, 1957.
9. Wyndham, C. H. and N. B. Strydom. The danger of an inadequate water intake during marathon running. *S. Afr. Med. J.* 43:893–896, 1969.

GUIDELINES FOR COLD WEATHER EXERCISE*

What guidelines should be followed for cardiac patients who exercise outdoors in cold weather? Is there a specific low temperature at which patients should be prohibited from exercising outdoors?

It has been the experience of the Toronto Rehabilitation Centre during the past 15 years that the vast majority of patients with coronary heart disease can safely walk, jog, or carry out equivalent outdoor exercise in temperatures as low as −10°C (15°F) or, in some cases, in temperatures as low as −12°C (10°F) if certain safeguards are taken.[1] Indeed, we find that summer conditions of high heat and humidity are a greater threat to patients.

PHYSIOLOGIC REACTIONS TO COLD

There is no doubt that the body's reaction to cold places stress on the cardiovascular system. Reflex constriction of the cutaneous blood vessels reduces heat loss through conduction, convection, and radiation and leads to an increase in peripheral resistance and myocardial oxygen consumption. This, in turn, may bring on angina prematurely. During exercise, mouth breathing becomes easier as the respiratory rate increases. The warming effect of the nasal blood vessels is bypassed, and cold air stimulates the tracheal nerve endings causing reflex coronary vasoconstriction, an additional factor in producing angina. Shallow breathing in the cold reduces venous return and, consequently, stroke volume. There is some suggestion that blood viscosity, as measured by hematocrit, increases as a result of exposure to lower temperatures.[2]

In addition, there are other associated problems when exercising in a winter climate. Snow-covered and icy surfaces require greater energy expenditure and increase the likelihood of injury. Head winds increase chilling

---

*Reprinted with permission from Kavanagh, T.: Guidelines for cold weather exercise. J. Cardiac Rehabil. *3:*70–73, 1983. *Note:* Figures 1 and 2 and the table from the original article are not reprinted. See Table 9–1 for information on the wind-chill factor.

effect and air resistance. Rain or wet snow reduces the insulating properties of clothing and allows body heat to "wick out" to the atmosphere. Paradoxically, dehydration can be as much of a problem in the winter as it is in the summer. Although heat loss by conduction, convection, and radiation is more efficient in a cold environment, the evaporative process continues, making excessive fluid loss by sweating possible. Moreover, exposure to cold air strongly suppresses the sense of thirst, and voluntary fluid replacement is often ignored.

With such a list of hazards, how could one even contemplate outdoor exercise in the winter? From the young to the elderly, however, tens of thousands of people do participate in finger-numbing jogging, cross-country skiing, and skating activities with considerable pleasure and exhilaration. The explanation lies in the fact that the body heat generated by physical activity balances heat that is lost to the surroundings, and a state of comfortable equilibrium is achieved.

For coronary heart disease patients who must live, work, and recreate in winter climates, part of the rehabilitation process is to advise and assist them in regard to cold weather exercise. A few considerations to bear in mind are:

ANGINA. When heat production balances heat loss, skin temperature is stabilized between 30°C and 35°C (86°F to 96°F). Cold-induced peripheral vasoconstriction does not occur, there is no increase in myocardial oxygen consumption, and cold weather angina is avoided. Of the two variables (heat loss and heat production), the ability to generate adequate body heat from exercise is the most difficult for the patient with ischemic heart disease. If effort angina precludes any appreciable level of caloric expenditure, then heat loss may exceed heat production. Body temperature falls, reflex peripheral resistance increases, and the additional load placed on the already ischemic myocardium leads to a lowering of the threshold for angina.

In practice, however, such a situation is relatively rare. Wearing as many as three or four layers of light clothing rather than a single heavy, bulky garment increases heat-retaining properties without adding to energy expenditure. This permits greater leeway in terms of exercise intensity. For instance, an additional energy expenditure of only five or six kilocalories per minute, i.e., walking one mile in 15 minutes, can be accomplished in −10 °C (15 °F) when the individual is suitably garbed. In those for whom even this level of exertion is impossible initially, an accurately prescribed indoor endurance training program used in conjunction with suitable antianginal medication when indicated will almost invariably result in a resting and exercise bradycardia, thus reducing double product, increasing anginal threshold, and eventually permitting a higher level of outdoor activity.

In patients who are capable of higher effort levels but who suffer angina within seconds of breathing cold air, the mechanism responsible is probably reflex coronary vasoconstriction.[3,4] Careful indoor warm-up exercise and the use of a woolen scarf of muffler covering the mouth is advised. In 1968, the Centre devised a simple plastic disposable oxygen mask that is attached to 12 inches of flexible tubing extending beneath the subject's T-shirt to about the level of the sternum. At a cost of about $5, this easily produced apparatus is highly effective in preventing cold-induced angina. (It is, incidentally, equally effective for patients with emphysema.)

CLOTHING. The purpose of clothing in cold weather is to insulate the surface of the skin from the surrounding environment and to prevent heat loss. Clothing traps air and modifies the skin's microclimate.[5] Layering garments and varying the closeness of the weave or knit allows considerable flexibility in achieving the desired level of heat retention. However, insulating properties may be changed drastically by the action of water or sweat. Tightly woven cotton with little interfiber air trapping sticks to the body when wet, eliminates large air pockets, and reduces insulation. Wool, on the other hand, retains its insulating properties with its natural oils and greater air-trapping interstices even when wet. In recent years, man-made fibers have been woven and knit in various ways to develop systems of functional clothing for cold weather activities of all types.

The layer next to the skin should be a tightly woven material that provides some insulation while allowing for evaporation during excessive sweating. The middle layer (loosely woven wool or a fishnet cotton and synthetic mix) should absorb some of this excess sweat but again allow for evaporation. The third layer (a tighter woven wool, wool/cotton combination, or synthetic fiber) should have some degree of stretch to permit variable insulation by opening and closing pores in the material in response to body movement. A fourth layer is needed only in conditions of high wind and extreme cold. It should protect against wind, rain, and snow and yet be permeable to body heat. Man-made materials have performed these functions with considerable success.

If possible, all upper-body garments should be zipped or buttoned in such a way that they can be loosened at the neck when the body overheats or closed up if chilling occurs. Dark or colored outer garments tend to conserve body heat; they should be adorned with reflective strip material so as to be visible in the darkness.

The legs rarely require more than two layers. Track suit pants over pantyhose will suffice on even the coldest days. Long underwear is fine, although it tends to restrict knee movement if it is not cut down. Socks should be a wool/cotton mixture or a ribbed and channeled, woven synthetic material. Hands, susceptible to cold because they are poorly muscled and used little in jogging, are best protected by wool mittens. Since considerable body heat is lost through the head, a woolen hat that pulls down over the ears to prevent frostbite is necessary. The exposed parts of the face should be protected from chapping and herpes simplex virus type 1 by applying petroleum jelly. Shoes with waffle soles give greater purchase on ice, and slightly flared heels provide greater stability on soft snow.

GENERAL CLIMATIC CONDITIONS. Air temperature is only one of the factors that should be taken into consideration when planning workouts in cold climates. Wind conditions, presence or absence of sunshine, and humidity levels all affect the body-cooling rate. A 24 km/hr wind can make a still-air temperature reading of 2 °C feel like –9 °C; thus, a windchill chart should always be consulted on windy days. Rain or wet snow will soak through unsuitable clothing, reducing or abolishing its thermal insulation qualities. The temperature difference between direct sunshine and an overcast sky can be as great as 7 °C (12 °F).

The danger of a combination of strong winds, heavy rain, and inadequate clothing was tragically underlined at the 8th Annual Four Inns Walking Competition (45 miles over high ground) in England in 1964. Only 22 of 240 healthy young competitors finished the race. Many competitors collapsed from exposure, three died, and four nearly died—yet the air temperatures never fell below 3 °C! In the final analysis, the competitors who finished where those who were fit enough to compensate for excessive body cooling by sustained high heat production, i.e., a hill-walking pace of 12 to 13 min/mile.

In the initial stages of the exercise program, our cardiac patients walk at a 20 min/mile pace or slower. Therefore, close attention to clothing and climatic conditions is mandatory. The following rules must be followed:

1. Always consult the windchill chart on windy days and use the effective temperature rather than the air temperature as a guideline.

2. Because wind and sun conditions can change rapidly, a short out-and-back course should be chosen, the furthest point of which should be no more than ¼ mile from the starting point. This is particularly important for the less fit.

3. In wet and cold conditions, the clothing layers should include a light outer garment that will provide up to two to three hours of protection against moisture.

4. Head winds must be taken into consideration and the pace adjusted downward to maintain the prescribed level of energy expenditure. Pulse rate during normal workout conditions should be used as a guideline. If this is not done, premature fatigue will ensue, a slower pace will lead to inadequate heat production, and symptoms from chilling may occur.

5. Frostbite is unusual but can occur in poorly protected hands, ears, and faces exposed to temperatures below –1 °C (30 °F). Failure to take windchill into account is usually the cause.

CONCLUSION

Coronary heart disease patients attend the Centre's exercise rehabilitation program for up to 18 months. They exercise once a week under supervision at the Centre and four times a week on their own. Every winter they are given a series of lectures covering the previously discussed factors. Their initial response to being told that most of them will be able to exercise outdoors throughout most of the winter is largely one of pleasure. Skiing, skating, and tobogganing are popular weekend family activities, and the unspoken fear that a heart attack will put an end to all of that must be taken into consideration. In our experience, no amount of complex testing can evaluate with greater accuracy those patients who function best in a cold environment than the simple question, "Do you like the cold?" This, together with careful observation during the weekly supervised sessions on the outdoor track, provides an effective initial screening.

Patients who are free from effort angina and whose exercise test is relatively uncomplicated (ST-segment depression < 2 mm, no critical cardiac arrhythmias, appropriate heart rate and blood pressure responses—to 80% of aerobic power) rarely, if ever, have problems exercising in the cold. Initially, they are asked to observe a lower temperature limit of –10 °C (15 °F); as they become more fit, the limit is reduced to –12 °C (10 °F). Permission to work out regularly at temperatures below this limit is only given to members of the Long Distance Marathon Group, each of whom is assessed by telemetry and/or Holter recording in trial conditions. For patients in whom effort angina develops or who have strongly positive exercise tests, the lower limit is explored by electrocardiographic monitoring and blood pressure responses on the outdoor track at successively lower and lower temperatures, commencing at about –5 °C (23 °F). With time and increasing fitness, these patients are often able to exercise safely at –10 °C (15 °F).

Obviously, there are individuals who are not capable of any activity in cold weather as well as severely cold days when few would venture outdoors any more than is absolutely essential. On the other hand, we find that these patients are rare in the average postcoronary disease population, and such days amount to only 30 or so a year in most of the large population centers in North America.

For more than 15 winters, a high percentage of some 4,500 patients have trained outdoors on all but the severest days without ill effects. At the same time we have maintained a creditable overall low incidence of fatal MI recurrence and episodes of ventricular fibrillation.[6] This, we feel, amply vindicates our approach.

REFERENCES

1. Kavanagh T: *The Healthy Heart Program.* Toronto, Van Nostrand, 1980.
2. Shephard RJ: *Alive Man! The Physiology of Physical Activity.* Springfield, Ill., Charles C Thomas, 1972.
3. Murray MJ: The effect of inhalation of cold air on the circulation in dogs. *Am J Cardiol* 1965; 15:141.
4. Murray MJ: Effect of inspiration of cold air on electrocardiograms of normal humans with angina pectoris (abstract). *Circulation* 1962; 26:765.
5. Fourt L, Hollies NRS: *Clothing: Comfort and Function.* New York, Marcel Dekker, 1970.
6. Kavanagh T: The Toronto Rehabilitation Centre's Cardiac Exercise Program. *J Cardiac Rehab* 1982; 6:496–502.

INDEX

Page numbers in *italics* indicate illustrations.
Page numbers followed by t indicate tables.